Pharmacy Labs

for Technicians

Second Edition

Pharmacy Labs

for Technicians

Second Edition

Jason Sparks, MEd, CPhT
Lisa McCartney, MEd, CPhT, PhTR

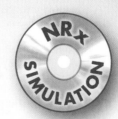

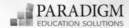

PARADIGM
EDUCATION SOLUTIONS

St. Paul

Managing Editor	Brenda M. Palo
Developmental and Production Editor	Stephanie Schempp
Cover and Text Designer	Jaana Bykonich
Production Specialist	Sara Schmidt Boldon
Indexer:	Ina Gravitz, I. Gravitz Indexing Services
Photographer	George Brainard
Illustrations	Rolin Graphics, Inc.
Cover Images:	Shutterstock/Shannon Heryet (top left), Paradigm Publishing/George Brainard (middle), Paradigm Publishing/George Brainard (top right).

ISBN 978-0-76385-239-9 (text and NRx Simulation CD)
ISBN 978-0-76385-236-8 (text)
ISBN 978-0-76385-238-2 (eBook)

© 2013 by Paradigm Publishing, Inc.
875 Montreal Way
St. Paul, MN 55102
E-mail: educate@emcp.com
Web site: www.emcp.com

Brief Contents

Contents

Preface

Pharmacy Labs for Technicians is the first comprehensive lab manual developed for pharmacy technician education. It is intended for students preparing to become pharmacy technicians in community, institutional, and other pharmacy settings. The role of the pharmacy technician in today's pharmacy is both challenging and rewarding. Pharmacy technicians are asked to perform many critical tasks, and they must perform these tasks responsibly and correctly. This laboratory manual provides students the opportunity to practice key skills in the areas of using drug references, managing patient records and prescriptions, compounding medications, working with crash carts and cart-fill requests, and preparing oral syringes and aseptic parenteral dosage forms. *Pharmacy Labs for Technicians* may be used for a stand-alone Pharmacy Labs course or to support lab activities that are taught as part of a Pharmacy Practice course.

Organization of the Lab Manual

The activities in this text are presented in 34 labs that are grouped into five sections (Units 1 through 5) according to the type of activity (research, software management, or material preparation) or the type of setting (community or institutional). Lab topics cover a wide variety of tasks that give instructors the flexibility to cover all 34 labs or to choose those labs that emphasize subjects they consider most important for their students.

Unit 1: Drug References, Labs 1–3

The first three labs provide students with experience researching and cross-referencing information in the most common reference sources used by pharmacy technicians.

Unit 2: Community Pharmacy Practice, Labs 4–14

These eleven labs teach skills that are commonly undertaken by pharmacy technicians who work in retail pharmacies. Labs 4, 5, 6, and 7 provide experience reviewing and verifying DEA numbers, information in patient profiles, submitted prescription forms, and filled prescription forms. Labs 8–14 are computer-based labs. These labs involve pharmacy software management skills that are increasingly necessary for pharmacy technicians working in community pharmacies, such as creating and maintaining patient records, managing prescriptions, and processing daily reports and insurance claims. To complete the computer labs, students use the software simulation on CD that accompanies this text.

Unit 3: Institutional Pharmacy Practice, Labs 15–21

This unit of seven labs offers students experience in pharmacy technician work within a hospital or other institutional pharmacy setting. Students practice the skills of completing a cart-fill request, checking floor stock, preparing oral syringes, processing a crash cart, filling an automated drug storage and dispensing system, and performing medication reconciliation.

Unit 4: Extemporaneous Compounding, Labs 22–27

In Labs 22–27, students prepare a variety of pharmaceutical products, including tablets, capsules, creams, and lozenges. Students also calculate doses, weigh and measure ingredients, compound a number of pharmaceuticals, and learn basic concepts in the on-demand preparation of custom pharmaceutical products in different dosage forms.

Unit 5: Aseptic Technique, Labs 28–34

Aseptic technique, which is governed by USP Chapter <797>, is addressed in the final unit of the book. Labs 28–30 provide explicit directions required for aseptic hand washing, garbing, and cleaning the horizontal laminar airflow hood, and prepare students for the critical techniques discussed in the final four labs. Labs 31–34 present in detail the use of ampules and the preparation of large- and small-volume parenteral dosage forms and sterile powder drug vials.

Lab Chapter Features

Each lab contains a list of objectives, a list of supplies, an introductory background discussion, step-by-step instructions on how to complete lab procedures, and a Lab Review, which reinforces concepts and skills taught in the lab. Many labs also include one or more worksheets that students will complete and submit to their instructor.

1 OBJECTIVES establish a clear set of goals for each lab.

2 SUPPLIES are listed to help students prepare prior to completing each lab.

3 BACKGROUND INFORMATION helps students connect lab activity with the practical work of a pharmacy technician.

4 KEY TERMS are set in bold and defined in the margin.

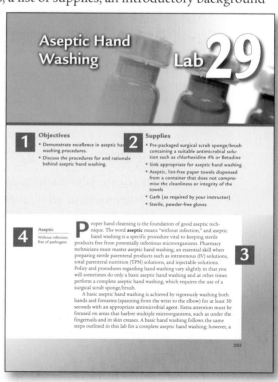

5 STEPS give clear instructions on how to perform lab tasks.

6 NUMBERED PHOTOS illustrate steps.

7 TIPS provide additional suggestions and warn of potential pitfalls within the steps themselves.

8 TAKE NOTE FEATURES offer additional suggestions and warn of potential pitfalls in the field of pharmacy practice.

A key feature of this text is the step-by-step instruction for every lab. These steps provide clear details on how to find information, prepare pharmaceutical compounds, and ensure aseptic conditions, among several other tasks. Many steps are illustrated with full-color photographs that help to demonstrate the technique being explained.

End-of-Chapter Features

All labs conclude with a Lab Review, which includes five multiple-choice Check Your Understanding questions and three Thinking Like a Pharmacy Tech discussion questions. Thus, students are challenged to both recall specific information and engage in critical thinking.

The third Thinking Like a Pharmacy Tech discussion question is marked by a special icon. This icon indicates that the question relates to job acquisition, professionalism, and soft skills while on the job as a pharmacy technician. Answers to these questions are not necessarily found in the text, and may require additional research. Students may be asked to prepare a résumé, research available pharmacy jobs in their area, or respond to on-the-job scenarios. Students can write their answers on a blank sheet of paper or use the Lab Review Answer Sheet. The answer sheet, which can be downloaded and printed, is available on the website for the book at www.paradigmcollege.net/pharmlabs2e.

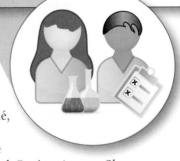

Additional Student Resources

In addition to the text, the following tools are available to students.

- Simulation of NRx software on CD
- Student Internet Resource Center

NRx Simulation CD

Becoming familiar with pharmacy management software is an important aspect of pharmacy technician training. One of the most commonly used programs is NRx, which is produced and sold by QS/1. Labs 8–14 require using a simulation of important NRx functions, which is offered on the CD packaged with each copy of this textbook. The skills gained in performing these computer labs are transferable to working with software programs used at any pharmacy.

In order for the computer simulations to work effectively, student computers should be equipped to meet the following minimum requirements:

Windows

- Intel® Pentium® III 1 GHz or faster processor, 512 MB of RAM (recommended: Pentium 4, 2 GHz or faster, 1 GB of RAM)
- Windows XP, Vista®, or Windows 7 operating system
- 50 MB of free disk space
- A connected printer to print reports, labels, and student performance results

Mac OS X

- Intel Core™ Duo 1.83 GHz or faster processor; PowerPC® G4, 1 GHz or faster processor
- Mac OS X operating system
- 512 MB of RAM
- 50 MB of free disk space
- A connected printer to print reports, labels, and student performance results

To install the software onto your computer, do the following:
- Insert the CD.
  - Mac users should then navigate to the CD and select PharmacyLabs.app.
  - PC users will observe that the CD will "auto run" and the Application Install dialog box will appear automatically.
- All users will then be asked to install Pharmacy Labs by Paradigm Publishing, Inc.
- Click "Install."
- Click "Continue."
- Wait for the application to install. (If your computer does not have the Adobe AIR application, you will next be prompted to review and accept the license agreement and then install it by clicking "I agree.")

Once the software is installed, the textbook will guide you through using the software for Labs 8–14, beginning with Step 1 of each of those labs.

Student Internet Resource Center

The Internet Resource Center for this title, located at www.paradigmcollege.net/pharmlabs2e, provides additional reference information and resources, such as Spanish for Pharmacy Technicians, a table of the most commonly prescribed drugs, guidelines for dispensing medications safely, and much more. Access to the site is free.

Resources for the Instructor

A printed Instructor's Guide and an Instructor's Internet Resource Center are provided with *Pharmacy Labs for Technicians* to help instructors plan their courses and assess student learning.

Instructor's Guide

The printed Instructor's Guide offers the following:

- Course objectives
- Syllabus for book used in a stand-alone Pharmacy Labs course
- Syllabus for book used in conjunction with a Pharmacy Practice book
- Teaching hints
- Lists of equipment needed for each lab
- Answers to questions in lab book
- Completed worksheets and other model answers
- Blank copies of worksheets used multiple times
- Lab Review answer sheets

Instructor Resources CD

Packaged with the printed Instructor's Guide is a CD that contains electronic versions of many of the Instructor's Guide features, including syllabuses, blank worksheets, and a Lab Review answer sheet. In addition, the CD includes Power-Point presentations and the EXAMVIEW Assessment Suite, a full-featured computerized test generator.

Instructor's Internet Resource Center

Many of the features that appear in the printed Instructor's Guide also are available on the password-protected instructor section of the Internet Resource Center for this title at www.paradigmcollege.net/pharmlabs2e.

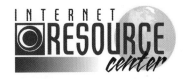

Textbooks in the Pharmacy Technician Series

In addition to *Pharmacy Labs for Technicians, Second Edition*, Paradigm Publishing, Inc. offers other titles designed specifically for the pharmacy technician curriculum:

- *Pharmacology for Technicians, Fifth Edition*
- *Pharmacology for Technicians Workbook, Fifth Edition*
- *Pharmacy Practice for Technicians, Fifth Edition*
- *Pharmacy Calculations for Technicians, Fifth Edition*
- *Certification Exam Review for Pharmacy Technicians, Third Edition*
- *Sterile Compounding and Aseptic Technique*

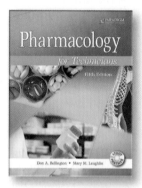
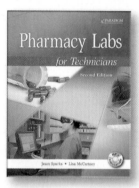
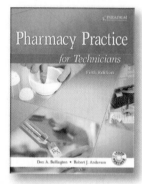
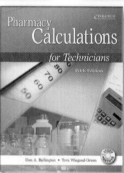
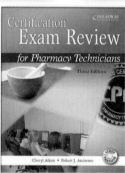
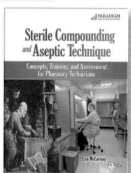

About the Authors

Jason P. Sparks, MEd, CPhT, is an experienced instructional and curriculum designer who has taught courses in pharmacy practice, pharmacy law, mathematics, and medical ethics. Formerly Coordinator of the Allied Health, Natural Sciences, and Emergency Management Division at Mid-South Community College, West Memphis, Arkansas; and an Associate Professor with the Department of Pharmacy Technology at Austin Community College, Austin, Texas, he continues to serve as an author, educator, and consultant in the field of pharmacy technology. Jason has also served as an item writer for PTCB's Pharmacy Technician Certification Exam. He is certified by the College of Pharmacy, University of Houston, as an ACPE Instructor in Aseptic Technique for Pharmacy Technicians. Jason has been working as a pharmacy technician in both community and institutional pharmacy settings since 2000. In 2007, he was named Pharmacy Technician of the Year by the Texas Pharmacy Association. Jason has delivered presentations across the United States, including for the Pharmacy Technician Educators Council, the Florida Society of Health-System Pharmacists, and the College of Pharmacy at the University of Texas at Austin. He has served on the Board of Directors of the Pharmacy Technician Educators Council, a national professional association, and on the Texas Pharmacy Association's Board of Directors (2006 to 2008). Jason has publications with the American Society of Health-System Pharmacists, American Pharmacists Association, *Journal of Developmental Education*, and CriticalPoint. He holds an AAS in pharmacy technology from Weatherford College, a BA in English with a minor in curriculum and instruction and in music from Texas State University–San Marcos, and a Master of Education in Management of Technical Education, also from Texas State University. Jason currently resides in Arlington, Virginia.

Lisa McCartney, MEd, CPhT, PhTR, is the department chair for the ASHP accredited pharmacy technician program at Austin Community College. She has been educating pharmacy technicians since 1999. Lisa has worked as a pharmacy technician for over 30 years. She is a subject matter expert in the area of sterile compounding and aseptic technique, and has been an ACPE-certified instructor in sterile product preparation and aseptic technique since 1997. Lisa has a wide range of pharmacy experience, including the community, hospital, and oncology pharmacy settings. She became a PTCB-certified pharmacy technician in 1995 and has been registered with the State of Texas since 2005. She received her AAS degree in Pharmacy Technology from Weatherford College in 2008. She received her BAAS Degree with an emphasis in Occupational Education from Texas State University in 2011. In 2013 she received her Master's Degree in Education from Texas State University. Lisa is a 2011 International NISOD Award winner for *Teaching and Leadership Excellence*. Lisa received the 2012 Roy Kemp award from the Pharmacy Technician Educator's Council, and in 2013, the Mike Knapp Pharmacy Technician of the Year award from the Texas Society of Health System Pharmacists. Lisa is currently serving on the USP <797> Expert Panel for the United States Pharmacopeia

Lisa is the author of the Paradigm book, *Sterile Compounding and Aseptic Technique: Concepts, Training, and Assessment for Pharmacy Technicians.*

Special Thanks

Jason Sparks: For every teacher who told me I can't, this is for you; for every teacher who told me I can, this is because of you. We can never doubt the value and the impact of the people who shape our lives through education. Value those who care to share their experience and knowledge with you. One day, you may find yourself thinking "I remember when my teacher told me about this." Thank you to all of my teachers and professors for helping me along the way.

Thank you...

- My Mother, Kathy, for meatloaf, baseball, swim team, choir practice, white cake with white icing, being there, unconditional love, and instilling in me her same strength, wisdom, and character. This is all because of you
- My brother, Steven, for saving my life in 2007—I wouldn't be here if it weren't for you. (Yes, literally)
- My father, Steve, and my brother, Rodney, for your continued love and support
- My friends for being ad hoc models (Travis, Chea, and Amanda), also for listening and supporting me during the crazy writing and revision process
- All of the wonderful people at Paradigm Publishing, past and present, for making my dream of this text a reality—Brenda, Spencer, Chris, Stephanie, Chuck, Nancy, Tim, Todd, Lara, Alison, Deanna, and the whole darn office
- W. Renée Acosta for my start in higher education at Austin Community College
- Lisa McCartney for being a great co-author, colleague, and friend
- Kelley for the friendship, entertainment, word scrambles of the day, and the chats during those long shifts at SNW
- My best friend, Larry... Buen Camino
- To every student who has learned something from this book—remember: you save lives every day

Lisa McCartney: I would to thank the following people for their encouragement and support during the creation of Pharmacy Labs for Technicians: my family, friends, and co-workers, my JUMP team and everyone at USM, Brenda Palo, George Brainard, Jason Sparks, all of my students, and all the educators who have inspired me to be the best educator that I can be. Most importantly, to my partner Liz, whose love and support make every day a blessing.

The outstanding photographs that appear in *Pharmacy Labs for Technicians, Second Edition,* were taken by renowned photographer George Brainard of Austin, Texas. The computer simulations on the accompanying CD were expertly prepared by Blue Earth Interactive LLC of St. Paul, Minnesota. We thank all of these participants for their contributions.

The authors and editorial staff invite your feedback on the text and its supplements. Please reach us by clicking the "Contact us" button at www.emcp.com. In addition, Jason Sparks and Lisa McCartney welcome questions and comments e-mailed to jsparks@emcp.com and lmccartney@emcp.com, respectively.

Acknowledgments

We are grateful to the many individuals who provided feedback by reviewing project ideas, drafts of manuscript, early versions of the text, and final pages. The following instructors reviewed *Pharmacy Labs for Technicians*:

Ann Barlow Oberg, BS, CPhT
Pharmacy Tech Consulting
Sioux Falls, South Dakota

Dr. Harold S. Bender, BS, RPh, DPh
National College of Business
and Technology
Nashville, Tennessee

Elizabeth Garcia, CPhT
San Joaquin Valley College
Visalia, California

Joseph P. Gee, PharmD
Professor and Program Director,
Pharmacy Technology
Cosumnes River College
Sacramento, California

Lisa Homburg, RPh
College of the Mainland
Texas City, Texas

Susan Howell, BS, CPhT
Ivy Tech Community College
Muncie, Indiana

Philip E. Johnston, RPh
Director of Pharmaceutical Services
St. David's Round Rock Medical Center
Round Rock, Texas
Associate Professor, Pharmacy Technician
Program
Austin Community College
Austin, Texas

Belva J. Matherly, BA, CPhT
National College
Salem, Virginia

Dr. Shawn McPartland, Dean
Harrison College
Indianapolis, Indiana

Lynda Melendez, CPhT
Texas State Technical College
Waco, Texas

Michael Mockler RPh, MBA
Heald College
Portland, Oregon

Elina Pierce, MSP, CPhT
Southeast Community College
Beatrice, Nebraska

Erika Plante-D'Arezzo, CPhT, BSSW
Sanford-Brown Institute
Cranston, Rhode Island

Vickey Rose, CPhT

Lisa L. Russell, CPhT
Program Director for Pharmacy Technicians
Pioneer Pacific College
Springfield, Oregon

Rebecca Schonscheck, BS-Biology
Phoenix, Arizona

Jacqueline T. Smith, RN, CPhT
National College
Princeton, West Virginia

Maureen C. Sparks, CPhT
Clover Park Technical College
Lakewood, Washington

Bobbi Steelman, MEd, CPhT
Pharmacy Technician Program Director
Daymar College
Bowling Green, Kentucky

Mary Ann Stuhan, PharmD, RPh
Cuyahoga Community College
Cleveland, Ohio

Dawn Tesner, DHEd, CPhT
Mid Michigan Community College
Mt. Pleasant, Michigan

Sandi Tschritter, MEd, CPhT
Spokane Community College
Spokane, Washington

Terry Walker (retired)
Selkirk College
British Columbia, Canada

Elaine Young, MEd, CPhT
Angelina College
Lufkin, Texas

Pharmacy Labs

for Technicians

Second Edition

Unit 1

Drug References

1

A day in the life of a pharmacy technician...

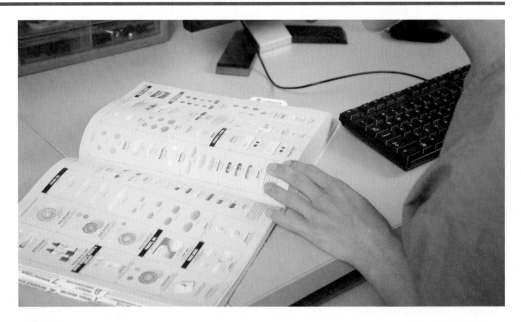

You arrive to the pharmacy and the pharmacist has a task for you: you are given a list of drugs and are asked to research the AWP for specific NDCs, identify any new labeling requirements, provide updates to any newly available dosage forms, identify a capsule found on the floor, determine if a particular NDC of Warfarin Sodium is at least an AB-rated therapeutic equivalent to Coumadin, and finally get the address for the nearest DEA office.

So, what do you do? Which references would you use? Is there a single comprehensive reference where all of this information is found? (hint: it's not a search engine on the Internet!)

A good pharmacy technician is a resourceful pharmacy technician: he or she knows how to get things done and where to locate valuable information at a moment's notice. Understanding how references work and organize information is a key skill for a pharmacy technician.

References come in a variety of types: printed books, online references, applications for personal computers, and apps for smart phones and tablets. Some of these are free while others require a subscription or annual purchase. A pharmacy technician should be familiar with using each reference type. You may find yourself in a pharmacy where only certain sources of information are available; for example, you may work in a pharmacy where only print references are available.

This unit guides you through some of the most commonly available print references used in pharmacy practice: *Drug Facts and Comparisons*, *United States Pharmacopoeia*, and *The Red Book*. These references were first published in print and are also now found online for an annual subscription fee. Some of these references are no longer being printed, but many pharmacies continue to use the last printed version of these texts. No matter which type of reference source you use in completing these labs, the importance of knowing how each of these references work is vital. You never know where and when you will be asked to research information in your daily work as a pharmacy technician.

Using *Drug Facts and Comparisons*

Lab 1

Objectives

- Describe the contents and organization of the *Drug Facts and Comparisons* reference text.
- Practice using *Drug Facts and Comparisons* as a pharmacy reference text.
- Identify how *Drug Facts and Comparisons* contributes to successful pharmacy practice and administration.

Supplies

- A copy of the most recent edition of *Drug Facts and Comparisons* or access to the online version (check with your instructor)

As a pharmacy technician, you must accurately research information to assist the pharmacist and contribute to patient safety. There are many research tools, known as clinical references, available to pharmacy professionals, including *Drug Facts and Comparisons, American Hospital Formulary Service, MicroMedex, United States Pharmacopoeia, Lexicomp,* and *Epocrates*. With so many references available, knowing which to use and when and how to use each one will increase your value as a pharmacy technician. This lab and the following two labs will show you how frequently consulted pharmacy references are organized and how to find the information you need within them.

Drug Facts and Comparisons, a reference of clinical information for both prescription and over-the-counter (OTC) products, is the focus of this lab. It provides important clinical and practical information for pharmacists and pharmacy technicians, ultimately enabling pharmacists to thoroughly and effectively counsel patients about their medication therapy.

Drug Facts and Comparisons is available in three separate editions: as a hardbound book, as a perpetually updated loose-leaf binder, and an online, or web-based, format. The hardbound edition (indexed at the back) is updated and published annually. The binder (indexed at the front) is updated by hand each month when a package of new and replacement pages is mailed to the pharmacy. A pharmacy staff member—most likely a pharmacy technician—follows the directions provided to remove some pages and to replace or add others. The online edition is updated more frequently because it is web-based. This lab offers you practice with all versions because you may have access to one or more forms of this reference at your pharmacy.

The printed and online versions of *Drug Facts and Comparisons* are organized in different ways. Both printed editions are organized by body system and then by drug classification. Each classification begins with a group **monograph**—a discussion of all the drugs in the group—and then presents the drugs one by one in individual product monographs. However, the online edition is organized differently. As is true of many websites, navigation among the different sections is fairly easy, and this lab will help you learn how to find what you need.

Because the world of pharmacy requires pharmacists and pharmacy technicians to stay current with pharmacy drug therapy and treatment, both printed editions of *Drug Facts and Comparisons* feature a "Keeping Up" section that provides the latest news on available and investigational medications, an appendix for supplemental information (such as controlled substance legislation, treatment guidelines, laboratory values, and calculations), and two indices—one that lists U.S. drug names, and another listing Canadian names. Access to both lists is not only crucial for pharmacy technicians working in Canada, but also helpful if you

Monograph

A detailed document containing specific information about a drug product

The hardbound and loose-leaf versions of *Drug Facts and Comparisons*.

practice pharmacy in the northern United States, where Canadian residents sometimes have prescriptions filled.

Comprehensive reference texts, by definition, contain large amounts of information. To keep the books a reasonable size, the data is efficiently organized and cross-references are used heavily. A **cross-reference** is usually a word or phrase placed at the end of an entry, directing you to another part of the text for related information. *Drug Facts and Comparisons* presents a great deal of information for your pharmacy research, including drug indications, administration and dosage, contraindications, warnings, adverse reactions, overdosage information, and patient information (a brief listing of counseling and safety information that pharmacists use to advise patients about their medications). To avoid listing the same information for an individual product or a family of products repeatedly, cross-references are placed at the end of individual product monographs and direct you to the group monograph.

When accessing large references such as *Drug Facts and Comparisons*, you will best benefit from your research by following cross-references. For example, when researching fluoxetine, you would find this cross-reference under the individual product listing: "For complete and comparative prescribing information, refer to the Selective Serotonin Reuptake Inhibitors group monograph." Follow such leads to make the most of the reference and to better assist the pharmacist. Remember, however, that the group monograph contains information about all drugs in the group and you must read carefully to make sure that you are providing the correct information about the specific drug with which you are working. Knowing how to use reference texts is a valuable skill when you are helping the pharmacist to research drugs or review prescription information. As a pharmacy technician, you must remember

Cross-reference

Directs a reader to another part of the text for related information

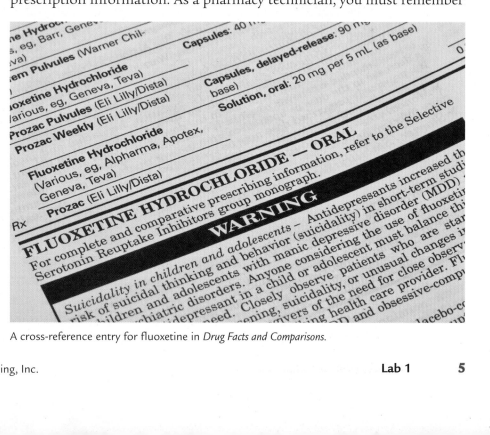

A cross-reference entry for fluoxetine in *Drug Facts and Comparisons*.

that you should never provide drug information or counselling to patients; all patient questions requiring professional judgement must be referred to a pharmacist.

It is very important that you always use the most up-to-date version of any reference text. Pharmacy drug therapy changes rapidly and using a **current edition** is crucial when relying on printed references. The most recent publication date of *Drug Facts and Comparisons* should be within the current year. To determine the publication date of your version, look on the cover of the hardbound edition or the update page located after the title page of the binder edition.

Current edition

Published within the most current year

Procedure

To complete this lab, either use the most recent printed version of *Drug Facts and Comparisons* available or access the online version, if your school has subscribed to it (ask your instructor). You will require additional copies of the worksheet located at the end of the lab, so you may make your own from that blank form, or your instructor may provide you with copies. Your instructor will tell you how many worksheets to complete for each version, based on the media you are able to access in your class.

Following the steps below, complete a worksheet for each drug listed in Step 2 and for one drug product of your choice. Note that the worksheet contains blanks near the top for you to fill in the brand and generic names of the drug. Step 2 provides you with some brand names and some generic names to research. However, be sure to fill in both drug name blanks, no matter which type of name you are initially given. Also, be careful when taking information from the group monographs—they contain information about all the drugs in the drug group.

1 Obtain the most current version of *Drug Facts and Comparisons* available to your classroom.

2 Using the information you find within the individual and group monographs, complete one worksheet for each of the following drugs: methylphenidate, Strattera, Lipitor, esomeprazole, Avandia, and one drug product of your choice.

3 Check cross-references for each drug and incorporate the information into your worksheet answers.

4 **Conclusion:** Make sure your name and today's date are on each worksheet. Turn in all completed worksheet pages to your instructor. On a separate sheet of paper, answer all questions in the following Lab Review section and turn in your answers to your instructor.

Lab Review

Check Your Understanding

1. Which of the following pieces of information may be found in *Drug Facts and Comparisons*?
   a. manufacturer procedures
   b. labeling procedures
   c. adverse reactions
   d. retail pricing

2. *Drug Facts and Comparisons* provides important ____ and ____ information.
   a. clinical; practical
   b. cost; dosage
   c. clinical; stability
   d. safety; preparation

3. To make the most of a comprehensive reference text like *Drug Facts and Comparisons*, be sure to check the ____ listed at the bottom of each entry.
   a. symbols
   b. condensed referencing
   c. signa abbreviations
   d. cross-references

4. Because pharmacy drug therapy and treatment change, it is important to use the ____ edition of the text.
   a. Web-based
   b. most recent
   c. perpetually updated
   d. hardbound

5. The group monograph contains potentially broad-ranging information on all drugs within the drug group. When researching information on a particular drug, you must ____ to ensure you are accessing pertinent information.
   a. cross-reference
   b. evaluate all monographs
   c. seek a secondary reference
   d. ask for review

Thinking Like a Pharmacy Tech

1. Why are comprehensive references such as *Drug Facts and Comparisons* necessary? That is, why can't a pharmacist just rely on his or her education to answer drug product questions that come up on the job?

2. Following cross-references can be time consuming. Why doesn't a reference text simply repeat the same information, saving the reader the trouble of flipping to another part of the text?

3. As you will learn reading this book, and through your studies to become a pharmacy technician, there are different settings you can practice in—namely community pharmacy (such as a chain pharmacy, independent pharmacy, etc.) and institutional (in a hospital). What appeals to you about each setting? What employers are in your area or the area you wish to live? Research two or three potential places where you may wish to seek employment once you become a pharmacy technician.

Name: _____ **Date:** _____

Lab 1　　　　　　　　　　　*Using* Drug Facts and Comparisons

Worksheet for *Drug Facts and Comparisons*

Brand name(s): _____ Generic name: _____

Available product dosage forms: _____

_____

_____

_____

Drug class: _____ Storage Requirements: _____

Control schedule: _____ Pronunciation: _____

Indication(s): _____

_____

Adult dosage: _____

_____

Pediatric dosage: _____

_____

Adverse effects: _____

_____

_____

Pregnancy category: _____

Drug interactions: _____

_____

Drug specific counseling information: _____

_____

Patient information: _____

_____

_____

Using the United States Pharmacopoeia: Drug Information

Lab 2

Objectives

- Describe the contents and organization of the *USP DI* reference texts.
- Practice using the *USP DI* as a pharmacy reference text serving both medical professionals and patients.
- Identify how *USP DI* contributes to successful pharmacy practice and administration.

Supplies

- Copies of the most recent editions of the *USP DI*, Volumes I and II, or access to the online version (check with your instructor)

The primary duty of any pharmacy technician is to process prescriptions. However, from time to time, you may also research drug information. In Lab 1, you became familiar researching in the reference text *Drug Facts and Comparisons*. In this lab, you will work with a multivolume reference, the *United States Pharmacopoeia: Drug Information (USP DI)*. A **pharmacopoeia** is an official compendium of drug products detailing their effects and directions for use.

The *USP DI* is a reference of clinical information for approved pharmaceutical products, including both prescription and over-the-counter (OTC) products. It is published in three concurrent volumes. Volume I is intended for use by healthcare professionals, such as pharmacists and pharmacy technicians, and is written for an audience that understands clinical and technical language. Volume II is intended for use by lay persons, such as your patients, and is written in non-technical, easier-to-understand language. Volume III is a listing of legal requirements used in prescribing and dispensing products. This lab will not require you to work with Volume III because pharmacy technicians infrequently use it and because legal requirements vary from state to state. In this lab, you will research information from only Volumes I and II so that you may learn the differences between them and understand how each serves its

Pharmacopoeia

An official compendium of drug products

11

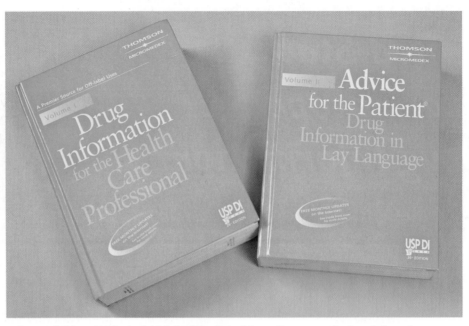

Volume I (left) and Volume II (right) of the *United States Pharmacopoeia: Drug Information.*

particular audience. The *USP DI* volumes are available in hardbound books and also in an online edition, retitled *DrugPoints*. (Ask your instructor if your school has online access via a subscription.)

The hardbound volumes are first organized alphabetically by generic name, and then by dosage form. Thus, when you are researching information, be sure that you are looking at the correct dosage form. Both Volume I and Volume II provide vital information on the safety and use of pharmaceutical products and consist of a series of pharmaceutical monographs. The monographs in Volume I contain information on indication, pharmacology and pharmacokinetics, precautions, side and adverse effects, overdose levels, patient considerations, general dosing guidelines, and separate dosage forms. Monographs in Volume II contain, in plain language, a drug description and information on brand and generic names, what to do prior to using the medication, proper use, precautions, side effects, and accompanying notes.

In addition to pharmaceutical monographs, both volumes provide supplemental information at the front and back of the text. Volume I contains several appendices, including a list of drug-induced effects, therapeutic guidelines, a cross-reference listing, the Veterans Health Administration medication classification system, a product identification chart, a listing of poison control centers, and a list of monographs no longer included in the printed text, but available in the online version, *DrugPoints*. (To save space, uncommon drugs are not listed in the *USP DI* but can be researched online.) The back of the book also includes an index of indications and off-label usage, and a general index. Volume II contains an alphabetical index in the front of the text. This index is designed to function as a table of contents for patients

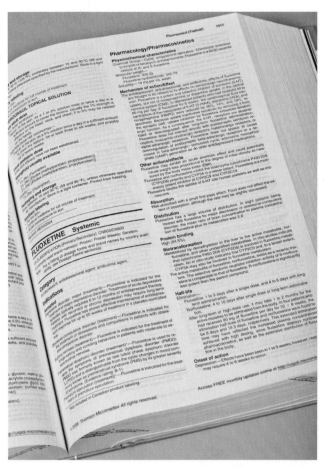

An example of a drug monograph from Volume I of the *USP DI*.

who may not be familiar with medical references. A listing of online monographs, poison control centers, categories of use, pregnancy categories, and breast-feeding precautions is located at the back of the book.

Knowing how to use both of these reference texts is a valuable skill when you are helping the pharmacist research drugs or review prescription information. As a pharmacy technician, you may also refer patients themselves to Volume II, particularly when they want to research details about their own prescriptions and also when they are simply taking advantage of waiting time at the pharmacy. Remember that you must never provide drug information or counselling to patients; all patient questions requiring professional judgment must be referred to a pharmacist.

Procedure

To complete this lab, you will need to search in both volumes of the *USP DI* or, if your school has access, use the web-based version, *DrugPoints*, to locate the requested information. You will require additional copies of both worksheets found at the end of the lab, so you may make your own from these blank forms or your instructor may provide you with copies. Note that one worksheet asks you to consult Volume I of the *USP DI,* and the other directs you to Volume II. Both worksheets have blanks near the top for you to fill in the brand and generic names of the drug. You should fill in both drug name blanks, no matter which type of name you are initially given.

1 Complete all sections of *both* worksheets for each of the following drugs: Accutane capsules, ciprofloxacin tablets, Lantus injectable insulin, and metformin tablets.

2 Complete all sections of *both* worksheets for another prescription product—your choice.

3 Ask your instructor if she or he wants to assign you additional drugs to research. If so, proceed to fill in all sections of *both* worksheets for each drug.

4 **Conclusion:** Make sure your name and today's date are on each worksheet. Turn in all completed worksheet pages to your instructor. On a separate sheet of paper, answer all questions in the following Lab Review section and turn in your answers to your instructor.

Lab Review

Check Your Understanding

1. *USP DI* stands for _____.
   a. United States Pharmacy: Drug Index
   b. United States Pharmacopoeia: Drug Index
   c. United States Pharmacopoeia: Drug Information
   d. United States Pharmacist: Drug Information

2. *USP DI*, Volume I, contains information for the health professional to use when researching pharmaceutical products.
   a. true
   b. false

3. The general index of Volume _____ is located in the front of the text because _____.
   a. I; health professionals need to locate information on drug products rapidly
   b. I; patients who may not be familiar with indices are probably familiar with a table of contents
   c. II; health professionals need to locate information on drug products rapidly
   d. II; patients who may not be familiar with indices are probably familiar with a table of contents

4. Monographs in Volume II contain information on the following topics, except _____.
   a. proper use
   b. side effects
   c. auxiliary labeling
   d. pharmacology

5. A pharmacy technician would probably have the opportunity to assist both pharmacists and _____ when researching drug information in the *USP DI*.
   a. physicians
   b. nurses
   c. office staff
   d. patients

Thinking Like a Pharmacy Tech

1. The *USP DI* and *Drug Facts and Comparisons* are both references that provide clinical information in a format that is convenient for quick research. What are the most significant differences and similarities between these texts?

2. Now that you have considered how the *USP DI* and *Drug Facts and Comparisons* compare, you may see an advantage to using one of these two references over the other. Other than the fact that one of the *USP DI* volumes contains information for the lay person, discuss key advantages to using the *USP DI*.

3. Have you explored the pharmacy technician certification exam, and what kinds of questions are on the exam? Visit the website for the Pharmacy Technician Certification Board, click Certification and then choose About the Exam. How will you study for this exam?

Name: _____   Date: _____

Lab 2   *Using the* United States Pharmacopoeia: Drug Information

Worksheet for *USP DI* Volume I

Brand name(s): _____ Generic name: _____

Category: _____

Mechanism of action: _____

_____

_____

_____

Pregnancy information: _____

_____

_____

_____

Side effects: _____

_____

_____

_____

Usual adult/pediatric dosage information: _____

_____

_____

Storage: _____

Auxiliary labeling: _____

_____

_____

Lab 2   *Using the* United States Pharmacopoeia: Drug Information

Worksheet for *USP DI* Volume II

Brand name(s): _____ Generic name: _____

Category: _____

Mechanism of action: _____

_____

_____

Pregnancy information: _____

_____

_____

Side effects: _____

_____

_____

Usual adult/pediatric dosage information: _____

_____

_____

Storage: _____

How do Volumes I and II compare in relation to the information presented for this drug?
Does each reference provide sufficient information for its target audience?

_____

_____

_____

_____

_____

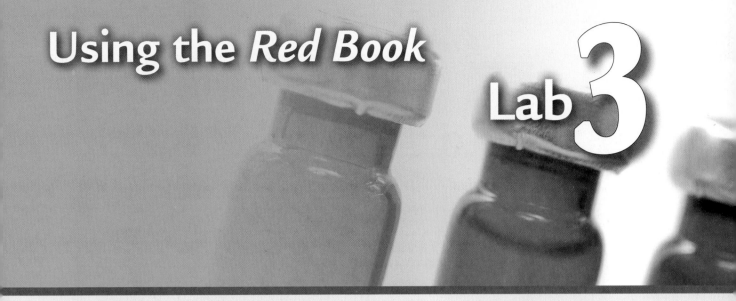

Using the *Red Book*

Lab 3

Objectives

- Describe the contents and organization of the *Red Book* reference text.
- Practice using the *Red Book* as a pharmacy practice text.
- Identify how the *Red Book* contributes to successful pharmacy practice and administration.

Supplies

- The most recent edition of the *Red Book*

The *Red Book*, like *Drug Facts and Comparisons* and the *USP DI*, is a reference text used by pharmacy technicians and pharmacists in pharmacy practice and administration. However, unlike the other two texts, the *Red Book* is not intended as a clinical reference. Rather, the *Red Book* is a hard-copy reference text specifically intended as an all-purpose compendium of product and pricing information for prescription products, over-the-counter (OTC) products, and medical supplies. One of the more commonly used references in pharmacy practice and administration, this book contains data on more than 100,000 products, organized within twelve labeled sections. The *Red Book* provides pharmacy employees with valuable information for pharmacy operations, including:

- **Average Wholesale Price (AWP):** The average price of products charged by wholesalers; using AWP in pharmacy pricing is standard practice in pharmacy reimbursement.
- **Federal Upper Limit Pricing (FUL):** The designation set by a federal agency, such as the Centers for Medicare and Medicaid (CMS), to limit cost and reimbursement amounts for specific drugs that are acquired from multiple sources.

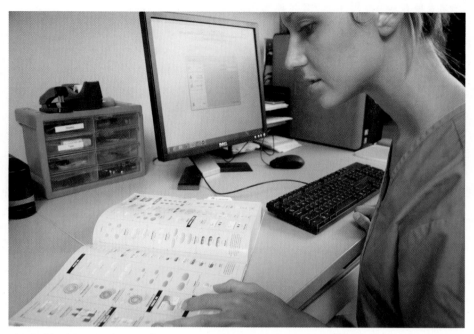

The *Red Book* is an indispensible source of information for pharmacy technicians.

- **Full-color product identification:** The *Red Book* also has full-color photographs of selected pharmaceutical products to aid your identification of the products when questions arise. (*Drug Facts and Comparisons* and *DrugPoints* also have detailed product identification databases.)
- **National Drug Code (NDC):** The unique number assigned to each Food and Drug Administration (FDA)-approved drug product.
- **Orange Book Code (Also known as OBC, Therapeutic Equivalency [TE] Code):** The *Orange Book* is a therapeutic equivalency guide published by the FDA. It was originally printed with an orange cover, which explains its name; however, it is no longer available in printed form. Although the OBC is available online (ask your instructor about access), the *Red Book* (printed with a red cover) also includes TE Codes to assist with determining which products a pharmacy needs and with order preparation.
- **Packaging information:** The data—often including strength, dosage form, size, and route of administration—printed on the packaging materials of retail drug products.
- **Pharmacy associations (state boards, buying groups, DEA offices, etc.):** The *Red Book* contains contact information for pharmacy wholesalers and buying groups, each State Board of Pharmacy, and your local office of the Drug Enforcement Administration (DEA). You may also find contact information for various disease management programs addressing conditions relating to cardiovascular disease, diabetes, HIV/AIDS, lupus, and others.
- **Suggested Retail Price (SRP):** The suggested retail price for OTC products.

Keep in mind that while knowing how to use reference texts is a valuable skill when you are helping the pharmacist research drugs or review prescription information, you should never provide drug information or counseling to patients. As a pharmacy technician, always refer all patient questions requiring professional judgement to a pharmacist.

Procedure

This lab will provide you with significant practice using the *Red Book*. You will become familiar with its numbered sections and information categories as you complete the worksheet at the end of the chapter. When researching and locating information for the worksheet, be sure to use the table of contents in the front of the book and the section tabs along the right side of the pages. Also remain aware of the manufacturer, NDC, and TE Codes when identifying products and product information in the *Red Book*.

1 Obtain the most current version of the *Red Book* available to your classroom.

2 Use the *Red Book* to carefully complete all worksheet questions.

3 **Conclusion:** Tear out and turn in the completed worksheet pages to your instructor. On a separate sheet of paper, answer all questions in the following Lab Review section and turn in your answers to your instructor.

Lab Review

Check Your Understanding

1. The acronym *AWP* stands for _____.
   a. Average Written Percentage
   b. Average Wholesale Price
   c. Annual Wholesale Purchase
   d. Annual Written Prescriptions

2. The *Red Book* contains information on over _____ products.
   a. 1,000
   b. 10,000
   c. 100,000
   d. 1,000,000

3. The *Red Book* contains all of the following information, except _____.
   a. federal pricing limits
   b. therapeutic equivalency
   c. buying groups
   d. third-party contracting

4. TE Codes are also found in the _____ *Book*.
   a. *Blue*
   b. *Orange*
   c. *Green*
   d. *Black*

5. The *Red Book* is a useful compendium of information aiding the pharmacist and pharmacy technician in pharmacy _____.
   a. administration
   b. location
   c. development
   d. compliance

Thinking Like a Pharmacy Tech

1. While the *Red Book* provides necessary AWP information, some of the other data contained in the *Red Book* is also available from additional sources such as *Drug Facts and Comparisons* and the *Orange Book*. What specific or general purpose does the *Red Book* serve?

2. As you have seen in Labs 1, 2, and 3, there is a variety of sources of information available to pharmacists and pharmacy technicians. In your opinion, is there a need for such variety? Explain why a single reference text would or would not be sufficient.

3. What qualities make a good pharmacy technician? Do they differ amongst pharmacy settings (community or hospital)? Which of these qualities do you possess? How might you strengthen the areas where you are weaker?

Lab 3 _____ *Using the* Red Book

Worksheet for the *Red Book*

1. Under which section of the *Red Book* may one find the *MedWatch* Reporting Form?

   _____

2. In Section 1, research the antidote for *Latrodectus mactans* poison and provide it here:

   _____

3. In what city is your closest Poison Control Center and what is the emergency phone number?

   _____

4. In which section of the *Red Book* is the generic availability guide?

   _____

5. Is a generic form of Andro Gel 1% available? _____

6. Is a generic form of Pepcid 40 mg/5 mL Oral Suspension available? _____

7. Is there a product listing for sugar-free products, alcohol-free products, and products

   that may cause photosensitivity? _____ If yes, in which section(s) are they

   found? _____

8. Which OTC vitamin product has a higher iron content, Centrum® or One-A-Day

   Active®? _____

9. What is the drug/alcohol interaction with sertraline?

   _____

   _____

10. For an adult male, what is the common laboratory test value for follicle-stimulating

    hormone (FSH)? _____

    _____

For an adult female? _____

_____

11. What is the meaning of the term *roborant*? In which section is this definition found?

_____

_____

12. What is the contact information for your nearest cardiovascular disease management program?

_____

_____

_____

13. One method to determine the value of a pharmacy listed for sale is known as the *Net Income* method. Look up this method and, using the provided formula, determine a sales price when the net profit of a pharmacy is $326,387, the owner's salary is $145,000, and the current inventory is valued at $276,472.

_____

_____

_____

14. Translate *Take as Needed* into Spanish. _____

15. List the contact information for your state's Board of Pharmacy.

_____

_____

_____

16. In what city is your closest DEA office? _____

17. a. What is the FUL price for diazepam 10 mg? $ _____

    b. What is the FUL price for prednisone 20 mg? $ _____

18. Describe the appearance and markings of Coumadin 4 mg tablets.

_____

_____

19. Describe the appearance and markings of Levothroid 125 mcg tablets.

_____

_____

20. What are the AWP and NDC of Ranbaxy Pharmaceutical's doxycycline monohydrate 100 mg? _____

21. What are the AWP and OBC for the following prescription products?

    a. Fentanyl citrate, Baxter, 10019-0035-74: _____

    b. Fluoxetine 10 mg, Major Pharmaceuticals, 00904-5784-61: _____

    _____

    c. Humulin-R U-100, Lilly, 55045-3506-01: _____

    d. Ipratropium bromide, Apotex Corp, 60505-0827-01: _____

    _____

    e. Ketoconazole, TEVA Pharmaceuticals, 00093-0900-05: _____

    _____

    f. Temazepam, Sandoz, 00781-2202-05: _____

22. What are the AWP and SRP for the following OTC products? _____

    a. Dermanail, Summers, 11086-0026-01: _____

    b. Good Neighbor Ibuprofen Junior Strength, 24385-0550-10: _____

    _____

    c. Orajel 7 g, Del, 10310-0222-40: _____

    d. Renu Multiplus Solution 355 mL, Bausch & Lomb, 10119-0031-22: _____

    _____

Unit

2

Community Pharmacy Practice

A day in the life of a pharmacy technician...

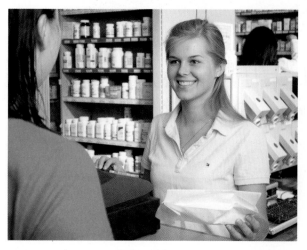

It's the first of the month. It seems like every single person in town wants to fill a prescription—some have refills, some don't, some are expired, some are too early, some have mistakes on the prescription form, and others have issues with the third party provider. You have to make a phone call on each prescription, which takes time. Overnight, over 100 people requested a refill online or via the telephone system. You've been open for 15 minutes and the wait to fill a prescription is already over an hour—and the phone just keeps ringing.

What are you going to do?

The important thing to remember is that you should not panic. This is a common day for many pharmacy technicians working in a community or retail pharmacy across the country. The knowledge to effectively process prescriptions, handle any sort of issue (called exceptions), and work as a member of the healthcare team to provide accurate and efficient pharmacy services is all acquired with practice and experience. As a new pharmacy technician, you will gain the skills to multitask and resolve complex issues encountered in the pharmacy on a daily basis.

From reviewing a patient profile for completeness and accuracy to working with the pharmacy team to accurately process each prescription, you play a vital role in the foundation of pharmacy operations. The pharmacy technician is an essential member of the pharmacy team. While you do a lot of work and engage frequently with customers, it is important to remember your central goal: to help everyone feel better and improve their health.

Pharmacy technicians must also be adaptable. Many aspects of the job are constantly changing—new laws are enacted, new brand name drugs come to the market, generics become available for popular drugs, and technology changes, such as doctors writing more e-prescriptions instead of patients bringing in hand-written forms. Pharmacy technicians should always be ready to learn new skills.

Task management (effective management of the assigned task) and working to meet the needs of each patient are keys to success as a pharmacy technician. The skills in this unit help you acquire the foundational knowledge of patient data management, prescription processing and management, as well as knowledge on how to resolve some of the more common situations encountered in the daily work of a pharmacy technician.

While it may seem like a lot at first, practice and repetition will help you build the skills you need to ensure smooth operations and provide the best service possible to each patient at the pharmacy.

Verifying DEA Numbers

Lab 4

Objectives

- Describe the purpose of a DEA number
- Describe the components and features of a DEA number
- Determine the validity of a prescriber's DEA number

Supplies

- *Pharmacy Labs for Technicians* textbook
- Calculator

A DEA number is a unique identifier assigned to prescribers, pharmacies, hospitals, and other entities (such as drug wholesalers and manufacturers) by the United States Drug Enforcement Administration, a branch of the Department of Justice. This number allows for tracking the authorized prescribing, preparation, and dispensing of controlled substances.

In accordance with law of the state in which the practitioner resides, having a DEA number grants them the ability to work with controlled substances pursuant to their area of responsibility. In other words, a prescriber with a DEA number may write prescriptions, a pharmacy with a DEA number may store and distribute controlled substances pursuant to a prescription order, and a hospital may do likewise in response to medication orders.

The DEA number consists of two letters and seven numbers. The first letter indicates the level of practice and responsibility. For example, physicians, dentists, podiatrists, veterinarians, pharmacies, and hospitals will have a DEA number that begins with the letters A, B, or F. Midlevel practitioners, such as a nurse practitioner, physician assistant, or optometrist, will be assigned a DEA number starting with the letter M. As noted above, other DEA numbers exist for manufacturers (E), /importer (J), and exporters (K); however, as a pharmacy technician, you will primarily work with those who prescribe, so this lab focuses only on those roles with prescriptive and housing authority (DEA numbers staring with A, B, F, and M).

The second letter represents one of two things: If assigned to a business, the second letter of the DEA number will be the first letter of the name of the business or the company that owns the business. If the number is assigned to an individual, the second letter will be the first letter of the last name of that individual.

The next six numbers are used as part of a checksum equation to verify the validity of the DEA number itself. The seventh number is used as the verification number for the checksum equation.

Procedure

Using the process described below, verify the DEA numbers on the following worksheet. If the number is correct, mark it as valid. If the number is incorrect, mark it as invalid and describe the corrections needed to make it a valid number.

To verify a DEA number, follow this checksum equation:

1 Add the first, third and fifth digits;

2 Add the second, fourth, and sixth digits, and then multiply the sum by 2;

3 Add the results from steps 1 and 2;

4 The last number of this final sum should be the same as the seventh number of the DEA number.

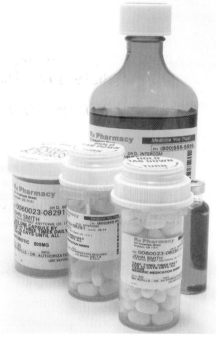

A DEA number allows a pharmacy to house and distribute controlled substances pursuant to a prescription order.

Example 1: Pollard's Pharmacy has been assigned DEA number FP1234563

The pharmacy has the authority to order, store, and dispense controlled substances. They have been assigned a "primary level of practice" DEA number starting with the letter F. The name of the business starts with the letter P, so that is the second letter in the DEA number. Using the equation above, the DEA number can be verified:

$$1 + 3 + 5 = 9$$
$$2 + 4 + 6 = 12 \times 2 = 24$$
$$9 + 24 = 33$$

The last number in the DEA number (3) matches the last number in the last step of the checksum equation, 3. The DEA number is valid.

Example 2: Spencer Brown, PA, has been assigned DEA number MB1178690

Mr. Brown, a physician assistant, has been assigned a DEA number starting with the letter M because he is a midlevel practitioner. Depending on state law, a physician assistant may have limited authority to write a prescription for a controlled substance. The prescriber's last name starts with the letter B, which is the second letter in the DEA number. Using the equation above, the DEA number can be verified:

$$1 + 7 + 6 = 14$$
$$1 + 8 + 9 = 18 \times 2 = 36$$
$$14 + 36 = 50$$

The last number in the DEA number (0) matches the last number in the last step of the checksum equation, 0. The DEA number is valid.

Example 3: Lisa Tierny, DDS, has been assigned DEA number AT6379241

Ms. Tierny, a dentist, has been assigned a DEA number starting with the letter A because she is a primary practitioner. A primary practitioner may write a prescription, in accordance with state regulations, for medications on schedules II to V. The prescriber's last name starts with the letter T, which is the second letter in the DEA Number. Using the equation above, the DEA number can be verified:

$$6 + 7 + 2 = 15$$
$$3 + 9 + 4 = 16 \times 2 = 32$$
$$15 + 32 = 47$$

The last number in the DEA number (1) does not match the last number in the last step of the checksum equation, 7. The DEA number is invalid.

Take Note

Schedule I drugs are not legally dispensed in the United States due to their high potential for abuse and addiction. Schedule II narcotics are the most highly regulated and sudden increases in usage in a particular pharmacy (or prescribed by a particular doctor) may cause the DEA to investigate. Schedule II drugs have no refills. Schedule III, IV, and V drugs have less abuse and addiction potential than Schedule II drugs and have no limits on refills. See Table 4.1

Take Note

In the case of an invalid DEA number, alert the pharmacist and seek guidance on how to proceed. There is a high level of liability in acting on a possible prescription forgery. Contacting local law enforcement should be handled by appropriate personnel, and only after consulting the pharmacist on duty and/or the pharmacy manager. Be sure to comply with company policies on the detection of prescription forgeries.

TABLE 4.1

Drug Schedules under the Controlled Substances Act of 1970

Schedule	Manufacturer's Label	Abuse Potential	Accepted Medical Use	Examples
Schedule I	C-I	highest potential for abuse	for research only; must have license to obtain; no accepted medical use in the United States	heroin, lysergic acid diethylamide (LSD)
Schedule II	C-II	high possibility of abuse, which can lead to severe psychological or physical dependence	dispensing severely restricted; cannot be prescribed by telephone except in an emergency; no refills on prescriptions	morphine, oxycodone, meperidine, hydromorphone, fentanyl, methylphenidate, dextroamphetamine
Schedule III	C-III	less potential for abuse and addiction than C-II	prescriptions can be refilled up to five times within 6 months if authorized by physician	codeine/hydrocodone with aspirin, codeine/hydrocodone with acetaminophen, anabolic steroids
Schedule IV	C-IV	lower abuse potential than C-II and C-III; associated with limited physical or psychological dependence	same as for Schedule III	benzodiazepines, meprobamate, phenobarbital
Schedule V	C-V	lowest abuse potential	some sold without a prescription depending on state law; if so, purchaser must be over 18 and is required to sign log and show driver's license	liquid codeine combination cough preparations, diphenoxylate/atropine

Lab Review

Check Your Understanding

1. A DEA number is assigned by the __B__.
   - a. Drug Enforcement Agency
   - b. Drug Enforcement Administration
   - c. Drug Enumeration Alliance
   - d. Department of Enforcement

2. A podiatrist will have a DEA number starting with which of the following letters?
   - a. F
   - b. J
   - c. K
   - d. M

3. A nurse practitioner will have a DEA number starting with which of the following letters?
   - a. A
   - b. F
   - c. M
   - d. Y

4. The second step of the DEA number verification process includes adding the __1__, __3__, and __5__ numbers.
   - a. first, third, and sixth
   - b. first, third, and fifth
   - c. second, fourth, and seventh
   - d. second, fourth, and sixth

5. The second letter of a dentist's DEA number whose name is Laura McKinney would be __M__.
   - a. A
   - b. L
   - c. M
   - d. K

[Handwritten notes:]
1st Letter = Profession
2nd Letter = First Letter in the Last name
Add the 1st, 3rd, & 5th #
Add 2nd, 4th, & 6th # the X2
now add the
sum of both #'s
last # should match last # in DEA code.

Thinking Like a Pharmacy Tech

1. Midlevel practitioners often have more limited prescription authority than primary practitioners. Many states limit the classes of controlled substances of which a midlevel practitioner may prescribe. Why do you think that is? Why can't a midlevel practitioner write for all levels in all states? In answering your question also think about why do states differ in prescriptive authority?

2. In addition to your answer above, use the following website and identify three states where a midlevel practitioner can prescribe for schedules II to V, and three where they cannot:
   www.paradigmcollege.net/pharmlabs2e/dea

 3. A résumé communicates your strengths, skills, and work experience to a potential employer. What qualities make up a strong résumé? Draft a résumé highlighting your own education and work history.

Lab 4   *Reviewing DEA Numbers*

Worksheet 1 *Reviewing DEA Numbers*

Directions: Certify the DEA numbers below. If the number is valid, mark it as "valid." If the number is invalid, mark it as "invalid" and describe the corrections needed to make it a valid number.

Example:

Lisa Tierny, DDS   AT6379241

_____ Valid   _X_ Invalid   Corrections: The last number should be 7.
6 + 7 + 2 = 15; 3 + 9 + 4 = 16 x 2 = 32; 15 + 32 = 47. Since the last number of the checksum is 7, the last number of the DEA number should be 7, not 1.

1. Floyd's Pharmacy   FP1743263

    _____ Valid   _X_ Invalid   Corrections: *the last number should be a 7 when all calculations are done not 9.*

    [handwritten: 1+4+2=7; 7+3+6=16 x 2 = 32; =39]

2. Michela Zuckerman, FNP   AZ6321474

    ~~Valid~~   ~~Invalid~~   Corrections: *His letters arent correct. It should be M not A*

    [handwritten: 6+2+4=12; 3+1+7=11 x 2 = 22; =34]

3. Robert Montague, DPM   FM4721362

    _____ Valid   _X_ Invalid   Corrections: *Last number on the DEA # is 2. It should be 7.*

    [handwritten: 4+2+3=9; 7+1+6=14 x 2 = 28; =37]

4. Albert Pickerman, MD   BP3419202

    _X_ Valid   _____ Invalid   Corrections: _____

    [handwritten: 3+1+2=6; 4+9+0=13 x 2 = 26; =32]

5. Vivek Rajeev, PA MR1842005 *1+4+0 = 5, 8+2+0 = 10×2 = 20 = 25*

$\times$ Valid ___ Invalid Corrections: _____

THIS DEA # IS valid. The letters match up & so does the last digit.

6. Kitty Corners Animal Hospital AK7249089

$\times$ Valid ___ Invalid Corrections: _____

_____

_____

7. Roberta Goodson, DDS FR1720617

___ Valid $\times$ Invalid Corrections: *Second letter doesn't match the first letter in last name. Should be G not R.*

8. Jason van Alstyne, OD (M)V3621148

___ Valid $\times$ Invalid Corrections: _____

First letter should be an A, B, or F. *= 33*

9. Curtis Longbottom, MD FL6392423 *1 1 1 6+9+4 = 19, 3+2+2 = 7×2 = 14*

$\times$ Valid ___ Invalid Corrections: _____

_____

10. Silvia Romero, DO *? what's DO?* BR9007469

~~___~~ Valid $\times$ Invalid Corrections: _____

_____

_____

Reviewing a Patient Profile

Lab 5

Objectives

- Demonstrate an understanding of the importance of a patient profile in pharmacy practice.
- Gain skill in reviewing a patient profile form for complete, accurate information.
- Demonstrate an understanding of the types of problems that missing or inaccurate patient information can introduce to pharmacy practice.
- Demonstrate strategies to resolve problems arising from incomplete patient profile forms.

Supplies

- None

Transcribing

Transferring information between documents, in electronic or other form

When patients first visit a pharmacy, they usually complete a hard-copy patient profile form. This form establishes a patient record with the pharmacy. Once the form is signed and submitted to the pharmacy, the pharmacy technician is often responsible for **transcribing**—transferring information from the completed paper form to the electronic patient record in the pharmacy management software. The technician's transcription work plays an important role in ensuring and maintaining patient safety. You must be vigilant and verify that the information provided by the patient is both accurate and complete. If the patient profile is not complete, you may have the added responsibility of interviewing the patient to solicit further data.

The patient profile form itself is a simple document that includes basic demographic information, such as name, address, birth date, telephone numbers (home, work, and "other"), and email address. The form requests other crucial information, including medications currently being taken, current or long-term health conditions, and allergies. All of this data has a

Best practice

A highly effective process, technique, or activity designed to deliver the best results with little or no margin of error

direct impact on the patient's drug therapy and some important cautions are in order. While it is not necessary to push for more than one phone number, it is a **best practice** to have multiple means of contacting a patient. You do need to record a street address for a patient, in case you must make contact in an emergency and because state regulations may require one when you fill certain prescriptions, such as those for controlled substances. In addition, when a parent or guardian is providing information for a child, ensure that the information the adult writes down is, indeed, about the child. Dosage and review guidelines for a pediatric patient are of high importance and accurate information is crucial to the child's safety.

While a physician has the knowledge to prescribe safely, pharmacy staff can fully review a patient's prescriptions for safety when the pharmacy is equipped with a complete and accurate patient record. Pharmacy staff can screen the requested medications against the patient's other current medications, check for errors caused by incorrect prescriptions, and respond competently if something undesired should result. Complete patient records provide a "big picture" view of a patient's medication program, enabling pharmacists and pharmacy technicians to serve patients well and protect their welfare.

One final note in patient safety is to consider the use of two very similar phrases, "No Known Drug Allergies" (NKDA) and "No Known Allergies" (NKA). NKDA implies that the pharmacy staff has asked only about *drug* allergies and has specifically identified that the patient has no known allergies to drug products. NKA is a more broad claim, implying that the pharmacy has established that the patient has no known allergies whatsoever, in any allergy category (such as drug allergies, food allergies, pet allergies, or plant allergies). As a pharmacy technician, you must ensure that you are using the proper phrase in the patient's pharmacy record.

As healthcare practitioners, pharmacy technicians are entrusted with personal data from each person receiving prescriptions and must protect that data. Always keep in mind the ethical implications of having access to **confidential** patient information and the necessity of not disclosing such information outside the pharmacy. The Health Insurance Portability and Accountability Act of 1996 (HIPAA) regulates the use and disclosure of Protected Health Information (PHI). For example, consider this scenario:

Confidentiality

The ethical practice of keeping patients' personal and private information safe and secure

You are transcribing Miguel Esparza's profile (Worksheet 4) when you notice he lives on the 7500 block of East 11th Street. Your Aunt Pamela lives on the 7600 block of the same street, so you strike up a conversation with the patient on how that neighborhood is slated for a street-paving project, according to your aunt. You also notice that Miguel has come in for a prescription antihistamine and, later that night, call your Aunt Pamela to tell her that Miguel has a bad cold and she should warn her friends that a cold or flu bug is circulating on East 11th Street.

While not intentional, your actions constitute a breach of ethical conduct, and are also a violation of HIPAA, which has potential legal implications. You have disclosed a patient's personal health information to a person not otherwise involved in his care and violated the trust between you and your patient, Miguel. As a pharmacy technician, you must strictly respect your patients' privacy when handling their protected health information.

Procedure

Several patients have filled out new patient profile forms as shown in Figures 5.1 and Worksheets 1–4. The form in Figure 5.1 is completely and accurately filled out, whereas those in the worksheets may be incomplete. In this lab, you will check the new patient profile forms in Worksheets 1 through 4 for completeness and accuracy.

As you proceed through the steps below, work thoughtfully and consider questions such as: Are all blank areas fully filled in? What kind of information is missing? Is the missing information required or not? Are allergies noted? Is medical information present? Is the form signed? When you encounter missing or incorrect data that requires resolution, you should ask yourself how you would handle such circumstances if they arose at your pharmacy. That is, identify a best practice to solicit the missing information from the patient, to discuss items that appear inaccurate, or to bring these issues to the pharmacist's attention. What would or should you do? What should you avoid doing or saying? Should you interview the patient at the pharmacy drop-off counter or pull the patient aside to the counseling window if the question is quite personal? How do you determine what a particular patient may consider "personal" information? Discuss all topics that you are unsure of with your instructor.

To complete the worksheets, follow the steps outlined to review each patient profile form for accuracy and completeness. Because this is a practice scenario, there is no patient present for you to speak with should you have questions about the profile form. Nonetheless, when a procedure step asks you to communicate with a patient, imagine the patient is in front of you and either whisper quietly to yourself as if having that conversation or imagine the patient's response. If your instructor permits it and time allows, you might also partner with another student to role-play these "pharmacy technician and patient" conversations. Remember that not all information is required. Clearly circle all errors that you discover on each worksheet and then describe the action you, as a pharmacy technician, would take to correct the error.

1 Carefully read over the completed, accurate profile, Figure 5.1 on the next page, noticing how the various sections are thoroughly and completely filled out.

FIGURE 5.1 Sample of a fully completed new Patient Profile

PATIENT PROFILE

Patient Name

Wilkins (Last) — Marquita (First) — ____ (Middle Initial)

6901 Westminster Chase (Street or PO Box)

Providence (City) — RI (State) — 02908 (ZIP)

Date of Birth: 02/29/1984 (MM / DD / YYYY)
Gender: ☐ Male ☒ Female
Social Security No.: 000-00-0000
E-mail: marquita@email.com

Home Phone: (401) 555-1212
Work Phone: (401) 555-1313
Other Phone: ( ) ____

☑ Yes, I would like medication dispensed in a child-resistant container.
☐ No, I do not want medication dispensed in a child-resistant container.

Medication Insurance: ☑ Yes ☐ No

Cardholder Name: same
☑ Cardholder ☐ Spouse ☐ Child ☐ Dependent Parent ☐ Disabled Dependent ☐ Full-Time Student
(Please provide the pharmacy with your card.)

MEDICAL HISTORY

HEALTH
- ☐ No Known Medical Conditions
- ☐ Anemia
- ☐ Arthritis
- ☐ Asthma
- ☐ Attention-Deficit Hyperactivity Disorder
- ☐ Blood Clotting Disorders
- ☐ Cancer
- ☐ Depression
- ☐ Diabetes Mellitus
- ☐ Epilepsy
- ☐ Esophagitis
- ☐ Generalized Anxiety Disorder
- ☐ Heart Condition
- ☐ Hypertension
- ☐ Kidney Disease
- ☐ Liver Disease
- ☐ Lung Disease
- ☐ Ulcers

ALLERGIES AND DRUG REACTIONS
- ☐ No Known Drug Allergies
- ☐ Aspirin
- ☐ Cephalosporins
- ☐ Codeine
- ☐ Erythromycin
- ☑ Penicillin G Potassium
- ☐ Sulfa
- ☐ Tetracyclines
- ☐ Xanthines

ICD-9 for Checked Condition(s): ____
Details for Checked Allergy(ies): ____

Medication(s) Currently Being Taken: ____

Primary Care Physician: Geoff Taylor

Comments: ____

Health information changes periodically. Please notify the pharmacy of any new medications, allergies, drug reactions, or health conditions.

Signature: Marquita Wilkins Date: 2/17/15 ☐ I choose not to fill out this form.

2 Go to the profile in Worksheet 1. Read the patient name and verify the spelling, confirming that it is legible. Be aware of gender-ambiguous names. In such cases, double-check the patient's gender by politely asking the patient if the prescription is for the patient or someone else. You might also ask to see a driver's license and discreetly seek your answer there.

3 Review the street address and verify spelling, city name, state, and zip code.

4 Verify the patient's date of birth—especially the year.

5 If a Social Security number is required for patient identification, be sure to get the entire number and explain that the number is required for insurance purposes only. Due to increasing identity theft, many patients are understandably hesitant to provide the number. Similarly, if the patient hesitates on providing an e-mail address, explain how and when your pharmacy plans to use the e-mail.

6 Look over the phone number section, ensuring you have at least one contact number for the patient.

7 If the box for child-resistant caps is checked, verify that this is correct.

8 If the patient has medication insurance, make sure the cardholder name is filled in and a relationship box is checked.

9 Ensure that the patient has indicated whether he or she has health conditions or allergies (medication or other types). If the patient writes in "No Known Drug Allergies" or checks a box indicating NKDA, keep in mind that you will have to record this designation carefully when you get to the computerized profile data-entry stage (Lab 8).

10 Verify whether the patient has taken any prescription or over-the-counter (OTC) medications recently or whether he or she takes any on a regular basis.

11 Check that the patient has signed the form. If not, ask the patient to do so.

12 Repeat Steps 2 through 11 for the remaining worksheets, completing Worksheets 1 through 4. When you have completed all four worksheets, proceed to Step 13.

13 **Conclusion:** Verify that you have written your name and the date, circled all errors, and written in your explanations on all four worksheets. Tear out the worksheets and turn them in to your instructor. On a separate sheet of paper, answer all questions in the following Lab Review section and turn in your answers to your instructor.

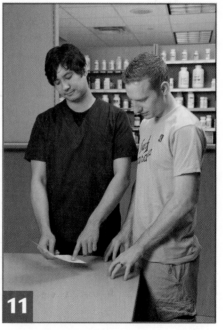

Pharmacy technician asking a customer to sign the patient profile form.

Lab Review

Check Your Understanding

1. Not entering a patient's allergy data into the computer system can have _____ consequences.
   a. no
   b. deadly
   c. minimal
   d. acceptable

2. Once a patient fills out a new patient profile form, a pharmacy technician can _____.
   a. translate the information loosely, as he or she sees fit
   b. transfer the information to the prescribing physician for approval
   c. transgress ethical boundaries without consequences
   d. transcribe the written information into an electronic patient record

3. Some states require _____ when filling a prescription.
   a. a P.O. box
   b. an e-mail address
   c. a street address
   d. an informal address

4. The phrases "No Known Allergies" and "No Known Drug Allergies" have different meanings, but using one for the other shouldn't present much of a problem.
   a. true
   b. false

5. By thoroughly reviewing a patient's profile, the pharmacy technician helps ensure patient _____.
   a. compliance
   b. health for a lifetime
   c. safety
   d. happiness with no chance of future complaints

Thinking Like a Pharmacy Tech

1. A patient must provide a written patient profile form to the pharmacy staff when establishing a patient record. Why shouldn't the patient save time and just orally communicate the information to the pharmacy staff while standing at the counter?

2. Suppose that a patient has submitted an incomplete patient profile form. Think about what a pharmacy technician must do to get complete information—such as for allergies, medical conditions, or insurance information—for this form. With a partner, role-play a scenario like this one in which one of you, as technician, must interview the other, as patient, to complete a blank patient profile form.

3. A cover letter is one of the first items a potential employer will see from you, and writing a good one can be tricky. Research cover letters and list three keys to a successful cover letter, and three things that will cause your letter to go to the bottom of the pile.

Lab 5

Reviewing a Patient Profile

Worksheet 1 New Patient Profile

PATIENT PROFILE

Patient Name

DONALDSON   VANCE
Last   First   Middle Initial

12 MAPLE LEAF TRAIL
Street or PO Box

ROUND ROCK   TX   78644
City   State   ZIP

Date of Birth   Gender   Social Security No.   E-mail
                     ☒ Male   000-00-0000 VDONALDSON@EMAIL.COM
MM/DD/YYYY   ☐ Female

Home Phone   Work Phone   Other Phone
(512) 555-1212   (512) 555-1313   (   )

☐ Yes, I would like medication dispensed in a child-resistant container.
☒ No, I do not want medication dispensed in a child-resistant container.

Medication Insurance   Cardholder Name SAME
☒ Yes   ☒ Cardholder   ☐ Child   ☐ Disabled Dependent
☐ No   ☐ Spouse   ☐ Dependent Parent   ☐ Full-Time Student
                            (Please provide the pharmacy with your card.)

MEDICAL HISTORY

HEALTH   ALLERGIES AND DRUG REACTIONS
☐ No Known Medical   ☐ Diabetes Mellitus   ☐ No Known Drug Allergies
   Conditions   ☐ Epilepsy   ☐ Aspirin
☐ Anemia   ☐ Esophagitis   ☐ Cephalosporins
☐ Arthritis   ☐ Generalized Anxiety Disorder ☐ Codeine
☐ Asthma   ☐ Heart Condition   ☐ Erythromycin
☐ Attention-Deficit   ☒ Hypertension   ☐ Penicillin G Potassium
   Hyperactivity Disorder ☐ Kidney Disease   ☐ Sulfa
☐ Blood Clotting Disorders ☐ Liver Disease   ☐ Tetracyclines
☐ Cancer   ☐ Lung Disease   ☐ Xanthines
☐ Depression   ☐ Ulcers

ICD-9 for Checked Condition(s): _____   Details for Checked Allergy(ies): _____

ICD-9: 401.9

Medication(s) Currently Being Taken: ASPIRIN 81 MG, ACCUPRIL 10 MG

Primary Care Physician: _____

Comments: _____
Health information changes periodically. Please notify the pharmacy of any new medications, allergies,
drug reactions, or health conditions.

Signature V. Donalds   Date 2/11/15   ☐ I choose not to fill out this form.

Circle the error(s) on this patient profile form.

Describe below the action(s) you would take to correct the error(s):

Missing the patients date of birth &
Primary care physician name.

Lab 5

Reviewing a Patient Profile

Worksheet 2 New Patient Profile

PATIENT PROFILE

Patient Name
Gupta   *Amala*
Last   First   Middle Initial

5473 W 10th Street
Street or PO Box

Cedar Rapids   *IA*   *52401*
City   State   ZIP

Date of Birth   Gender   Social Security No.   E-mail
08/24/1949   ☐ Male   *000-00-0000*   *guptaamala@email.com*
MM / DD / YYYY   ☑ Female

Home Phone   Work Phone   Other Phone
(319) 555-1212   ( )   ( )

☐ Yes, I would like medication dispensed in a child-resistant container.
☑ No, I do not want medication dispensed in a child-resistant container.

Medication Insurance   Cardholder Name *Same*
☑ Yes   ☑ Cardholder   ☐ Child   ☐ Disabled Dependent
☐ No   ☑ Spouse   ☐ Dependent Parent   ☐ Full-Time Student
     (Please provide the pharmacy with your card.)

MEDICAL HISTORY

HEALTH
☑ No Known Medical   ☐ Diabetes Mellitus
   Conditions   ☐ Epilepsy
☐ Anemia   ☐ Esophagitis
☐ Arthritis   ☐ Generalized Anxiety Disorder
☐ Asthma   ☐ Heart Condition
☐ Attention-Deficit   ☐ Hypertension
   Hyperactivity Disorder   ☐ Kidney Disease
☐ Blood Clotting Disorders   ☐ Liver Disease
☐ Cancer   ☐ Lung Disease
☐ Depression   ☐ Ulcers

ALLERGIES AND DRUG REACTIONS
☑ No Known Drug Allergies
☐ Aspirin
☐ Cephalosporins
☐ Codeine
☐ Erythromycin
☐ Penicillin G Potassium
☐ Sulfa
☐ Tetracyclines
☐ Xanthines

ICD-9 for Checked Condition(s): _____

Details for Checked Allergy(ies): _____

Medication(s) Currently Being Taken: _____

Primary Care Physician: *Sunita Patel*

Comments: _____

Health information changes periodically. Please notify the pharmacy of any new medications, allergies, drug reactions, or health conditions.

Signature _____ Date *2/16/15*   ☐ I choose not to fill out this form.

Circle the error(s) on this patient profile form.

Describe below the action(s) you would take to correct the error(s):

This prescription is missing the patients signature.

Lab 5

Worksheet 3 New Patient Profile

PATIENT PROFILE

Patient Name

Riley   *Cas*
Last   First   Middle Initial

72u50 Okade Court
Street or PO Box

Orlando   *FL*   *32810*
City   State   ZIP

Date of Birth	Gender	Social Security No.	E-mail
01 / 22 / 1998 MM / DD / YYYY	☑ Male ☐ Female	*000-00-0000*	*Casr@email.com*

Home Phone   Work Phone   Other Phone

(407) 555-1212   (   )   (   )

☑ Yes, I would like medication dispensed in a child-resistant container.
☐ No, I do not want medication dispensed in a child-resistant container.

Medication Insurance   Cardholder Name *Molly Riley*
☑ Yes   ☐ Cardholder   ☑ Child   ☐ Disabled Dependent
☐ No   ☐ Spouse   ☐ Dependent Parent   ☐ Full-Time Student
                        (Please provide the pharmacy with your card.)

MEDICAL HISTORY

HEALTH   ALLERGIES AND DRUG REACTIONS
☐ No Known Medical   ☐ Diabetes Mellitus   ☐ No Known Drug Allergies
  Conditions   ☐ Epilepsy   ☐ Aspirin
☐ Anemia   ☐ Esophagitis   ☐ Cephalosporins
☐ Arthritis   ☐ Generalized Anxiety Disorder ☐ Codeine
☐ Asthma   ☐ Heart Condition   ☐ Erythromycin
☑ Attention-Deficit   ☐ Hypertension   ☐ Penicillin G Potassium
  Hyperactivity Disorder ☐ Kidney Disease   ☐ Sulfa
☐ Blood Clotting Disorders ☐ Liver Disease   ☐ Tetracyclines
☐ Cancer   ☐ Lung Disease   ☐ Xanthines
☐ Depression   ☐ Ulcers

ICD-9 for Checked Condition(s): _____   Details for Checked Allergy(ies): _____

ICD-9 : 314.01

Medication(s) Currently Being Taken: ____ *Ritalin 10 mg* _____

Primary Care Physician: ____ *Philip McCracken* _____

Comments: _____

Health information changes periodically. Please notify the pharmacy of any new medications, allergies, drug reactions, or health conditions.

Signature *Molly Riley*   Date *2/1/15*   ☐ I choose not to fill out this form.

Circle the error(s) on this patient profile form.

Describe below the action(s) you would take to correct the error(s):

_____

_____

Lab 5

Reviewing a Patient Profile

Worksheet 4 New Patient Profile

PATIENT PROFILE

Patient Name

Esparza   *Miguel*
Last   First   Middle Initial

7583 E. 11th Street
Street or PO Box

Austin   *TX*   *78705*
City   State   ZIP

Date of Birth   Gender   Social Security No.   E-mail

09/12/1953   ☒ Male   *000-00-0000*
MM/DD/YYYY   ☐ Female

Home Phone   Work Phone   Other Phone

(512) 555-1212   (   )   (   )

☒ Yes, I would like medication dispensed in a child-resistant container.
☒ No, I do not want medication dispensed in a child-resistant container.

Medication Insurance   Cardholder Name   *same*
☒ Yes   ☒ Cardholder   ☐ Child   ☐ Disabled Dependent
☐ No   ☐ Spouse   ☐ Dependent Parent   ☐ Full-Time Student
                        (Please provide the pharmacy with your card.)

MEDICAL HISTORY

HEALTH   ALLERGIES AND DRUG REACTIONS
☐ No Known Medical   ☒ Diabetes Mellitus   ☐ No Known Drug Allergies
  Conditions   ☐ Epilepsy   ☐ Aspirin
☐ Anemia   ☐ Esophagitis   ☐ Cephalosporins
☐ Arthritis   ☐ Generalized Anxiety Disorder ☐ Codeine
☐ Asthma   ☐ Heart Condition   ☐ Erythromycin
☐ Attention-Deficit   ☐ Hypertension   ☐ Penicillin G Potassium
  Hyperactivity Disorder   ☐ Kidney Disease   ☐ Sulfa
☐ Blood Clotting Disorders ☐ Liver Disease   ☐ Tetracyclines
☐ Cancer   ☐ Lung Disease   ☐ Xanthines
☐ Depression   ☐ Ulcers

ICD-9 for Checked Condition(s): _____   Details for Checked Allergy(ies): _____

ICD-9 : 250.9

Medication(s) Currently Being Taken: _____

Primary Care Physician: _____

Comments: _____

Health information changes periodically. Please notify the pharmacy of any new medications, allergies, drug reactions, or health conditions.

Signature *Miguel Esparza*   Date *1/1/15*   ☐ I choose not to fill out this form.

Circle the error(s) on this patient profile form.

Describe below the action(s) you would take to correct the error(s):

missing Physician information

Reviewing a Prescription Form

Lab 6

Objectives

- Evaluate unprocessed prescriptions for completeness and accuracy.
- Learn the additional checking steps for reviewing controlled-substances prescriptions.

Supplies

- None

A written prescription is the primary form of communication between a prescribing healthcare provider and pharmacy staff in community pharmacies, while hospitals and institutional pharmacies tend to use medication orders instead. A prescription establishes the appropriate therapy protocol in an effort to relieve the patient of symptoms or illness.

A pharmacy technician's first responsibility is to process prescriptions—from receiving them from patients at the drop-off counter, to interpreting the data, to labeling the bottles. Prescription data is presented in the form of a **signa**, a series of abbreviations that begins with an action verb and communicates dispensing and patient directions in this order: dose, quantity, route of administration, time interval, and additional information. As a pharmacy technician, you will notice that prescriptions arrive in a variety of ways. Traditionally, you would only have seen handwritten, or hard copy, prescriptions, but today you also see prescriptions in other formats, including faxed and typewritten. As technology progresses, you will increasingly see electronic prescriptions sent in a manner resembling email.

Accurate filling of a prescription begins with a careful review of the form. Thus paying attention to detail is imperative. You must develop expertise in reviewing prescriptions for complete and accurate components including the patient, physician, and pharmacy data; the signa; and the

Signa

A series of abbreviations to communicate prescription and patient directions

49

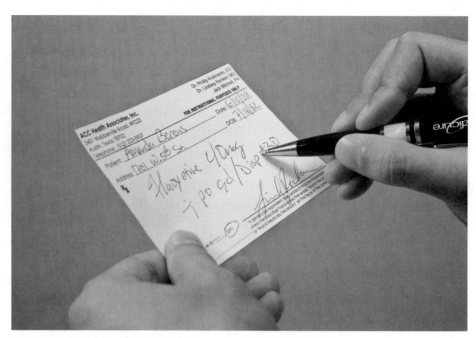
Pharmacy technician verifying information on a prescription form.

DEA number. You must also check adherence to additional state regulations for prescription drugs and controlled substances and verify any data specific to electronic prescriptions, which currently require information about the receiving pharmacy and a transmit date.

When preparing prescriptions, it is always a best practice to be mindful of the type of prescription that you are filling. When filling a prescription for a controlled substance, use added caution because regulations governing the preparation and dispensing of controlled substances are much stricter than are those for noncontrolled substances because of abuse potential. Remember that the quantity prescribed must be written in *both* numeral form and word form (e.g., "30, thirty") to prevent alteration of a prescribed quantity. If one of the two forms is missing, alert the pharmacist and contact the prescriber's office to verify the prescription. Also remember that federal regulations limit the quantity of refills on most controlled substances to five, for a maximum number of six total fills in six months (180 days). Lastly, be sure that a *valid* DEA number is on the prescription. See Lab 4 for more information on verifying DEA numbers.

Take Note

The laws regulating the practice of pharmacy and filling of prescriptions vary from state to state. Check with your instructor regarding any special exceptions concerning laws, rules, and regulations discussed in this text. Prescriptions for noncontrolled substances are valid for 1 year, while those for controlled substances are valid for 6 months. Prescriptions for noncontrolled substances can be refilled for up to 1 year, while those for controlled substances can be refilled only 5 times in a six-month period.

Procedure

This lab helps you develop your skills in reviewing prescriptions for completeness and accuracy. The worksheets at the end of the lab contain forms for unprocessed prescriptions. Using your current knowledge of pharmacy practice, information from your classroom textbook, and the instructions in the steps below, you will evaluate and comment on each prescription to ensure that the required information is included.

As you proceed through the numbered steps, you will use Checklist A for each worksheet prescription form. However, be aware that there may be more information to verify on some of the forms. In cases where the prescription was sent as an electronic prescription, you must also take the additional steps listed in Checklist B. In cases where the prescription is for a controlled substance, you must also take the additional steps listed in Checklist C. In some cases, you may need to use all three checklists. It is your responsibility to determine which checklists to consult for each prescription form. Checklists A, B, and C follow Step 6.

1 Read carefully over the prescription form and the Scenario included below the form.

2 Verify on each worksheet the information bulleted under Checklist A. If you find any errors or questionable components, mark them by clearly circling them on the prescription form itself.

3 In the space provided under the prescription form, explain the error(s) and then the best practice to correct the error(s) or resolve the issue(s).

4 If the prescription was sent as an electronic prescription, also check the bulleted items under Checklist B. As you did for Checklist A, mark the errors clearly on the prescriptions and write your explanations on the blank lines provided.

5 If the prescription is for a controlled substance, also check the bulleted items under Checklist C. As you did for Checklist A, mark the errors clearly on the prescriptions and write your explanations on the blank lines provided.

6 **Conclusion:** Tear out and turn in the completed worksheets to your instructor. On a separate sheet of paper, answer all questions in the following Lab Review section and turn in your answers to your instructor.

Checklist A, for all prescriptions on the worksheets:

- Check the physician information: name, address, phone number, and handwritten signature.
- Check the patient information: date of birth, name, and address.
- Check the prescription information: date written, drug name, strength, quantity, and refill information.
- Check the directions to the patient (the signa): dose quantity, route of administration, time interval, and additional information.

Checklist B, for electronic prescriptions on the worksheets:

- Check the receiving pharmacy information for your pharmacy's name, address, and phone number.
- Check whether the transmit date is different from the written date. If it is, you may need to call to verify the prescription's validity.
- Check that an electronic signature is on file.
- Check whether this electronic prescription is also for a controlled substance. If it is, verify with your instructor whether your state allows electronic transmission for such prescriptions and respond accordingly on the worksheet.

Checklist C, for controlled-substances (Schedules C-III and C-IV) prescriptions on the worksheets:

- Check that today's date, as presented in the scenario, is within 6 months (180 days) of when the prescription was written.
- Check the validity of the DEA number.
- Check that the quantity is written in both numeral form and word form.
- Check that the maximum number of refills is 5.
- Check the quantity, verify with your instructor whether your state places limitations on this substance, and respond accordingly on the worksheet.
- C-V prescriptions have no federal limit; be sure to check the regulations in your state.

Take Note

Because each state regulates the prescribing and dispensing of prescription drugs, especially C-II medications, differently, be sure to ask your instructor how these prescriptions are prepared and regulated in your state.

Lab Review

Check Your Understanding

1. A prescription for a controlled substance can have a maximum of _____ refills in 180 days.
   a. 12
   b. 6
   c. 5
   d. PRN

2. A prescription for a noncontrolled substance will usually contain patient name and date of birth; physician name, signature, and contact information; drug name, strength, and quantity; directions to the patient; and _____.
   a. a state license number
   b. refill information
   c. a written-out quantity
   d. the generic name

3. Which of the following choices lists the *correct* order of some of the components of a prescription signa?
   a. dose, route of administration, time interval, additional information
   b. route of administration, dose, time interval, action verb, additional information
   c. action verb, dose, route of administration, time interval, additional information
   d. dose, time interval, route of administration, additional information

4. A prescriber is required to hand sign all written prescriptions.
   a. true
   b. false

5. In most states, a prescription for a noncontrolled substance is valid for _____.
   a. 7 days
   b. PRN
   c. 6 months
   d. 12 months

Thinking Like a Pharmacy Tech

1. Since the pharmacist assumes the final professional responsibility for the accuracy of a prescription, why should a pharmacy technician take such care to evaluate the prescription? Why not let the pharmacist evaluate each form?

2. Why are controlled-substances prescriptions limited to a maximum number of six fills in a 6-month period? Since licensed practitioners are supposed to monitor prescriptions for controlled substances, why not allow prescriptions to remain valid for a full year?

3. The saying, "it's all about who you know," is especially true when it comes to searching for a job. Who do you know that might help you land a job as a pharmacy technician? If you do not personally know many people in the field, research other ways you could network, such as networking sites like LinkedIn. LinkedIn has many pharmacy-related groups one can join, such as the Pharmacy Technician Certification Board group or the National Pharmacy Technician Association group.

Lab 6

Worksheet 1 Prescription

℞ John Ashfield, MD
Greta Zlatoski, FCNP
Gregory Smythe, MD
44 Medical Pkwy.
Austin, TX 78704
(512) 555-1212   fax: (512) 555-1313

DOB *May 15, 1975* DEA# (?)

Pt. name *Vance Donaldson*   Date (?)

Address *12 Maple Leaf Trail*
Round Rock, TX 78664

Accupril
10 mg
30
i po QD

Refill *PRN* times (no refill unless indicated)

_____ MD

_____ License #

Scenario: This prescription was brought into the pharmacy with worn edges and creases. Explain the error(s) on this prescription: *This script is missing a DEA number and the date the script was written.*

What is a best practice to correct the error(s) or resolve the issue(s)?

Contact the physician to make sure it is a valid prescription.

Lab 6   *Reviewing a Prescription Form*

Worksheet 2 Prescription

R̫ Sunjita Patel, MD
7612 N. HWY 27
Cedar Rapids, IA 52404
(319) 555-1212 fax: (319) 555-1313

DOB *Aug 24, 1949* DEA# *AP4756687*

Pt. name _____ Date *2/16/2015*

Address *5473 W 104th St*
        Cedar Rapids, Ia 52401

Lorazepam
0.5 mg
120
i po q4-6 h prn anxiety

Refill___*5*___times (no refill unless indicated)

_____*Sunjita Patel, MD*_____ MD
_____ License #

Scenario: This prescription was presented to the pharmacy on February 16, 2015.
Explain the error(s) on this prescription: *This prescription is missing the patients name.*

What is a best practice to correct the error(s) or resolve the issue(s)?

look up the system to see if the address matches the name & will throw system verify who they wrote prescription can not be used.

Lab 6

Reviewing a Prescription Form

Worksheet 3 Prescription

Rx

Todd Jackson, MD
Anita Johnson, MD
Kunal Gupta, MSN, FCNP
5730 Congress Avenue
Boise, ID 83702
(208) 555-1212 fax: (208) 555-1313

DOB *Oct 18, 1978* DEA# _____

Pt. name *LILY NGUYEN* Date *02/12/2015*

Address *2934 ANDERSON LANE*
BOISE, ID 83722

ALPRAZOLAM
2 MG
120 (ONE HUNDRED TWENTY)
i po q6h prn anxiety

Refill *5* times (no refill unless indicated)

_____ MD

_____ License #

Scenario: This prescription was presented to the pharmacy at 7:45 p.m. on February 16, 2015. Explain the error(s) on this prescription: *Although it was written on the 12th its ok to fill on the 16th. Missing DEA number & the physicians signature.*

What is a best practice to correct the error(s) or resolve the issue(s)?

Call the physician to make sure the prescription is valid.

Lab 6
Reviewing a Prescription Form

Worksheet 4 Prescription

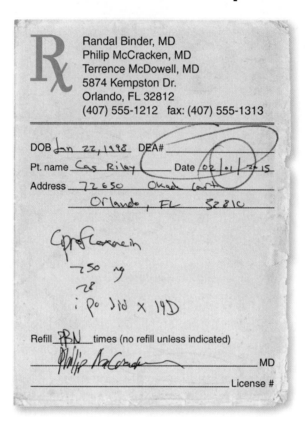

Scenario: This tattered prescription was presented to the pharmacy on Saturday, February 17, 2015.

Explain the error(s) on this prescription: _The prescription is missing a DEA number & is dated for the first_

What is a best practice to correct the error(s) or resolve the issue(s)?

Call and verify that this prescription can still be filled.

Lab 6   *Reviewing a Prescription Form*

Worksheet 5 Prescription

R℞ Simona Brushfield, MD
2222 IH-35 South
Austin, TX 78703
(512) 555-1212   fax: (512) 555-1313

DOB *Sep 12, 1952* DEA# _____

Pt. name *Miguel Espana* Date *01/15/2015*

Address *7583 E 11th St.*

Humalog
100 units/mL Vial
1 vial
12 units Sub Q qAM;
18 units sub Q qPM pc

Refill *PRN* times (no refill unless indicated)

_____ MD

_____ License #

Scenario: This prescription was delivered to the pharmacy by hand.
Explain the error(s) on this prescription: *Missing*
This prescription is ~~DEA~~ the DEA
number.

What is a best practice to correct the error(s) or resolve the issue(s)?
Contact the physician to see if
this is a valid prescription.

Lab 6

Reviewing a Prescription Form

Worksheet 6 Prescription

R
Frieda Nadal, MD
67 Savin Hill Ave
Boston, MA 02109
(617) 555-1212   fax: (617) 555-1313

DOB *Jun 23, 1988*   DEA# *⟨scribble⟩*
Pt. name *Kimberly Jackson*   Date *02/19/2015*
Address *4590 Settling Glen Dr*
Boston, MA 02109

Amoxicillin
150 mL
1 tsp po TID x 10 D

Refill *0* times (no refill unless indicated)

Frieda Nadal _____ MD
_____ License #

Scenario: This prescription was delivered to the pharmacy by hand.
Explain the error(s) on this prescription: _____

prescription is missing the physicians DEA number.

What is a best practice to correct the error(s) or resolve the issue(s)?

contact physician to make sure the prescription is valid.

Lab 6 *Reviewing a Prescription Form*

Worksheet 7 Prescription

R℞ Geoff Taylor, MD
67 Whitford Avenue
Providence, RI 02908
(401) 555-1212   fax: (401) 555-1313

DOB _Feb 29, 1984_ DEA# _____
Pt. name _Marquita Wilkins_ Date _02/19/2015_
Address _6901 Westminster Chase_
Providence, RI 02908

Patanol
_5 ml_
_i - ij_

Refill _0_ times (no refill unless indicated)
_Geoff Taylor_____ MD
_____ License #

Scenario: This prescription was delivered to the pharmacy by hand.
Explain the error(s) on this prescription: _This prescription is_
missing DEA number
_____

What is a best practice to correct the error(s) or resolve the issue(s)?
Call physician to make sure this is
a valid prescription.
_____

Lab 6 *Reviewing a Prescription Form*

Worksheet 8 Prescription

```
--------------------------------------------------------------
!!! -- START SECURED ELECTRONIC PRESCRIPTION TRANSMISSION -- !!!
--------------------------------------------------------------
FROM THE OFFICES OF PHIL JACKSON, MD; ETHEL JACOBSON, MD;
                    PETER JARKOWSKI, PA; EUGENE JOHNSON, DO

OFFICE ADDRESS:            67 EAST ELM
                          CEDAR RAPIDS, IA 52411
OFFICE TELEPHONE:         (319) 555-1212   TRANSMIT DATE:
OFFICE FAX:               (319) 555-1313   WRITTEN DATE:  FEB 20, 2015
--------------------------------------------------------------
TRANSMITTED TO            THE CORNER DRUG STORE
PHARMACY ADDRESS:

PHARMACY TELEPHONE:       (319) 555-1414
--------------------------------------------------------------
PATIENT NAME:             JEFFREY KLEIN     D.O.B.: OCT 18, 1979
PATIENT ADDRESS:          1157 NORTH PLAZA AVE
                          CEDAR RAPIDS, IA 52411
--------------------------------------------------------------
PRESCRIBED MEDICATION:    FLUOXETINE 20 MG
SIGNA:                    i PO QD
DISPENSE QUANTITY:        30
REFILL(S):                PRN
--------------------------------------------------------------
PHYSICIAN SIGNATURE:      [[ ELECTRONIC SIGNATURE ON FILE ]]
                          [[ FOR DR. ETHEL JACOBSON ]]

--------------------------------------------------------------
!!! -- END SECURED ELECTRONIC PRESCRIPTION TRANSMISSION -- !!!
--------------------------------------------------------------
```

Scenario: This prescription was received by the pharmacy on May 1, 2015. Explain the error(s) on this prescription: *prescription sent in t) days after given missing DEA number, complete pharm. address & patients number*

What is a best practice to correct the error(s) or resolve the issue(s)?

_____

_____

_____

Reviewing a Filled Prescription Lab 7

Objectives

- Gain skill in comparing a processed prescription to a printed label for completeness and accuracy.
- Identify practices to correct errors on printed labels generated from prescriptions.

Supplies

- None

The prescription is the primary means by which a prescriber communicates with pharmacy staff. Always keep in mind that accurate interpretation of the prescription is crucial in your work as a pharmacy technician because patient safety is of highest importance.

During the filling process, the prescription must be frequently reviewed to ensure that it is properly interpreted and the information is accurately transcribed from the prescription paper into the patient profile in the computer system. Though the pharmacist is ultimately accountable for any prescription dispensed to a patient, recently more states are also holding pharmacy technicians responsible for errors made on prescriptions. Therefore, it is important that whenever you are presented with a prescription—no matter what stage of the filling process you are focused on—you review the prescription for accuracy.

In the daily work of verifying prescriptions at the pharmacy, special attention is given to the following nine items in a process known as the "9-point check":

9-point check

A systematic approach to verifying prescription data during the filling process, often done first by a pharmacy technician and again by a pharmacist

1. Patient name
2. Patient date of birth
3. Date the prescription was written
4. Prescription drug name
5. Prescription drug strength
6. Prescription drug quantity

7. Label instructions
8. Prescriber information (name, DEA number, etc)
9. Refill information

When the prescription is first received, the staff member accepting it at the drop-off window reviews it for accuracy and completeness, using the 9-point check. After the prescription is transcribed, it should be reviewed again. Next, after the label is generated, the technician filling the prescription should focus on comparing the information on the prescription to the information on the label.

The **filling technician** plays a vital role in prescription processing because he or she is the last person to see the prescription prior to final verification and dispensing by the pharmacist. Before filling the prescription, the filling technician should closely examine the prescription and compare it to the printed label for accuracy. If a mistake is caught, the incorrect information must be circled or highlighted and brought to the attention of the technician who prepared the label. That technician must correct the error, or, if that original technician is unavailable or unable to correct the error at that time, the filling technician should correct the information and print a new label. The filling technician then verifies that the corrected label is accurate, fills the prescription, and passes it on to the pharmacist for final verification.

When you review prescriptions for controlled substances, remember that they have special characteristics that you must verify, including a DEA number and restrictions on refills, dates, and how the quantity is indicated.

Filling technician

Pharmacy technician responsible for prescription counting or pouring, packaging, and labeling during the filling process

> ### Take Note
>
> The number of refills on prescriptions is legally regulated. According to federal law, controlled Schedule II substances can never be refilled without a new prescription (except in emergency situations, when a pharmacist must handle the situation). Substances controlled on Schedules III and IV may have up to five refills within a 6-month period. Noncontrolled prescriptions and controlled substances on Schedule V have no limitation on refills (stated as "PRN"), provided the prescription is not 365 days old and expired. Note that with both controlled and noncontrolled medications, the prescriber can choose to prohibit refills or stipulate a maximum number of refills. **You may have additional regulations in your state.**

Keep in mind: The more people assigned to verify a prescription, the less likely an error will occur.

Procedure

In this lab, you will review a series of prescriptions and printed labels, grouped together on Worksheets 1 through 6 at the end of this lab. Your task is to verify that the information on the printed label corresponds to that on the written prescription. This textbook is written with federal regulations in mind. However, you should ask your instructor about standards and regulations in your state prior to completing the following steps.

1 Perform the 9-point check by comparing the printed label with the prescription for each of these nine items:

1. Patient name
2. Patient date of birth
3. Date the prescription was written
4. Prescription drug name
5. Prescription drug strength
6. Prescription drug quantity
7. Label instructions
8. Prescriber information (name, DEA number, etc)
9. Refill information

2 If an error is present on the label, circle the error and clearly write in the correct information on the blank lines provided.

3 **Conclusion:** When you are satisfied that you have verified the prescriptions and noted corrections for all label errors on the blank lines of the worksheets, tear out the worksheet pages and submit them to your instructor. On a separate sheet of paper, answer all questions in the following Lab Review section and turn in your answers to your instructor.

Lab Review

Check Your Understanding

1. What is the primary means of communication between a prescriber and the pharmacy?
   a. telephone
   b. letter
   c. email
   d. prescription

2. A _____ is often the last person to see a prescription before it is verified by the pharmacist.
   a. pharmacy clerk
   b. pharmacy customer
   c. pharmacy technician
   d. pharmacist

3. Only the pharmacist can be held accountable for a medication error.
   a. true
   b. false

4. "The _____ people assigned to _____ a prescription, the _____ likely an error will occur."
   a. more, transcribing, more
   b. more, verify, less
   c. fewer, transcribing, more
   d. fewer, verifying, less

5. Which of the following pieces of information is verified in the 9-point check?
   a. drug strength
   b. drug interactions
   c. therapeutic rating
   d. allergies

Thinking Like a Pharmacy Tech

1. Many states now hold pharmacy technicians accountable for medication errors. If final verification is the ultimate responsibility of the pharmacist, why are pharmacy technicians held accountable?

2. Contact your State Board of Pharmacy and request available statistics on the number of pharmacist-related and pharmacy-technician-related errors. What is your response to these statistics? Does anything surprise you about any reported statistics?

3. If you are interviewing for a technician job where you will wear scrubs most of the time, why does dressing well for an interview matter?

Lab 7 — *Reviewing a Filled Prescription*

Worksheet 1 Prescription and Label

R︎x

John Ashfield, MD
Greta Zlatoski, FCNP
Gregory Smythe, MD
44 Medical Pkwy.
Austin, TX 78704
(512) 555-1212 fax: (512) 555-1313

DOB *May 15, 1975* DEA# _____

Pt. name *Vance Donaldson* Date *2/11/2015*

Address *12 Maple Leaf Trail*
Round Rock, TX 78664

Accupril
10 mg
30
i po QD

Refill *PRN* times (no refill unless indicated)

_____ MD

_____ License #

THE CORNER DRUG STORE
17 Main Street - Austin, TX 78704
phone: (512) 555-1212 fax: (512) 555-1313

RX **6001012**

DATE FILLED: 02/13/2015
ORIGINAL DATE: FEB 13, 2015

DONALDSON, VANCE
12 Maple Leaf Trail; Round Rock, TX 78664 – DOB: May 15, 1975

TAKE 1 TABLET BY MOUTH ONCE A DAY.

QUINAPRIL 20 MG TABLETS - MYLAN **QTY: 30**
GENERIC SUBSTITUTION FOR ACCUPRIL 20MG TABLET

Prescriber: GREGORY SMYTHE, MD

REFILLS: PRN   **JPS/LAM**

Circle the error(s) on this label.
Write the correct label information below:

NO DEA number on the script. The Mg on the script & the label dont match. 2 different dates.

_____

_____

_____

Lab 7

Reviewing a Filled Prescription

Worksheet 2 Prescription and Label

Sunjita Patel, MD
7612 N. HWY 27
Cedar Rapids, IA 52404
(319) 555-1212 fax: (319) 555-1313

DOB *Aug 24, 1949* DEA# *AP4756680*

Pt. name *Amala Gupta* Date *02/16/2015*

Address *5473 W 70th Street*
Cedar Rapids, IA 52401

Lorazepam
0.5 mg
120 (one hundred twenty)
i po q4-6 h prn anxiety

Refill *5* ___times (no refill unless indicated)

Sunjita Patel, MD _____ MD

_____ License #

[handwritten notes: 4756687, 4+5+6=15, 7+6+8=21 x2, 42, 15, 57, x2]

THE CORNER DRUG STORE
17 Main Street - Cedar Rapids, IA 52404
phone: (319) 555-1212 fax: (319) 555-1313

RX **4001008**   DATE FILLED: 02/16/2015
ORIGINAL DATE: FEB 16, 2015

GUPTA, AMALA
27 Cherry Hill Blvd; Cedar Rapids, IA 52401 – DOB: FEB 16, 2015

i po q4-6 h prn anxiety.

LORAZEPAM 0.5 MG TABLETS-MYLAN   **QTY: 120**

Prescriber: SUNJITA PATEL, MD
REFILLS: 5   **JPS/LAM**

Circle the error(s) on this label.
Write the correct label information below:

_____

_____

_____

_____

_____

_____

Lab 7

Reviewing a Filled Prescription

Worksheet 3 Prescription and Label

R℞

Todd Jackson, MD
Anita Johnson, MD
Kunal Gupta, MSN, FCNP
5730 Congress Avenue
Boise, ID 83702
(208) 555-1212   fax: (208) 555-1313

DOB *OCT 18, 1978*   DEA# *FJ1234563*
Pt. name *LILY NGUYEN*   Date *02/12/2015*
Address *2934 ANDERSON LANE*
BOISE, ID 83702

ALPRAZOLAM
2 MG
120 (ONE HUNDRED TWENTY)
i po q6h prn anxiety

Refill *5* times (no refill unless indicated)
_____ MD
_____ License #

(handwritten: 1234563 = 7 a+24 33 4+3+5=7 2+4+6=12 x 2 / 24)

THE CORNER DRUG STORE
17 Main Street - Boise, ID 83702
phone: (208) 555-1212   fax: (208) 555-1313

RX **4001009**   DATE FILLED: 02/16/2015
                                   ORIGINAL DATE: FEB 12, 2015

NGUYEN, LILY
2934 Anderson Lane; Boise, ID 83722 – DOB: Oct 18, 1978

**TAKE 1 TABLET BY MOUTH EVERY
6 HOURS AS NEEDED FOR ANXIETY.**

ALPRAZOLAM 2 MG TABLETS-RNBXY   **QTY: 120**

Prescriber: ANITA JOHNSON, MD
REFILLS: 5   **JPS/LAM**

Circle the error(s) on this label.
Write the correct label information below:

_____

_____

_____

_____

_____

_____

Lab 7   *Reviewing a Filled Prescription*

Worksheet 4 Prescription and Label

℞ Randal Binder, MD
Philip McCracken, MD
Terrence McDowell, MD
5874 Kempston Dr.
Orlando, FL 32812
(407) 555-1212   fax: (407) 555-1313

DOB *Jan 22, 1998* DEA# _____

Pt. name *Cas Riley* ____ Date *02/9/2015*

Address *72650 Okade Court*

Orlando, FL 32810

Ciprofloxacin

250 mg

28

: po bid x 14D

Refill *0* ____ times (no refill unless indicated)

_____ MD

_____ License #

℞ **THE CORNER DRUG STORE**
17 Main Street - Orlando, FL 32812
phone: (407) 555-1212   fax: (407) 555-1313

RX **6001012**   DATE FILLED: 02/17/2015
ORIGINAL DATE: FEB 1, 2015

RILEY, CAS
72650 Okade Court; Orlando, FL 32810 – DOB: Jan 22, 1998

**TAKE 1 TABLET BY MOUTH EVERY
6 HOURS AS NEEDED FOR ANXIETY.**

CIPROFLOXACIN 250 MG TABLETS-APTH   QTY: 28

Prescriber: PHILIP MCCRACKEN, MD
REFILLS: 0   **JPS/LAM**

Circle the error(s) on this label.
Write the correct label information below:

Missing DEA number.

_____

_____

_____

_____

_____

Lab 7   *Reviewing a Filled Prescription*

Worksheet 5 Prescription and Label

Simona Brushfield, MD
2222 IH-35 South
Austin, TX 78703
(512) 555-1212 fax: (512) 555-1313

DOB *Sept 12, 1953* DEA# _____

Pt. name *Miguel Esparza* Date *01 / 15 / 2015*

Address *7583 E 11th St*
Austin, TX 78705

Humalog
100 units/mL Vial
1 vial
12 units sub Q qAM;
18 units sub Q qPM pc

Refill *PRN* times (no refill unless indicated)

_____ MD

_____ License #

THE CORNER DRUG STORE
17 Main Street - Austin, TX 78703
phone: (512) 555-1212 fax: (512) 555-1313

RX **6001014**   DATE FILLED: 02/17/2015
                          ORIGINAL DATE: JAN 15, 2015

ESPARZA, MIGUEL
7583 E 11th St.; Austin, TX 78705 – DOB: Sep 12, 1953

**INJECT 12 UNITS SUBCUTANEOUSLY EACH MORNING
AND 18 UNITS SUBCUTANEOUSLY EACH EVENING
BEFORE MEALS.**

HUMALOG INSULIN, 100 UNITS/ML VIAL   QTY: 20 mL

Prescriber: SIMONA BRUSHFIELD, MD
REFILLS: PRN   **JPS/LAM**

Circle the error(s) on this label.
Write the correct label information below:

Missing DEA number

_____

_____

_____

_____

Lab 7 *Reviewing a Filled Prescription*

Worksheet 6 Prescription and Label

Frieda Nadal, MD
67 Savin Hill Ave
Boston, MA 02109
(617) 555-1212 fax: (617) 555-1313

DOB *Jun 23, 1988* DEA# _____

Pt. name *Kimberly Jackson* Date *02/19/2015*

Address *4590 Settling Glen Dr*
Boston, MA 02109

Amoxicillin
250 mg / 5 mL
150 mL
1 tsp po TID x 10 D

Refill *0* times (no refill unless indicated)

Frieda Nadal _____ MD

_____ License #

THE CORNER DRUG STORE
17 Main Street - Boston, MA 02109
phone: (617) 555-1212 fax: (617) 555-1313

RX **6001027**   DATE FILLED: 02/19/2015
                        ORIGINAL DATE: FEB 19, 2015

JACKSON, KIMBERLY
4590 Settling Glenn Dr; Boston, MA 02109 – DOB: Jun 23, 1988

**TAKE 1 TEASPOONFUL BY MOUTH
3 TIMES A DAY FOR 10 DAYS.**

AMOXICILLIN 250 MG/5 ML SUSP. QTY: 100 mL

Prescriber: FRIEDA NADAL, MD
REFILLS: **JPS/LAM**

Circle the error(s) on this label.
Write the correct label information below:

_____

_____

_____

_____

_____

_____

Lab 7
Reviewing a Filled Prescription

Worksheet 7 Prescription and Label

Geoff Taylor, MD
67 Whitford Avenue
Providence, RI 02908
(401) 555-1212   fax: (401) 555-1313

DOB _Feb 29, 1984_ DEA# _____

Pt. name _Marquita Wilkins_ Date _02/19/2015_

Address _6901 Westminster Chase_
Providence, RI 02908

Patanol
_5 ml_
i-ii gtts au BID

Refill _0_ times (no refill unless indicated)

Geoff Taylor MD

_____ License #

THE CORNER DRUG STORE
17 Main Street - Providence, RI 02908
Phone: (401) 555-1212   Fax: (401) 555-1313

RX **6001018**

DATE FILLED: 02/19/2015
ORIGINAL DATE: FEB 19, 2015

WILKINS, MARQUITA
6901 Westminster Chase; Providence, RI 02908 – DOB: Feb 29, 1984

INSTILL 1 TO 2 DROPS IN THE LEFT EAR TWO TIMES A DAY.

PATANOL 0.1% EYE DROPS   **QTY: 5 mL**

Prescriber: GEOFF TAYLOR, MD
REFILLS: 0   **JPS/LAM**

Circle the error(s) on this label.
Write the correct label information below:

_____

_____

_____

_____

_____

_____

Lab 7   *Reviewing a Filled Prescription*

Worksheet 8 Prescription and Label

```
------------------------------------------------------------------------
!!! -- START SECURED ELECTRONIC PRESCRIPTION TRANSMISSION -- !!!
------------------------------------------------------------------------
FROM THE OFFICES OF PHIL JACKSON, MD; ETHEL JACOBSON, MD;
                    PETER JARKOWSKI, PA; EUGENE JOHNSON, DO

OFFICE ADDRESS:          67 EAST ELM
                         CEDAR RAPIDS, IA 52411
OFFICE TELEPHONE:        (319) 555-1212   TRANSMIT DATE: FEB 20, 2015
OFFICE FAX:              (319) 555-1313   WRITTEN DATE:  FEB 20, 2015
------------------------------------------------------------------------
TRANSMITTED TO           THE CORNER DRUG STORE
PHARMACY ADDRESS:        875 PARADIGM WAY
                         CEDAR RAPIDS, IA 52410
PHARMACY TELEPHONE:      (319) 555-1414
------------------------------------------------------------------------
PATIENT NAME:            JEFFREY KLEIN    D.O.B.: OCT 18, 1979
PATIENT ADDRESS:         1157 NORTH PLAZA AVE
                         CEDAR RAPIDS, IA 52411
------------------------------------------------------------------------
PRESCRIBED MEDICATION:   FLUOXETINE 20 MG
SIGNA:                   i PO QD
DISPENSE QUANTITY:       30
REFILL(S):               PRN
------------------------------------------------------------------------
PHYSICIAN SIGNATURE:     [[ ELECTRONIC SIGNATURE ON FILE ]]
                         [[ FOR DR. ETHEL JACOBSON ]]
------------------------------------------------------------------------
!!! -- END SECURED ELECTRONIC PRESCRIPTION TRANSMISSION -- !!!
------------------------------------------------------------------------
```

 THE CORNER DRUG STORE
17 Main Street - Cedar Rapids, IA 52411
phone: (319) 555-1212 fax: (319) 555-1313

RX **6001019**   DATE FILLED: 02/20/2015
                                     ORIGINAL DATE: FEB 20, 2015

KLEIN, JEFFREY
1157 North Plaza Avenue; Cedar Rapids, IA 52411 – DOB: Oct 18, 1979

**TAKE 1 CAPSULE BY MOUTH
FOUR TIMES DAILY.**

FLUOXETINE   QTY: 30

Prescriber: ETHEL JACOBSON, MD
REFILLS: 0   **JPS/LAM**

Circle the error(s) on this label.
Write the correct label information below:

Label doesn't say how many Mg are in each tablet.

Entering Patient Data

Lab 8

Objectives

- Begin using and learning from the CD that accompanies your lab manual.
- Become more familiar with the patient profile—now in computer form—as a means of recording patients' personal and health information for access by pharmacy staff.
- Learn to navigate efficiently within a model patient profile software system.
- Increase skills in identifying standard patient profile information and evaluating profiles for completeness and accuracy.

Supplies

- NRx-Based Training Software

The patient profile is the first bit of information a pharmacy collects. As one of the chief means of recording patient information in the pharmacy, the profile is initiated when patients first patronize a pharmacy and complete a paper form. Because you will work with patients to establish their profiles on paper, remember to be as empathetic as possible. New patients must divulge information that is private and very personal.

Like the paper file in a doctor's office, the computerized profile contains all of a patient's medical information. The pharmacy must always have easy access to viewing or updating the profile, particularly when patients wish to update their information, such as by listing new allergies or changing their address or insurance information. The computerized profile provides such access at your fingertips. Your role in entering and keeping accurate, up-to-date computerized patient profiles is vital to helping the pharmacy manage patients' medication therapy.

This lab is the first of seven that will simulate use of the NRx pharmacy management software produced by QS/1. Your textbook includes a CD containing a simulation of the NRx software, which closely resembles the programs that you are likely to encounter in your pharmacy work. The purpose of these software-related labs is to familiarize you with the essential steps leading up to and including prescription preparation—an electronic or computer-based process in most pharmacies. The principles of practice on which pharmacy management software programs operate are generally the same. However, several brands of software programs are used in pharmacy practice and will differ from pharmacy to pharmacy. Therefore, your focus is not to master any particular software system. Instead, your goal is to master the *principles* of using software to serve your patients effectively and accurately.

Procedure

In order to complete this lab and the remaining labs (Labs 9–14) in this Community Pharmacy Practice Unit, you must insert the CD accompanying your textbook into your computer, follow the installation instructions on the CD packaging label, and work your way through the outlined steps.

Take Note

As you perform each of the NRx-based software simulation labs (Labs 8–14), be aware that you can choose "Print this screen" in the upper-right corner of any open screen. This printing option may be necessary under unusual circumstances, such as if you have to stop performing a lab in mid-stream due to closure of a campus computer lab, personal emergency, or similar circumstance. You may print the screen to demonstrate to your instructor just how far you progressed on the lab. Under ordinary circumstances, you will be printing only the final screen of the lab, the results screen that shows your numerical score and accuracy percentage. You will be clearly instructed when and how to print the results screen within the final steps of each lab.

For entering your first patient profile in this lab, imagine that Vance Donaldson has just moved into the neighborhood and would like to have his prescriptions filled at your pharmacy. Vance has given you his completed profile, insurance card, and a new prescription to fill. Using his profile and insurance card (see Figure 8.1 on page 79) and the steps below, add the patient's information into the NRx software simulation. When you reach the end of the procedure for Vance Donaldson, you will be instructed to repeat the main steps for additional patients.

1 First install the NRx Simulation CD that accompanied your textbook by following the installation directions on page xii of the Preface. Begin this lab by clicking the PharmacyLabs icon that should now be on your

desktop. When the sign-in fields appear, type in your First Name and Last Name and click OK.

2 When the menu for all available labs appears on the left, click the dark purple tab of the lab number and lab title you wish to perform. When the list of sub-labs (for example Lab 8.1, Lab 8.2, Lab 8.3, and so on) appears below the main lab tab, click the sub-lab you wish to perform.

Tip: The sub-labs represent the different patients you will be processing through the lab procedures. Most labs present several sub-labs for processing; however, some labs have only one sub-lab.

3 When the NRx Security screen appears, log in to the NRx-based training software as the Primary User by typing "Student" as the Login ID and "Training" as the Password. Press Tab or click Log In.

Tip: After you have completed this log-in step for the first listed sub-lab (for example, Lab 8.1, Lab 9.1, Lab 10.1, and so on), you will not be prompted to log in again for the remaining sub-labs in that listing and may skip this log-in step.

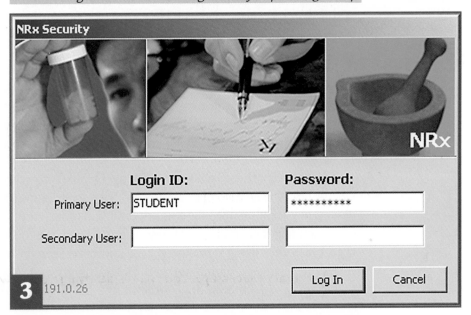

4 On the Rx Processing Tasks menu, click Search or press F3.

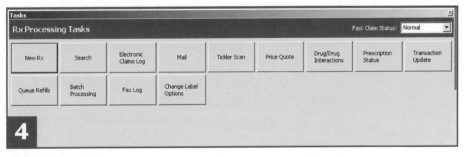

5 When the Rx/Patient Search screen appears, type the patient's name in Lastname, Firstname format in the Search Criteria field (for the first profile,

you will use Figure 8.1 and enter Donaldson, Vance). Click Find or press Enter. *Tip: Some pharmacy management software systems are case sensitive, and in your pharmacy work you will need to be careful about using upper case (capital) or lower case letters when typing in patient names and other data. However, for the purposes of these labs (Labs 8–14), you will not have to be concerned about case sensitivity.*

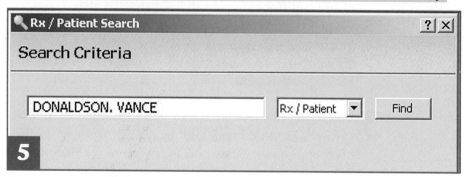

6 The Patient Scan screen will appear. Because this is the only patient with this name and the patient is new to the pharmacy, no names will appear in the search results. Click the New Patient icon on the top toolbar or press CTRL+N to begin the process of adding this patient.

7 Continue using Figure 8.1 to enter into the NRx system, in order, the following categories of Mr. Donaldson's personal data: Last Name, First Name, full and *exact* Address, Phone number(s), Birth Date, and E-mail, pressing Tab to move between fields. After entering the final item—the E-mail, or the Birth Date, if the patient has no E-mail—press Tab.

8 To add the primary care physician, click the Double Arrows to the right of the Doctor field. When the Prescriber Record Scan screen appears, look for the desired physician's name. If it is listed, double-click it or press the corresponding function key (or F-key, as explained in the following Take Note). If the physician's name is not listed, type it into the Search Criteria field in Lastname, Firstname format and click Find or press Enter. When the desired physician's name appears, double-click it or press the corresponding F-key.

Take Note

As you work with the simulation of the NRx pharmacy software and with the pharmacy software program at your job, you will often have the option of using function keys, or F-keys. On your keyboard, the F-keys are F1, F2, F3, and so on, and are usually found along the top row of your keyboard. On your screen, the F-keys are listed within a field that offers you a choice of items. One F-key is associated with each item line in the field and is usually found in the far-left column of the screen. You may have the option of pressing the corresponding F-key or double-clicking on the item you want. While using F-keys can speed up your process quite a bit, accuracy should always be your first priority.

FIGURE 8.1
Patient Profile and Insurance Card

PATIENT PROFILE

Patient Name
Donaldson   Vance
Last   First   Middle Initial

12 Maple Leaf Trail
Street or PO Box

Round Rock   TX   78664
City   State   ZIP

Date of Birth   Gender   Social Security No.   E-mail
05/15/1975   ☑ Male   000-00-0000   vdonaldson@email.com
MM / DD / YYYY   ☐ Female

Home Phone   Work Phone   Other Phone
(512) 555-1212   (512) 555-1313   (   )

☐ Yes, I would like medication dispensed in a child-resistant container.
☑ No, I do not want medication dispensed in a child-resistant container.

Medication Insurance   Cardholder Name _same_
☑ Yes   ☑ Cardholder   ☐ Child   ☐ Disabled Dependent
☐ No   ☐ Spouse   ☐ Dependent Parent   ☐ Full-Time Student
                         (*Please provide the pharmacy with your card.*)

MEDICAL HISTORY

HEALTH   ALLERGIES AND DRUG REACTIONS
☐ No Known Medical   ☐ Diabetes Mellitus   ☐ No Known Drug Allergies
   Conditions   ☐ Epilepsy   ☐ Aspirin
☐ Anemia   ☐ Esophagitis   ☐ Cephalosporins
☐ Arthritis   ☐ Generalized Anxiety Disorder ☐ Codeine
☐ Asthma   ☐ Heart Condition   ☐ Erythromycin
☐ Attention-Deficit   ☑ Hypertension   ☑ Penicillin G Potassium
   Hyperactivity Disorder ☐ Kidney Disease   ☐ Sulfa
☐ Blood Clotting Disorders ☐ Liver Disease   ☐ Tetracyclines
☐ Cancer   ☐ Lung Disease   ☐ Xanthines
☐ Depression   ☐ Ulcers

ICD-9 for Checked Condition(s): _____   Details for Checked Allergy(ies): _____

ICD-9: 401.9

Medication(s) Currently Being Taken: _aspirin 81 mg, Accupril 10 mg_

Primary Care Physician: _Gregory Smythe_

Comments: _____

Health information changes periodically. Please notify the pharmacy of any new medications, allergies, drug reactions, or health conditions.

Signature _Vance Donaldson_   Date _2/11/15_   ☐ I choose not to fill out this form.

Cobalt Care
Insurance card

VANCE DONALDSON
BIN: 00123
ID: ZVD996274638

GROUP: 11770
RELATIONSHIP: 01, CARDHOLDER

MEMBER SERVICES: 1-800-555-3232
CLAIMS/INQUIRIES: 1-800-555-6363

9 The Patient Information screen will return. Compare the information on screen with the information on the Patient Profile form. When you are satisfied that the new electronic profile is complete and accurate, click Save on the top toolbar or press CTRL+S.

Take Note

Remember to save your work frequently. You can do this by clicking Save or pressing CTRL+S on the keyboard.

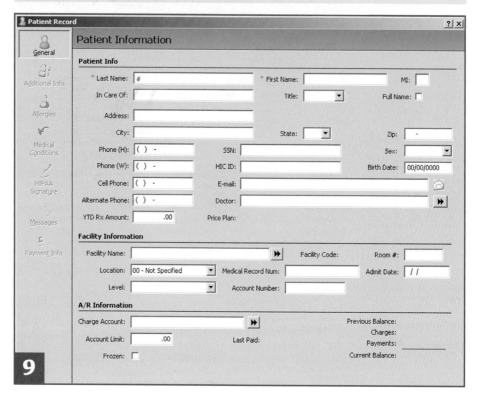

10 Click the Allergies button on the left menu bar. In cases where the patient has indicated having no known drug allergies, type in the exact phrase No Known Drug Allergies, press Enter, and proceed to Step 11. However, because Mr. Donaldson *does* have allergies, you will do the following for him and all patients declaring allergies on their forms. In the Search for Allergy field, type in the exact word or words following the checked box under ALLERGIES AND DRUG REACTIONS. Press Enter. If the allergy does not appear, check your spelling and revise as needed.

Tip: As you gain experience on the job, you will become familiar with the most common allergies and the abbreviations used to designate some of them. For example, common allergies include Penicillin (PCN), Aspirin (ASA), Acetaminophen (APAP), Codeine (no standard abbreviation), and Sulfonamides (no standard abbreviation).

Take Note

The CD that accompanies your textbook provides you with a simulation of the NRx software. However, because it is a simulation only, it does not fully replicate all functions of the software itself. When you are working with a fully operational software system at the pharmacy, you will notice that when typing into a field, you will often need to type only the first few letters of the phrase or word you are entering. To save you time, the software will pull up a complete phrase or word matching the first few characters you have entered and, after verifying that what is filled in is exactly what you want, you will simply press Enter to complete your task without having to type all the characters.

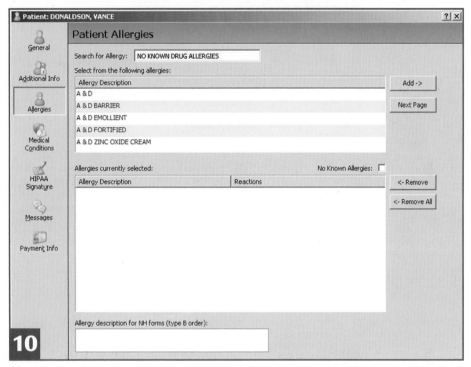

11 When the Allergy Description field appears, either click the correct allergy name (using any additional Patient Profile form details provided below the checked box), or click the phrase NO KNOWN DRUG ALLERGIES, as is appropriate for the patient. Click Add.

Tip: At the pharmacy, if you encounter patients listing more than one allergy on their forms, you would need to repeat Steps 10 and 11 as necessary to enter all listed allergies.

12 Cross-check that the allergies on the Patient Profile form are the same as those now listed on screen in the Allergies currently selected field. Click Save on the top toolbar or press CTRL+S.

Tip: In the actual NRx software, if an incorrect allergy were still present at this point, you would have one more chance to remove it and replace it with the correct allergy. For the purposes of this lab, you have only one chance to verify allergy spelling and correctness, which you did in Step 10.

13 Click the Medical Conditions button on the left menu bar. In the Search for ICD-9 or Medical Condition field, type the name of the patient's condition or the *exact* phrase No Known Medical Conditions if the patient has checked that item on the Patient Profile form. Press Enter. If the condition does not appear, check your spelling and revise as needed.

14 When the appropriate medical condition appears in the Select from the following medical conditions field, click the correct phrase or condition name and click Add.

Tip: If more than one entry appears on screen for the same medical condition, compare the ICD-9 code on the Patient Profile form with the on-screen ICD-9 codes, and select the correct condition based on the code.

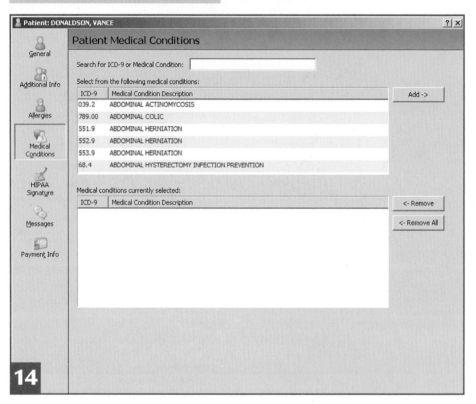

15 Cross-check the reported medical conditions on the Patient Profile form with those listed on screen in the Medical Conditions currently selected field. When you are satisfied it is complete, click Save on the top toolbar or press CTRL+S.

Tip: In the actual NRx software, if an incorrect medical condition were still present at this point, you would have one more chance to remove it and replace it with the correct condition. For the purposes of this lab, you have only one chance to verify condition spelling and correctness, which you did in Step 13.

16 To add payment information to the patient's record, you will need to have the patient's insurance card, which is provided to the patient by the insurance carrier. (See Figure 8.1 for an example of what an insurance card may look like; for the purposes of this lab, the payment plan name appears above the title "Insurance Card.") Click the Payment Info button on the left menu bar. Click New on the top toolbar, and a blank Patient Insurance Record will appear. Click the Double Arrows to the right of the Payment Plan field for a list of available price plans.

Tip: Be aware that not all insurance cards will look alike. Also note that not all patients will have an insurance card; some may pay the cash price (covered in Step 17).

17 In the Price Plan Scan screen, select the desired price plan by double-clicking the plan name or by pressing the corresponding F-key. If the desired price plan is not shown in the alphabetical list currently on screen, you may search within the available plans by typing the full plan name (or the word Cash for cash plan patients) in the blank Search Criteria field. Leave Description in the adjacent drop-down menu and click Find or press Enter. When your choices appear, double-click the correct plan name (or the category Cash Pricing) or press the corresponding F-key.

Tip: Many pharmacy management software systems will also allow you to search for the price plan by entering the Bank Identification Number (BIN number) located on the Insurance Card (see Figure 8.1 for an example of a card with a BIN number). For the purposes of this lab, however, you may search only by entering the plan name.

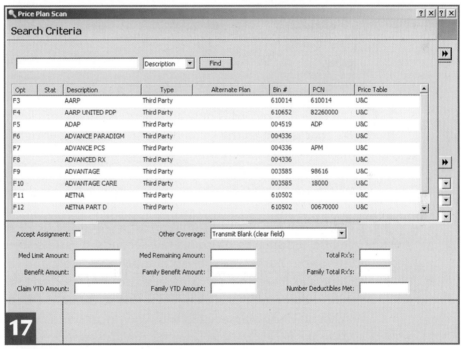

18 The Patient Insurance Record screen has returned and you will enter three additional items from the patient's Insurance Card (Figures 8.1 through 8.8). However, if you are processing a cash plan patient and selected Cash Pricing in the previous step, you should simply click Save on the top toolbar or press CTRL+S and proceed to Step 19. For all other patients, first click in the Policy ID Number field, type in the ID number, and press Tab. Next, type the Group name or number in the Group Number field and press Tab (unless the Insurance Card indicates "None" for the Group, in which case you should leave the blank Group Number field as is). Then, for the Relationship data, click on the Relationship drop-down menu and select the corresponding code number and name (if the Relationship on the Insurance Card is "00-Not Specified," leave the field as is). Click Save on the top toolbar or press CTRL+S.

18

19 The patient's record is now complete. Press Esc or click the small black "X" that is next to the small black "?" in the upper-right corner of the Insurance Record screen.

*Tip: Be careful! Do **not** click the large red "X" found in the upper-right corner of the lab window. Doing so will (always) close the entire lab and your work will be lost.*

20 The Patient Payment Information screen and the newly added plan will be briefly displayed. Within a few seconds, a results screen will appear, listing your name, the sub-lab number, your start and finish times, your numerical score and a maximum score, and your accuracy percentage. Print these results by clicking Print this screen in the upper-right corner. (A small window associated with your local printer options will appear. Make the necessary selections for the local printer you wish to use and click as required to print the screen.) When you are sure the screen has printed, retrieve it and set it aside to be turned in at the end of the lab. Click Close this lab in the upper-right corner of the screen.

Tip: Do not close the lab until you are absolutely certain that your results screen has printed successfully. You will not be able to retrieve your results once you click Close this lab.

21 Repeat Steps 2 through 20 with the seven remaining patient profiles given in Figures 8.2 through 8.8 on pages 86–92 and represented as Labs 8.2 through 8.8 in the sub-labs listing. As you complete the procedure steps for those profiles, you should ignore the initial references to Vance Donaldson and substitute the name and data from each subsequent patient profile. As you print the results screens for the sub-labs, set them aside in a stack for turning in at the end of the lab. When you have processed the last patient (sub-Lab 8.8), proceed to Step 22 to conclude the lab.

22 **Conclusion**: Turn in the complete stack of eight results screens to your instructor. On a separate sheet of paper, answer all questions in the following Lab Review section and turn in your answers to your instructor.

FIGURE 8.2
Patient Profile and Insurance Card

PATIENT PROFILE

Patient Name
Gupta _Amala_
Last _____ First _____ Middle Initial

5473 W 10th Street
Street or PO Box

Cedar Rapids _IA_ _52401_
City _____ State _____ ZIP

Date of Birth | Gender | Social Security No. | E-mail
_08/24/1949_ | ☐ Male | _000-00-0000_ | _guptaamala@email.com_
MM / DD / YYYY | ☑ Female | |

Home Phone | Work Phone | Other Phone
(_319_) _555-1212_ | ( ) | ( )

☐ Yes, I would like medication dispensed in a child-resistant container.
☑ No, I do not want medication dispensed in a child-resistant container.

Medication Insurance | Cardholder Name _same_
☑ Yes | ☑ Cardholder | ☐ Child | ☐ Disabled Dependent
☐ No | ☐ Spouse | ☐ Dependent Parent | ☐ Full-Time Student
| *(Please provide the pharmacy with your card.)*

MEDICAL HISTORY

HEALTH
☑ No Known Medical Conditions
☐ Anemia
☐ Arthritis
☐ Asthma
☐ Attention-Deficit Hyperactivity Disorder
☐ Blood Clotting Disorders
☐ Cancer
☐ Depression

☐ Diabetes Mellitus
☐ Epilepsy
☐ Esophagitis
☐ Generalized Anxiety Disorder
☐ Heart Condition
☐ Hypertension
☐ Kidney Disease
☐ Liver Disease
☐ Lung Disease
☐ Ulcers

ALLERGIES AND DRUG REACTIONS
☑ No Known Drug Allergies
☐ Aspirin
☐ Cephalosporins
☐ Codeine
☐ Erythromycin
☐ Penicillin G Potassium
☐ Sulfa
☐ Tetracyclines
☐ Xanthines

ICD-9 for Checked Condition(s): _____

Details for Checked Allergy(ies): _____

Medication(s) Currently Being Taken: _____

Primary Care Physician: _Sunjita Patel_

Comments: _____

Health information changes periodically. Please notify the pharmacy of any new medications, allergies, drug reactions, or health conditions.

Signature _Amala Gupta_ Date _2/16/15_ ☐ I choose not to fill out this form.

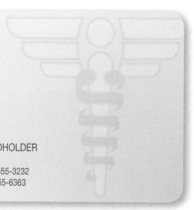

PublicAid
Insurance card

AMALA GUPTA
BIN: 100009
ID: 778342987

GROUP: NONE
RELATIONSHIP: 01, CARDHOLDER

MEMBER SERVICES: 1-800-555-3232
CLAIMS/INQUIRIES: 1-800-555-6363

FIGURE 8.3
Patient Profile and Insurance Card

PATIENT PROFILE

Patient Name
Klein **Jeffrey**
Last / First / Middle Initial

1157 North Plaza Ave
Street or PO Box
Cedar Rapids **IA** **52411**
City / State / ZIP

Date of Birth: **10/18/1979** MM/DD/YYYY
Gender: ☑ Male ☐ Female
Social Security No.: **000-00-0000**
E-mail: **kleinj@email.com**

Home Phone: (**319**) **555-1212**
Work Phone: (**319**) **555-1313**
Other Phone: ( )

☐ Yes, I would like medication dispensed in a child-resistant container.
☑ No, I do not want medication dispensed in a child-resistant container.

Medication Insurance
☑ Yes
☐ No

Cardholder Name **Katja Klein**
☐ Cardholder ☐ Child ☐ Disabled Dependent
☑ Spouse ☐ Dependent Parent ☐ Full-Time Student
(*Please provide the pharmacy with your card.*)

MEDICAL HISTORY

HEALTH
☐ No Known Medical Conditions
☐ Anemia
☐ Arthritis
☐ Asthma
☐ Attention-Deficit Hyperactivity Disorder
☐ Blood Clotting Disorders
☐ Cancer
☑ Depression

☐ Diabetes Mellitus
☐ Epilepsy
☐ Esophagitis
☐ Generalized Anxiety Disorder
☐ Heart Condition
☐ Hypertension
☐ Kidney Disease
☐ Liver Disease
☐ Lung Disease
☐ Ulcers

ALLERGIES AND DRUG REACTIONS
☐ No Known Drug Allergies
☐ Aspirin
☐ Cephalosporins
☑ Codeine
☐ Erythromycin
☐ Penicillin G Potassium
☐ Sulfa
☐ Tetracyclines
☐ Xanthines

ICD-9 for Checked Condition(s): _____
ICD-9: 309.0

Details for Checked Allergy(ies): _____

Medication(s) Currently Being Taken: _____

Primary Care Physician: **Ethel Jacobson**

Comments: _____

Health information changes periodically. Please notify the pharmacy of any new medications, allergies, drug reactions, or health conditions.

Signature **Jeffrey Klein** Date **2/19/15** ☐ I choose not to fill out this form.

ApolloHealth
Insurance card

JEFFREY KLEIN
BIN: 459872
ID: 882646507

GROUP: NONE
RELATIONSHIP: 02, SPOUSE

MEMBER SERVICES: 1-800-555-3232
CLAIMS/INQUIRIES: 1-800-555-6363

FIGURE 8.4
Patient Profile and Insurance Card

PATIENT PROFILE

Patient Name
Nguyen   *Lily*
Last   First   Middle Initial

2934 Anderson Lane
Street or PO Box

Boise   *ID*   *83722*
City   State   ZIP

Date of Birth   Gender   Social Security No.   E-mail
10/18/1978   ☐ Male   *000-00-0000*   *lilyflower@email.com*
MM / DD / YYYY   ☑ Female

Home Phone   Work Phone   Other Phone
(*208*) *555-1212*   (*208*) *555-1313*   ( )

☐ Yes, I would like medication dispensed in a child-resistant container.
☑ No, I do not want medication dispensed in a child-resistant container.

Medication Insurance   Cardholder Name
☐ Yes   ☐ Cardholder   ☐ Child   ☐ Disabled Dependent
☑ No   ☐ Spouse   ☐ Dependent Parent   ☐ Full-Time Student
    (*Please provide the pharmacy with your card.*)

MEDICAL HISTORY

HEALTH   ALLERGIES AND DRUG REACTIONS

☐ No Known Medical   ☐ Diabetes Mellitus   ☑ No Known Drug Allergies
   Conditions   ☐ Epilepsy   ☐ Aspirin
☐ Anemia   ☐ Esophagitis   ☐ Cephalosporins
☐ Arthritis   ☑ Generalized Anxiety Disorder   ☐ Codeine
☐ Asthma   ☐ Heart Condition   ☐ Erythromycin
☐ Attention-Deficit   ☐ Hypertension   ☐ Penicillin G Potassium
   Hyperactivity Disorder   ☐ Kidney Disease   ☐ Sulfa
☐ Blood Clotting Disorders   ☐ Liver Disease   ☐ Tetracyclines
☐ Cancer   ☐ Lung Disease   ☐ Xanthines
☐ Depression   ☐ Ulcers

ICD-9 for Checked Condition(s): _____   Details for Checked Allergy(ies): _____
ICD-9: 300.02

Medication(s) Currently Being Taken: _____

Primary Care Physician: *Todd Jackson*

Comments: _____

Health information changes periodically. Please notify the pharmacy of any new medications, allergies, drug reactions, or health conditions.

Signature *Lily Nguyen*   Date *2/12/15*   ☐ I choose not to fill out this form.

No insurance card presented; patient on cash plan.

FIGURE 8.5
Patient Profile and Insurance Card

PATIENT PROFILE

Patient Name
Riley _____ Cas _____
Last | First | Middle Initial

72650 Okade Court
Street or PO Box

Orlando _____ FL _____ 32810
City | State | ZIP

Date of Birth
01/22/1998
MM / DD / YYYY

Gender
☑ Male
☐ Female

Social Security No.
000-00-0000

E-mail
casr@email.com

Home Phone
(407) 555-1212

Work Phone
( )

Other Phone
( )

☑ Yes, I would like medication dispensed in a child-resistant container.
☐ No, I do not want medication dispensed in a child-resistant container.

Medication Insurance
☑ Yes
☐ No

Cardholder Name Molly Riley
☐ Cardholder   ☑ Child   ☐ Disabled Dependent
☐ Spouse   ☐ Dependent Parent   ☐ Full-Time Student
(Please provide the pharmacy with your card.)

MEDICAL HISTORY

HEALTH
☐ No Known Medical Conditions
☐ Anemia
☐ Arthritis
☐ Asthma
☑ Attention-Deficit Hyperactivity Disorder
☐ Blood Clotting Disorders
☐ Cancer
☐ Depression

☐ Diabetes Mellitus
☐ Epilepsy
☐ Esophagitis
☐ Generalized Anxiety Disorder
☐ Heart Condition
☐ Hypertension
☐ Kidney Disease
☐ Liver Disease
☐ Lung Disease
☐ Ulcers

ALLERGIES AND DRUG REACTIONS
☐ No Known Drug Allergies
☐ Aspirin
☐ Cephalosporins
☐ Codeine
☐ Erythromycin
☐ Penicillin G Potassium
☑ Sulfa
☐ Tetracyclines
☐ Xanthines

ICD-9 for Checked Condition(s): _____
ICD-9: 314.01

Details for Checked Allergy(ies): _____
Sulfa (Sulfonamides)

Medication(s) Currently Being Taken: Ritalin 10mg

Primary Care Physician: Philip McCracken

Comments: _____
Health information changes periodically. Please notify the pharmacy of any new medications, allergies, drug reactions, or health conditions.

Signature Molly Riley   Date 2/1/15   ☐ I choose not to fill out this form.

Wellness Institute
Insurance card

CAS RILEY
BIN: 776520
ID: YPJ75113

GROUP: RXCare
RELATIONSHIP: 03, CHILD

MEMBER SERVICES: 1-800-555-3232
CLAIMS/INQUIRIES: 1-800-555-6363

FIGURE 8.6
Patient Profile and Insurance Card

PATIENT PROFILE

Patient Name
Esparza _____ *Miguel* _____
Last   First   Middle Initial

7583 E 11th St.
Street or PO Box
Austin _____ *TX* *78705*
City   State   ZIP

Date of Birth   Gender   Social Security No.   E-mail
09/12/1953   ☑ Male   *000-00-0000*
MM / DD / YYYY   ☐ Female

Home Phone   Work Phone   Other Phone
(*512*) *555-1212*   (   )   (   )

☑ Yes, I would like medication dispensed in a child-resistant container.
☐ No, I do not want medication dispensed in a child-resistant container.

Medication Insurance   Cardholder Name *same*
☑ Yes   ☑ Cardholder   ☐ Child   ☐ Disabled Dependent
☐ No   ☐ Spouse   ☐ Dependent Parent ☐ Full-Time Student
                         (*Please provide the pharmacy with your card.*)

MEDICAL HISTORY

HEALTH   ALLERGIES AND DRUG REACTIONS
☐ No Known Medical   ☑ Diabetes Mellitus   ☑ No Known Drug Allergies
   Conditions   ☐ Epilepsy   ☐ Aspirin
☐ Anemia   ☐ Esophagitis   ☐ Cephalosporins
☐ Arthritis   ☐ Generalized Anxiety Disorder ☐ Codeine
☐ Asthma   ☐ Heart Condition   ☐ Erythromycin
☐ Attention-Deficit   ☐ Hypertension   ☐ Penicillin G Potassium
   Hyperactivity Disorder ☐ Kidney Disease   ☐ Sulfa
☐ Blood Clotting Disorders ☐ Liver Disease   ☐ Tetracyclines
☐ Cancer   ☐ Lung Disease   ☐ Xanthines
☐ Depression   ☐ Ulcers

ICD-9 for Checked Condition(s): _____   Details for Checked Allergy(ies): _____
ICD-9: 250.9

Medication(s) Currently Being Taken: _____

Primary Care Physician: *Simona Brushfield* _____

Comments: _____
Health information changes periodically. Please notify the pharmacy of any new medications, allergies,
drug reactions, or health conditions.

Signature *Miguel Esparza* _____ Date *1/15/15* ☐ I choose not to fill out this form.

FederalAide
Insurance card

MIGUEL ESPARZA
BIN: 999990
ID: 119875639

GROUP: B
RELATIONSHIP: 00, NOT SPECIFIED

MEMBER SERVICES: 1-800-555-3232
CLAIMS/INQUIRIES: 1-800-555-6363

FIGURE 8.7
Patient Profile and Insurance Card

PATIENT PROFILE

Patient Name
Jackson   _Kimberly_
Last   First   Middle Initial

4590 Settling Glen Dr
Street or PO Box

Boston   _MA_   _02109_
City   State   ZIP

Date of Birth: _06/23/1988_ (MM/DD/YYYY)
Gender: ☐ Male   ☑ Female
Social Security No.: _000-00-0000_
E-mail: _jacksok@email.com_

Home Phone: (_617_) _555-1212_
Work Phone: (_617_) _555-1313_
Other Phone: (___) _____

☐ Yes, I would like medication dispensed in a child-resistant container.
☑ No, I do not want medication dispensed in a child-resistant container.

Medication Insurance
☑ Yes
☐ No

Cardholder Name _Chris Redcedar_
☐ Cardholder   ☐ Child   ☐ Disabled Dependent
☑ Spouse   ☐ Dependent Parent   ☐ Full-Time Student
(*Please provide the pharmacy with your card.*)

MEDICAL HISTORY

HEALTH
☐ No Known Medical Conditions
☐ Anemia
☐ Arthritis
☐ Asthma
☐ Attention-Deficit Hyperactivity Disorder
☐ Blood Clotting Disorders
☐ Cancer
☐ Depression
☐ Diabetes Mellitus
☐ Epilepsy
☑ Esophagitis
☐ Generalized Anxiety Disorder
☐ Heart Condition
☐ Hypertension
☐ Kidney Disease
☐ Liver Disease
☐ Lung Disease
☐ Ulcers

ALLERGIES AND DRUG REACTIONS
☐ No Known Drug Allergies
☑ Aspirin
☐ Cephalosporins
☐ Codeine
☐ Erythromycin
☐ Penicillin G Potassium
☐ Sulfa
☐ Tetracyclines
☐ Xanthines

ICD-9 for Checked Condition(s): _____
ICD-9: 530.10

Details for Checked Allergy(ies): _____

Medication(s) Currently Being Taken: _____

Primary Care Physician: _Frieda Nadal_

Comments: _____

Health information changes periodically. Please notify the pharmacy of any new medications, allergies, drug reactions, or health conditions.

Signature _Kimberly Jackson_   Date _2/19/15_   ☐ I choose not to fill out this form.

PublicAid
Insurance card

KIMBERLY JACKSON
BIN: 100009
ID: 711937589

GROUP: NONE
RELATIONSHIP: 02, SPOUSE

MEMBER SERVICES: 1-800-555-3232
CLAIMS/INQUIRIES: 1-800-555-6363

FIGURE 8.8
Patient Profile and Insurance Card

PATIENT PROFILE

Patient Name
Wilkins   *Marquita*
Last   First   Middle Initial

6901 Westminster Chase
Street or PO Box

Providence   *RI*   *02908*
City   State   ZIP

Date of Birth   Gender   Social Security No.   E-mail
02/29/1984   ☐ Male   *000-00-0000*   *marquita@email.com*
MM / DD / YYYY   ☑ Female

Home Phone   Work Phone   Other Phone
(*401*) *555-1212*   (*401*) *555-1313*   ( )

☑ Yes, I would like medication dispensed in a child-resistant container.
☐ No, I do not want medication dispensed in a child-resistant container.

Medication Insurance   Cardholder Name *same*
☑ Yes   ☑ Cardholder   ☐ Child   ☐ Disabled Dependent
☐ No   ☐ Spouse   ☐ Dependent Parent   ☐ Full-Time Student
                              (Please provide the pharmacy with your card.)

MEDICAL HISTORY

HEALTH   ALLERGIES AND DRUG REACTIONS
☑ No Known Medical   ☐ Diabetes Mellitus   ☐ No Known Drug Allergies
  Conditions   ☐ Epilepsy   ☐ Aspirin
☐ Anemia   ☐ Esophagitis   ☐ Cephalosporins
☐ Arthritis   ☐ Generalized Anxiety Disorder   ☐ Codeine
☐ Asthma   ☐ Heart Condition   ☐ Erythromycin
☐ Attention-Deficit   ☐ Hypertension   ☑ Penicillin G Potassium
  Hyperactivity Disorder   ☐ Kidney Disease   ☐ Sulfa
☐ Blood Clotting Disorders   ☐ Liver Disease   ☐ Tetracyclines
☐ Cancer   ☐ Lung Disease   ☐ Xanthines
☐ Depression   ☐ Ulcers

ICD-9 for Checked Condition(s): _____   Details for Checked Allergy(ies): _____

Medication(s) Currently Being Taken: _____

Primary Care Physician: _____*Geoff Taylor*_____

Comments: _____

Health information changes periodically. Please notify the pharmacy of any new medications, allergies, drug reactions, or health conditions.

Signature *Marquita Wilkins*   Date *2/17/15*   ☐ I choose not to fill out this form.

Wellness Institute
Insurance card

MARQUITA WILKINS
BIN: 776520
ID: GHT88729

GROUP: RXCare
RELATIONSHIP: 01, CARDHOLDER

MEMBER SERVICES: 1-800-555-3232
CLAIMS/INQUIRIES: 1-800-555-6363

Lab Review

Check Your Understanding

1. To save information you've entered into the system, you should _____.
   a. click Save or press CTRL+S
   b. press CTRL+N
   c. press F3
   d. press Esc

2. Common patient drug allergies include all of the following *except* _____.
   a. penicillin
   b. codeine
   c. Zoloft
   d. sulfonamides

3. You may search for a patient's insurance plan by _____ number.
   a. PIN
   b. BIN
   c. SIN
   d. DIN

4. You enter patient profile information into the computer system by transcribing it from the _____.
   a. patient at the counter
   b. patient's prescription
   c. patient profile form
   d. insurance card

5. What would you do if what the patient wrote on the form did not exactly match the field choices on your computer screen?
   a. Make your best guess.
   b. Ask the pharmacist or another technician to advise you.
   c. Choose the field's suggested word or phrase that is closest to what is written.
   d. Text the patient's cell phone to obtain more information.

Thinking Like a Pharmacy Tech

1. Changes in patient information (address, phone number, insurance information, medical conditions, and allergies) can happen frequently. The prescribing practitioner may not always make a note of such changes when writing the prescription. Discuss why it is important for patients to communicate such changes to the pharmacy, and if they don't, make suggestions how you would become aware of the changes.

2. Is the paper copy of the patient profile necessary? If not, describe your rationale for having the patient simply state this information to the pharmacy technician. If so, describe your rationale for having the patient continue to write this information on the patient profile form.

3. Sometimes when interviewing for a pharmacy technician job, the interviewer will ask you a difficult question. He or she may ask about working with a difficult person, or an ethics question that you are unsure of the answer to. What do you do when you are asked a difficult question? What are some possible strategies to giving an honest answer that puts you in a good light?

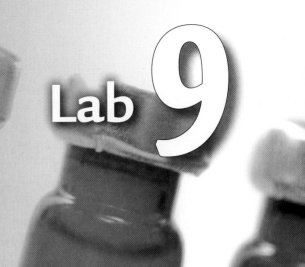

Processing a Prescription

Lab 9

Objectives

- Accurately process patient prescriptions.
- Accurately process serialized prescription forms used in prescription monitoring programs.
- Practice using pharmacy management software for prescriptions and monitored prescriptions.

Supplies

- NRx-Based Training Software

Signa

A series of abbreviations to communicate prescription and patient directions

One of the primary duties of pharmacy technicians is prescription processing. To be successful, you must accurately interpret and process prescriptions so that the patient receives the proper medication in the correct dosage form and strength, accompanied by the appropriate instructions. Knowing how to transcribe information accurately, including interpreting **signa** abbreviations and keeping current on legal requirements for prescriptions in your state, is fundamental to your pharmacy technician work. Signa abbreviations follow a specific order, always beginning with an action verb and continuing through dose quantity, route of administration, time interval, and additional information.

Also key to your career success is familiarity with pharmacy software. As technology and computer software, such as pharmacy management systems, are further integrated into pharmacy practice, pharmacy technicians must become more technology-savvy. Pharmacies use pharmacy management software products such as NRx in the daily practice of serving patients. Gaining experience using such a system is important and this lab will build your general awareness of pharmacy software systems. However, because pharmacies can choose from numerous software products, once in the field you will need to gain expertise with the specific functions of your

95

workplace software.

Regardless of the particular software system at your pharmacy, some prescriptions will require careful, close monitoring. In response to the increase in prescription-drug abuse, many states have adopted regulations known as prescription monitoring programs (PMPs) for monitoring prescribed controlled substances. These programs were originally designed to monitor Schedule II (C-II) prescriptions through mandatory reporting of specific information, such as prescriber, pharmacy, and patient information, as well as drug name, strength, quantity, National Drug Code (NDC), and number of days supplied. In recent years, however, many states have expanded these programs to include specific drug classes such as benzodiazepines, or specific drug products such as carisoprodol and tramadol. In addition, some states have expanded these programs to require mandatory reporting on *all* controlled substance prescriptions (Schedules II, III, IV, and V).

To monitor such prescriptions more accurately, several states, including Texas and New York, require that each monitored prescription be written on a specially designed, tamper-proof prescription blank. The blanks are serialized, or individually numbered, with a specific **control number**. The control number must be entered into the pharmacy management software at different points for different software systems. For tracking purposes, the number is then electronically reported—along with specific prescriber, pharmacy, patient, and prescription information—to the state regulatory agency enforcing controlled substance monitoring. The agency responsible for these state-level programs is typically a law enforcement agency, such as the Department of Public Safety, in Texas, and the Department of Health, in New York, rather than the state's Board of Pharmacy.

When filling prescriptions, you may process them in one of two ways. For most prescriptions, whether for controlled or noncontrolled substances, you may either fill them immediately—the most common practice—or you may add them to the profile and place them "on hold" to be filled at a later date. When you fill a prescription for immediate use, the label will print with a "last filled" date and monograph, which will then be passed on to the next station for counting and pouring, either by you or another technician. When the patient simply wants to add the prescription to his or her profile for later use, a label will still print. However, the "last filled" date and the monograph will not print, indicating that the prescription is not being dispensed, but simply placed on file for filling at another time.

In your pharmacy practice, you will at times be asked to partially fill a prescription. A partial fill might be necessary when a pharmacy does not have enough of the medication in stock or when a patient does not have enough money to pay for the entire prescription. Should these events occur, the pharmacy may fill only a few days' or a week's worth of medication. The patient would return to pick up the remaining fill quantity at a later date—when the pharmacy has acquired the rest of the

Control number

Unique number assigned to any monitored prescription for management and tracking purposes stock or when the patient is able to pay for the rest of the prescription. Pharmacy management software systems, such as the NRx system, enable pharmacies to account for partial fills.

Procedure

Take Note

As you perform each of the NRx-based software simulation labs (Labs 8–14), be aware that you can choose "Print this screen" in the upper-right corner of any open screen. This printing option may be necessary under unusual circumstances, such as if you have to stop performing a lab in mid-stream due to closure of a campus computer lab, personal emergency, or similar circumstance. You may print the screen to demonstrate to your instructor just how far you progressed on the lab. Under ordinary circumstances, you will be printing only the final screen of the lab, the results screen that shows your numerical score and accuracy percentage. You will be clearly instructed when and how to print the results screen within the final steps of the lab.

In the previous lab, you set up a computer profile for a new patient, Vance Donaldson. After his profile was created, Mr. Donaldson gave you his prescription to fill. Using the following steps, fill his prescription (Figure 9.1 on page 99 in this lab, corresponding to sub-lab 9.1 in the software) and continue practicing by filling the prescriptions included for other patients (Figures 9.2 through 9.9 on pages 106–109 in this lab, corresponding to sub-labs 9.2–9.9 in the software). When you encounter a monitored prescription, you must enter the control number. For the NRx-based training software, control number entry occurs at the end of the filling process.

This lab provides you with practice processing prescriptions using a particular feature of the NRx software system: short codes. This NRx feature, found in many similar software products, allows you to enter prescription directions using a shorthand system. Short codes are designed to ensure that spelling is consistent and directions are standardized within the pharmacy, from prescription to prescription and patient to patient. Short codes also save pharmacy technicians considerable time because entering prescription directions with short codes is quicker than free-typing each full word of the entire set of directions. Imagine typing "Take 1 to 2 tablets by mouth every 4 to 6 hours as needed for pain" multiple times a day when, instead, you could use short codes and simply type "t 1-2 tab po q 4-6h prn fp". Short codes alleviate the burden of lengthy repetition and also save time. In this lab, you will be directed at Step 7 to use the short codes found in Table 9.1 on the next page to enter prescription directions into the software.

TABLE 9.1 Signa Short Codes

Action Verb		Quantity		Dosage Form		Route of Administration		Time Interval		Additional Information	
Word	Short Code	Word	Short Code	Word	Short Code	Word	Short Code	Word	Short Code	Word	Short Code
inject	inj	one	1	capsule	cap	both ears	au	once a day	qd	after meals	pc
instill	inst	one to two	1-2	drops	gtts	both eyes	ou	two times a day	bid	and	and
give	g	three	3	units	units	by mouth	po	three times a day	tid	anxiety	anx
take	t	four	4	tablet	tab	left ear	as	every 4 to 6 hours	q 4-6h	as needed	prn
		five	5	teaspoonful	tsp	right eye	od	every 6 hours	q6h	as needed for	asnf
		twelve	12			subcutane-ously	sc	each morning	qam	before	bef
		eighteen	18					each evening	qpm	breakfast	bkft
								30 minutes	30m	for 10 days	f 10d
										for 14 days	x14d
										for pain	fp
										6pm	6pm

Important Note: In some instances, portions of specific directions given to the patient cannot be entered using short codes. In such cases, as with Figure 9.9, you will need to enter free-text (fully type out) that portion of the signa. Use care when deciding when to use short codes and when to use free-text on each part of the signa. Maintaining uniformity in directions among prescriptions is important for preventing medication errors.

1 First install the NRx Simulation CD that accompanied your textbook by following the installation directions on page xii of the Preface. Begin this lab by clicking the PharmacyLabs icon that should now be on your desktop. When the sign-in fields appear, type in your First Name and Last Name and click OK.

2 When the menu for all available labs appears on the left, click the dark purple tab for Lab 9. When the list of sub-labs (for example, Lab 9.1, Lab 9.2, Lab 9.3, and so on) appears below the main lab tab, click the sub-lab you wish to perform, beginning with 9.1.

Tip: The sub-labs represent the different patients you will be processing through the lab procedures. Most labs present several sub-labs for processing; however, some labs have only one sub-lab.

3 When the NRx Security screen appears, log in to the NRx-based training software as the Primary User by typing "Student" as the Login ID and "Training" as the Password. Press Tab or click Log In.

Tip: After you have completed this log-in step for the first listed sub-lab (for example, Lab 8.1, Lab 9.1, Lab 10.1, and so on), you will not be prompted to log in again for the remaining sub-labs in that lab's listing and may then skip this log-in step.

FIGURE 9.1

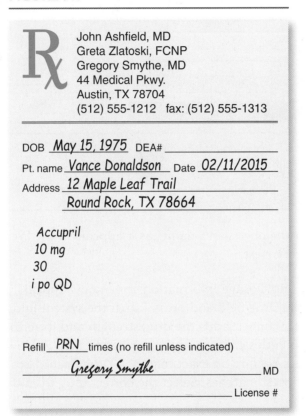

Rx

John Ashfield, MD
Greta Zlatoski, FCNP
Gregory Smythe, MD
44 Medical Pkwy.
Austin, TX 78704
(512) 555-1212   fax: (512) 555-1313

DOB *May 15, 1975* DEA# _____

Pt. name *Vance Donaldson* Date *02/11/2015*

Address *12 Maple Leaf Trail*
Round Rock, TX 78664

Accupril
10 mg
30
i po QD

Refill *PRN* times (no refill unless indicated)

Gregory Smythe _____ MD

_____ License #

4 On the Rx Processing Tasks menu, click New Rx or press F2. When the New Prescription screen appears, type the patient's name in the Patient field in Lastname, Firstname format and press Tab. The patient's payment information (either third party or cash) and primary prescriber will appear in the appropriate fields.

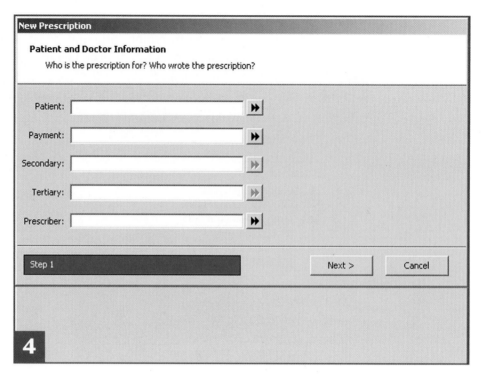

5 Verify that the physician's name, as it appears in the Prescriber field, is correct. Click Next.

6 The Drug and Dosage Information screen now appears. Type the drug name in the Drug field and press Tab. If the system finds an exact match to the drug name, it adds the drug strength and form to the name in the Drug field. In this case, you may proceed to Step 7. However, if the system does *not* find an exact match, a Drug Record Scan list appears with the closest matches. Select the correct drug from the list by double-clicking it.

Take Note

The CD that accompanies your textbook provides you with a simulation of the NRx software. However, because it is a simulation only, it does not fully replicate all functions of the software itself. When you are working with a fully operational software system at the pharmacy, you will notice that when typing into a field, you will often need to type only the first few letters of the phrase or word you are entering. To save you time, the software will pull up a complete phrase or word matching the first few characters you have entered and, after verifying that what is filled in is exactly what you want, you will simply press Enter to complete your task without having to type all the characters.

6

7 Refer to the prescriber's signa and to Table 9.1 and enter the short codes into the Sig field, beginning with the action verb short code and leaving a space between each of the six short code elements as you type. Press Tab. The software will translate your short codes into clear patient instructions, which will appear now in the Sig field and also be printed on the prescription label at the end of the lab.

Tip: If you need assistance translating the signa into short codes, ask your instructor for help. You might also take a moment to write out the full sentence translation of the signa on the prescription form represented in Figures 9.1–9.9. Then use your sentences and Table 9.1 to determine the short codes you should type into the Sig field on screen.

8 Type the quantity into the Quantity Authorized field and press Tab. Note that the same number automatically appears in the Quantity Dispensed field (and may also appear in the Days Supply field). When working in the pharmacy, you would change the Quantity Dispensed number only if you were going to fill the prescription partially rather than completely. For the purposes of this lab, you are completely filling all prescriptions, so leave the Quantity Dispensed field as is.

9 To decide what to enter in the Days Supply field, use the signa as your guide and calculate the number of days this prescription will last. If the field has already been populated with a number, verify that the quantity is correct according to your calculations, and proceed to Step 10. If there is no number in the Days Supply field, type in the quantity you have calculated and press Tab.

Tip: If you have not yet practiced calculating a day's supply, ask your instructor to demonstrate the process.

10 To enter the number of refills, you have two choices. If the physician has authorized a specific number of refills (including "0"), enter that numeral in the Refills Authorized field and press Tab. However, if PRN refills are authorized, instead click inside the small field, or box, next to the term PRN, causing a check mark to appear.

Take Note

The number of refills on prescriptions is legally regulated. According to federal law, controlled Schedule II substances can *never be refilled* without a new prescription (except in emergency situations, when a pharmacist must handle the situation). Substances controlled on Schedules III and IV may have *up to five refills* within a 6-month period. Noncontrolled prescriptions and controlled substances on Schedule V have *no limitation* on refills (stated as "PRN"), provided the prescription is not 365 days old and expired. Note that with both controlled and noncontrolled medications, the prescriber can choose to prohibit refills or stipulate a maximum number of refills. You may have additional regulations in your state.

11 Just above the PRN box is the Dispense as Written (DAW) field. When working in the pharmacy, you would need to look closely at the prescription to determine whether the prescriber has authorized a generic substitution or has mandated that the brand be dispensed. You would then type either Y (Yes) or N (No) into the DAW field. Since state laws vary, assume for the purposes of this lab that substitution is permitted. Notice that Y (Yes) is already present by default in the DAW field, and leave it as is.

Take Note

DAW code terminology may vary among different pharmacy software systems. However, some common DAW codes include: 0—Selection Permitted; 1—Physician requests Brand; and 2—Patient requests Brand.

12 Just above the DAW field, click your cursor in the Date Written field. Using numerals only, enter the date the prescription was written, and press Tab.

Tip: For the purposes of this lab, use only numerals to enter the date and use two digits for the month. For example, January would be 01, February would be 02, and so on.

13 The Rx Summary/General Information screen will appear and you should verify that all information is entered correctly. Review the patient, prescriber, and all prescription information. If there are no errors, simply click Save or press CTRL + S. (Notice that the question marks in the Rx number are updated and the prescription now has an assigned Rx number.)

Tip: While you might not have access to a stock bottle in your particular educational facility or pharmacy course lab, be aware that in pharmacy practice, verification of the stock bottle NDC number is a best practice and may also be required by law. Thus, when filling a prescription in pharmacy practice, you would look to the Messages field at the bottom left to note the NDC number and verify that it matches the NDC number on the stock bottle.

Take Note

In practice, at your pharmacy job, remember to save your work frequently. You can do this by clicking Save or pressing CTRL+S on the keyboard.

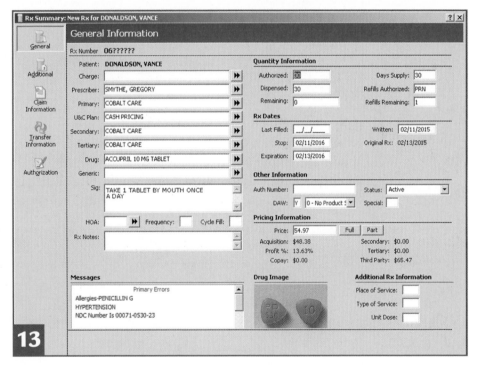

14 On this same screen, select your filling option. Mr. Donaldson wants his prescription filled immediately rather than placed on hold, so click Fill on the top toolbar. For the purposes of this lab, assume that all other patients want their prescriptions filled at this time, and when you reach this step for those patients, click Fill for each of them.

Tip: When working at the pharmacy, if you want to place the prescription into the patient profile but not fill it right away, you would click Profile Only on the top toolbar to be done with the patient's prescription for the time being.

15 A Filling Options dialog box pops up, asking how many labels you would like to print. The default quantity is one and appears automatically. On the job, you might choose to change the print quantity. For the purposes of this lab, leave the quantity as is and click Fill.

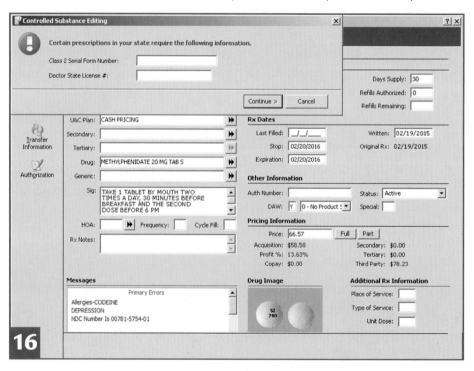

16 If the prescription is for a noncontrolled drug, proceed to Step 17. If the prescription is for a C-II drug, the Controlled Substance Editing dialog box will appear and require you to enter the Control Number and Doctor State License number. Transcribe this information from the face of the prescription into those two fields and click Continue or press Tab. Then proceed to Step 17.

17 If a Clinical Checking dialog box appears on the screen, you would have to alert the pharmacist while on the job, because possible adverse effects or contraindications may be present for this prescription. The pharmacist would inform you of the next steps to take. For the purposes of this lab, alert your instructor about the box, click Bypass on the top toolbar, and proceed to Step 18.

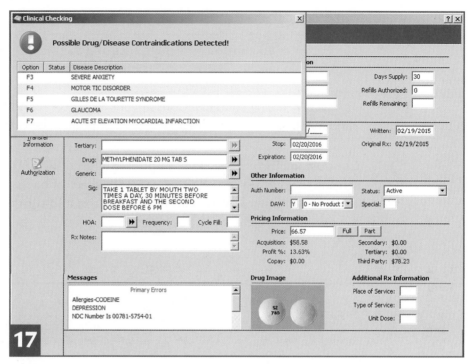

18 A window previewing the prescription label is now on screen. To print this prescription label at your local printer, click Print this screen in the upper-right corner. (A small window associated with your local printer options will appear. Make the necessary selections for the printer you wish to use and click as required to print the label.) Retrieve the printed prescription label and set it aside for your instructor to evaluate at the end of the lab.

19 Click Next at the bottom of the print-preview window. Within a few seconds, a results screen will appear, displaying your name, the lab number, your start and finish times, your numerical score and a maximum score, and your accuracy percentage. Print these results by clicking Print this screen in the upper-right corner. (Once again, a small window associated with your local printer will appear and you should take the steps necessary to print the screen.) When you are sure the screen has printed, retrieve it and set it aside to be turned in at the end of the lab. Click Close this lab in the upper-right corner of the screen.

Tip: Do not close the lab until you are absolutely certain that your results screen has printed successfully. You will not be able to retrieve your results once you click Close this lab.

20 Your screen will now display the main labs and sub-labs page. In numerical order, select the next sub-lab you wish to perform and repeat Steps 4 through 19 for all remaining prescriptions (Figures 9.2 through 9.9), setting aside all printed prescription labels and results screens in a stack. When you have processed all nine prescriptions, proceed to Step 21 to conclude the lab.

Take Note

According to your instructor's preference and the available lab time and capacity, you might now have the chance to prepare the prescription itself—not just process the data associated with the prescription—and label a bottle including contents. Consult your instructor for additional supplies and materials needed to prepare the prescription in laboratory practice.

21 **Conclusion:** Turn in the stack of printed prescription labels and results screens to your instructor. On a separate sheet of paper, answer all questions in the following Lab Review section and turn in your answers to your instructor.

FIGURE 9.2

Sunjita Patel, MD
7612 N. HWY 27
Cedar Rapids, IA 52404
(319) 555-1212 fax: (319) 555-1313

DOB _Aug 24, 1949_ DEA# _AP4756687_
Pt. name _Amala Gupta_ Date _02/16/2015_
Address _5473 W 10th Street_
Cedar Rapids, IA 52401

Lorazepam
0.5 mg
120 (one hundred twenty)
i po q4-6 h prn anxiety

Refill _5_ times (no refill unless indicated)
Sunjita Patel, MD _____ MD
_____ License #

FIGURE 9.3

Todd Jackson, MD
Anita Johnson, MD
Kunal Gupta, MSN, FCNP
5730 Congress Avenue
Boise, ID 83702
(208) 555-1212 fax: (208) 555-1313

DOB _Oct 18, 1978_ DEA# _FJ1234563_
Pt. name _Lily Nguyen_ Date _02/12/2015_
Address _2934 Anderson Lane_
Boise, ID 83722

Alprazolam
2 mg
120 (one hundred twenty)
i po q6 h prn anxiety

Refill _5_ times (no refill unless indicated)
Todd Jackson _____ MD
_____ License #

FIGURE 9.4

Rx

Randal Binder, MD
Philip McCracken, MD
Terrence McDowell, MD
5874 Kempston Dr.
Orlando, FL 32812
(407) 555-1212 fax: (407) 555-1313

DOB _Jan 22, 1998_ DEA# _____

Pt. name _Cas Riley_ Date _02/01/2015_

Address _72650 Okade Court_
Orlando, FL 32810

Ciprofloxacin
250 mg
28
i po bid x 14D

Refill _0_ times (no refill unless indicated)

Philip McCracken MD

_____ License #

FIGURE 9.5

Rx

Simona Brushfield, MD
2222 IH-35 South
Austin, TX 78703
(512) 555-1212 fax: (512) 555-1313

DOB _Sep 12, 1953_ DEA# _____

Pt. name _Miguel Esparza_ Date _01/15/2015_

Address _7583 E 11th St._
Austin, TX 78705

Humalog
100 Units/mL Vial
1 vial
12 units subQ qAM;
18 units subQ qPM pc

Refill _PRN_ times (no refill unless indicated)

Simona Brushfield, MD MD

_____ License #

FIGURE 9.6

Rx

Frieda Nadal, MD
67 Savin Hill Ave
Boston, MA 02109
(617) 555-1212 fax: (617) 555-1313

DOB _Jun 23, 1988_ DEA# _____

Pt. name _Kimberly Jackson_ Date _02/19/2015_

Address _4590 Settling Glen Dr_
Boston, MA 02109

Amoxicillin
250 mg/5 mL
150 mL
1 tsp po TID x 10D

Refill _0_ times (no refill unless indicated)

Frieda Nadal MD

_____ License #

FIGURE 9.7

Rx

Geoff Taylor, MD
67 Whitford Avenue
Providence, RI 02908
(401) 555-1212 fax: (401) 555-1313

DOB _Feb 29, 1984_ DEA# _____

Pt. name _Marquita Wilkins_ Date _02/19/2015_

Address _6901 Westminster Chase_
Providence, RI 02908

Patanol
5 mL
i-ii gtts ou BID

Refill _0_ times (no refill unless indicated)

Geoff Taylor MD

_____ License #

FIGURE 9.8

```
--------------------------------------------------------------------
!!! -- START SECURED ELECTRONIC PRESCRIPTION TRANSMISSION -- !!!
--------------------------------------------------------------------
FROM THE OFFICES OF PHIL JACKSON, MD; ETHEL JACOBSON, MD;
                    PETER JARKOWSKI, PA; EUGENE JOHNSON, DO

OFFICE ADDRESS:           67 EAST ELM
                          CEDAR RAPIDS, IA 52411
OFFICE TELEPHONE:         (319) 555-1212   TRANSMIT DATE: 02/20/2015
OFFICE FAX:               (319) 555-1313   WRITTEN DATE:  02/20/2015
--------------------------------------------------------------------
TRANSMITTED TO            THE CORNER DRUG STORE
PHARMACY ADDRESS:         875 PARADIGM WAY
                          CEDAR RAPIDS, IA 52410
PHARMACY TELEPHONE:       (319) 555-1414
--------------------------------------------------------------------
PATIENT NAME:             JEFFREY KLEIN      D.O.B.: OCT 18, 1979
PATIENT ADDRESS:          1157 NORTH PLAZA AVE
                          CEDAR RAPIDS, IA 52411
--------------------------------------------------------------------
PRESCRIBED MEDICATION:    FLUOXETINE 20 MG
SIGNA:                    i PO QD
DISPENSE QUANTITY:        30
REFILL(S):                PRN
--------------------------------------------------------------------
PHYSICIAN SIGNATURE:      [[ ELECTRONIC SIGNATURE ON FILE ]]
                          [[ FOR DR. ETHEL JACOBSON ]]


--------------------------------------------------------------------
!!! -- END SECURED ELECTRONIC PRESCRIPTION TRANSMISSION -- !!!
--------------------------------------------------------------------
```

FIGURE 9.9

State License # J76839   DEA # MJ1234563

Ethel Jacobson, MD
MONITORED PRESCRIPTION FORM
67 EAST ELM
CEDAR RAPIDS, IA 52411
PHONE: (319) 555-1212   FAX: (319) 555-1313

CTRL # 678290463718

Name *Jeffrey Klein*

Address *1157 North Plaza Avenue, Cedar Rapids, IA 52411*

Age or DOB *Oct 18, 1979*   Date *02/19/2015*

SECURITY FEATURES ON BACK

R *Methylphenidate*
20 mg
60 (sixty)
i po BID, 30 min a breakfast,
second dose a 6PM

Ethel Jacobson, MD

Practitioner Signature–Indicate if "Brand Medically Necessary"

Pharmacist Signature	
Rx Number	Date Filled

Lab Review

Check Your Understanding

1. The PRN box is used to indicate that this prescription may be filled on an as-needed basis.
   a. true
   b. false

2. The DAW Code 1 signifies which of the following?
   a. The patient requests the brand medication.
   b. The prescriber requests the brand medication.
   c. The patient requests the generic medication.
   d. The prescriber requests the generic medication.

3. The patient's name is entered into the NRx-based training software system in the Firstname, Lastname format.
   a. true
   b. false

4. Which of the following is not an acceptable delivery method as noted in the NRx-based training software system?
   a. electronic
   b. telephone
   c. written
   d. unspecified

5. According to federal law, C-III prescriptions may be refilled up to 5 times.
   a. true
   b. false

Thinking Like a Pharmacy Tech

1. Prior to the use of computerized pharmacy management software, pharmacy personnel typed prescription labels on typewriters and manually updated patient prescription profiles using paper files and Rolodexes. Discuss the advantages and disadvantages for both filing systems.

2. Reporting confidential information as a means to prevent fraud and theft of prescription drug products is becoming more common. Discuss the extent to which you think that the mandatory reporting of patient and prescription information is a violation of privacy.

3. Having good answers to an interviewer's questions is important, but just as important is the impression you give through your speech, mannerisms, and eye contact. Why would an interviewer care about these things? What are ways you can ensure you're communicating clearly with an interviewer, especially if you are nervous?

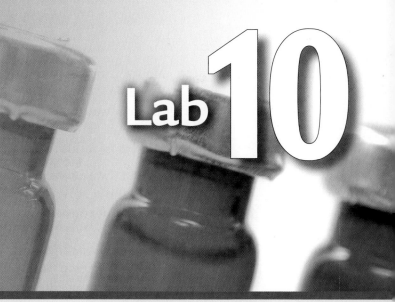

Processing a Refill

Lab 10

Objectives

- Demonstrate proficiency in the use of pharmacy management software for processing prescription refills.

Supplies

- NRx-Based Training Software

Chronic condition

A health concern that recurs frequently or lasts for an extended time

While many patients take prescription medications to cure symptoms and diseases, many more take them to treat chronic and ongoing medical conditions such as diabetes, hypertension, and depression. By definition, ongoing and **chronic conditions** require treatment over an extended period of time, and patients with such conditions will likely have prescriptions needing long-term refilling. A significant part of your work time as a pharmacy technician includes processing refill requests, often for such medical conditions. In fact, you will probably find that you process refill requests just as frequently as you process new prescription requests. Thus, knowing how to accurately and quickly process refills is critical to your pharmacy practice.

Accurate refill-request processing requires that you build awareness and skills beyond those necessary to process and fill new prescriptions. Always verify refill regulations for the state in which you practice. At the federal level, there are particular restrictions on refilling the various prescription categories. Knowledge of these restrictions will eventually become second nature to you in your pharmacy work. Start to learn these rules and eventually integrate them into your practice:

- Controlled Schedule II substances can *never be refilled* without a new prescription (except in an emergency situation, when a pharmacist must handle the situation).
- Substances controlled on Schedules III and IV may have *up to five refills* within a 6-month period.

113

- Noncontrolled prescriptions and controlled substances on Schedule V have *no limitation* on refills (stated as "PRN"), provided the prescription is not 365 days old and has not expired. Note that the prescriber can choose to prohibit refills or stipulate a maximum number of refills for both scheduled and non-scheduled medications.

Also be aware that in the NRx pharmacy management software system, but not necessarily in all similar programs, the prescription profile is color coded for easy reference. Pharmacy staff can take advantage of color coding to easily and quickly distinguish active prescriptions from prescriptions that are expired or placed on hold. (Note that an unfilled prescription can remain on hold for an unspecified period of time, but if it is not filled, it can still expire per legal limitations.) You will find the following color coding in the NRx system:

Black: Prescription is valid and has refills remaining.

Red: No refills remain or the prescription has expired.

Purple: Prescription was placed into profile and has not been filled.

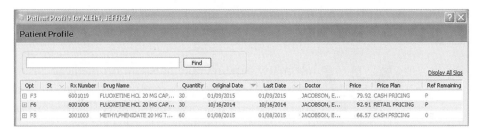

When patients telephone or come into the pharmacy seeking refills, some might have their prescription bottle in hand, some might simply have the prescription number or medication name written on a piece of paper, and others might know only the drug name or what the medication is supposed to treat. Knowing how to access and read a patient profile and understanding the use of a medication will help you to serve patients and provide them with the correct medication at the proper time. If you ever have a question about which medication to fill, ask your pharmacist before proceeding.

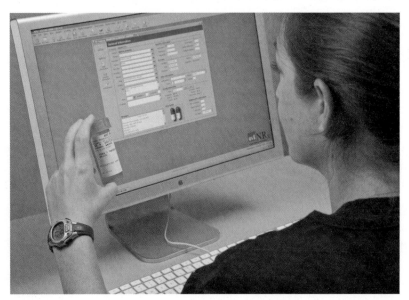

Pharmacy technician using patient's prescription bottle to process a refill request.

Procedure

Take Note

As you perform each of the NRx-based software simulation labs (Labs 8–14), be aware that you can choose "Print this screen" in the upper-right corner of any open screen. This printing option may be necessary under unusual circumstances, such as if you have to stop performing a lab in mid-stream due to closure of a campus computer lab, personal emergency, or similar circumstance. You may print the screen to demonstrate to your instructor just how far you progressed on the lab. Under ordinary circumstances, you will be printing only the final screen of the lab, the results screen that shows your numerical score and accuracy percentage. You will be clearly instructed when and how to print the results screen within the final steps of each lab.

In this lab, you will practice using the NRx-based training software to process refill requests for prescriptions filled in earlier labs. You will find the refill request data on the end-of-lab worksheet. Use the data to enter the requests into the software system. When you reach Step 5, you will be guided through filling out the Result column for each worksheet entry.

Scenario: Several of your regular patients have either phoned in requests or brought their used prescription bottles into the pharmacy and are requesting refills. You will encounter one of two conditions as you work through these refill requests: either patients will request a refill and have their prescription number on hand, or patients will request a refill but *not* have their prescription number with them.

As you follow the steps to practice processing refills and complete the worksheet, take care when you reach Step 4 and Step 5. At Step 4 you will need to choose either Step 4a or 4b for *each* refill request, based on whether the patient presents a prescription number. At Step 5, you will need to choose either Step 5a or 5b for *each* refill request, based on how the software responds to your request.

1 First install the NRx Simulation CD that accompanied your textbook by following the installation directions on page xii of the Preface. Begin this lab by clicking the PharmacyLabs icon that should now be on your desktop. When the sign-in fields appear, type in your First Name and Last Name and click OK.

2 When the menu for all available labs appears on the left, click the dark purple tab for Lab 10. When the list of sub-labs (for example, Lab 10.1, Lab 10.2, Lab 10.3, and so on) appears below the main lab tab, click the sub-lab you wish to perform, beginning with 10.1.

Tip: The sub-labs represent the different patients you will be processing through the lab procedures. Most labs present several sub-labs for processing; however, some labs have only one sub-lab.

3 When the NRx Security screen appears, log in to the NRx-based training software as the Primary User by typing "Student" as the Login ID and "Training" as the Password. Press Tab or click Log In.

Tip: After you have completed this log-in step for the first listed sub-lab (for example, Lab 9.1, Lab 10.1, Lab 11.1, and so on), you will not be prompted to log in again for the remaining sub-labs in that lab's listing and may then skip this log-in step.

4 At this point, you will choose to follow *either* Step 4a or 4b, depending on whether the patient has brought in a prescription number with the refill request. If the patient brought in the number, it is listed under the Rx Number, Prescription column of the worksheet.

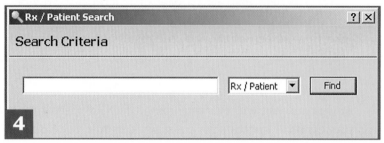

4a If the patient requests a refill *with* a prescription number:
- From the Rx Processing Tasks menu, click Search or press F3.
  Tip: F-keys, such as F3, F4, and so on, are usually found along the top row of your keyboard.
- Type the patient's prescription number into the Search field and press Enter or click Find.
- Proceed now to Step 5.

4b If the patient requests a refill *without* a prescription number:
- From the Rx Processing Tasks menu, click Search or press F3.
- Type the patient's name (in Lastname, Firstname format) in the empty field and click Find or press Enter.
- When the Patient Information screen appears, click the Rx Profile icon on the top toolbar.
- When the Patient Profile screen appears, find and double click the requested prescription or press the corresponding F-key.
  Tip: F-keys, such as F3, F4, and so on, are usually found along the top row of your keyboard.
- Proceed now to Step 5.

5 At this point, the Rx Summary screen should appear. However, one of two things will occur. Either the Rx Summary screen in fact will appear in full view (Step 5a) or that screen will appear but with the Refill Request Options dialog box popped up over it, alerting you to take further action because the prescription is no longer valid (Step 5b). According to what your screen displays, follow the associated step below for each refill request. When you have completed Step 5a or 5b for *all* of the refill requests and indicated each result on the worksheet, proceed to the final, step, Step 6, which is the Conclusion step for this lab.

5a If the Rx Summary screen appears, you *may be able* to process the refill request without incident. But first, verify patient name and medication name and compare the on-screen Last Filled date and Days Supply quantity with the Refill Request date on the worksheet.

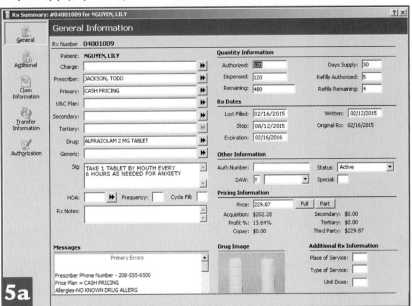

According to how the Last Filled date and Days Supply quantity compare with the Refill Request date, proceed with one of the following two bulleted "*If*" sections:

- **If** *too little time has passed since the Last Filled date and what the Days Supply had provided,* you are in a situation known as "refill too soon," and the patient's insurance plan might not cover the prescription. You *will be unable* to process this prescription during this lab.

  - Complete the worksheet entry for this refill request by circling Refill Too Soon in the Result column and also writing the number of days since the last fill date on the blank line provided.

  - Be aware that in the next lab, Lab 11, you will learn about seeking authorization and filling expired prescriptions. At this time, stop the refill request process for this particular prescription by pressing Esc.

  - When the results screen appears, displaying your name, the lab number, your start and finish times, your numerical score and a maximum score, and your accuracy percentage, click Print this screen in the upper-right corner. A small window associated with your printer options will appear. Make the necessary selections for the printer you wish to use, and click as required to print the screen.

- When you are sure the results screen has printed, retrieve it and set it aside to be turned in at the end of the lab. Click Close this lab in the upper-right corner of the screen.
  Tip: Do not close the lab until you are absolutely certain that your results screen has printed successfully. You will not be able to retrieve your results once you click Close this lab.

- When the main screen listing all labs and sub-labs appears, you may process the next refill request. First, double-check that you have marked the worksheet Result column for the patient you have just finished processing. Then, progress in numerical order down the worksheet by returning to Procedure Step 4a or 4b, according to the next patient's situation.

■ *If the amount of time that has passed is just a day or two before the supply is intended to run out or if the date exceeds the time span covered by the days supply, you will be able* to fill the prescription.

- Click the Fill icon on the top toolbar and a Filling Options dialog box will appear. Verify that the Print Label box is checked, and then click Fill.

- A window previewing the prescription label is now on screen. To print this label at your printer, click Print this screen in the upper-right corner. A small window associated with your printer options will appear. Make the necessary selections for the printer you wish to use, and click as required to print the label. Retrieve the printed label and set it aside to turn in at the end of the lab.

- Complete the worksheet entry for this refill request by circling Refill Processed in the Result column.

- Click Next at the bottom of the print-preview window. Within a few seconds, a results screen will appear, displaying your name, the lab number, your start and finish times, your numerical score and a maximum score, and your accuracy percentage. Click Print this screen in the upper-right corner. Once again, a small window associated with your local printer will appear and you should take the steps necessary to print the screen.

- When you are sure the results screen has printed, retrieve it and set it aside with the prescription label to be turned in at the end of the lab. Click Close this lab in the upper-right corner of the screen.
  Tip: Do not close the lab until you are absolutely certain that your results screen has printed successfully. You will not be able to retrieve your results once you click Close this lab.

- When the main screen listing all labs and sub-labs appears, you may process the next refill request. First, double-check that you have marked the worksheet Result column for the patient you have just finished processing. Then, progress in numerical order down the worksheet by returning to Procedure Step 4a or 4b, according to the next patient's situation.

Take Note

Controlled substances should *never* be refilled early. When the prescription is for a controlled substance, check the last fill date and the proper day's supply against today's date. Refills must be delayed until after the supply is exceeded or until the pharmacy receives permission after contacting the physician. If you encounter a request for early refill of a controlled substance, ask the pharmacist to intervene.

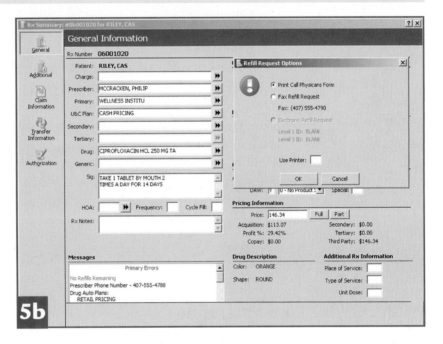

5b If the Refill Request Options dialog box pops up, alerting you that the prescription is no longer valid, you *will be unable* to process this prescription during this lab. For this refill request, do the following:

- Complete the worksheet entry for this refill request by circling Invalid Prescription in the Result column.

- Be aware that in the next lab, Lab 11, you will learn about seeking authorization and filling expired prescriptions. At this time, do not click anything in the Refill Request Options dialog box. Stop the refill request process for this particular prescription by pressing Esc twice to go through the Rx Summary screen to the results screen.

- When the results screen appears, displaying your name, the lab number, your start and finish times, your numerical score and a maximum score, and your accuracy percentage, click Print this screen in the upper-right corner. A small window associated with your local printer options will appear. Make the necessary selections for the printer you wish to use, and click as required to print the screen.

- When you are sure the results screen has printed, retrieve it and set it aside to be turned in at the end of the lab. Click Close this lab in the upper-right corner of the screen. **Tip:** *Do not close the lab until you are absolutely certain that your results screen has printed successfully. You will not be able to retrieve your results once you click Close this lab.*

- When the main screen listing all labs and sub-labs appears, you may process the next refill request. First, double-check that you have marked the worksheet Result column for the patient you have just finished processing. Then, progress in numerical order down the worksheet by returning to Procedure Step 4a or 4b, according to the next patient's situation.

6 **Conclusion**: Double-check that you have completed the Result column for all entries on the worksheet before concluding. Write your name and the date on the worksheet and tear it out. Attach all printed labels and the eight results screens to the worksheet and turn in the whole set to your instructor. On a separate sheet of paper, answer all questions in the following Lab Review section and turn in your answers to your instructor.

Lab Review

Check Your Understanding

1. According to federal regulations, a prescription for a C-II may _____.
   a. be refilled as needed for up to one year
   b. be refilled five times in a 6-month period
   c. be refilled as needed in a 6-month period
   d. not be refilled unless a new prescription is presented

2. "Chronic" conditions refer to conditions described as _____.
   a. short-term
   b. long-term
   c. acute
   d. incurable

3. Depression is a condition that is usually treated and cured within a week's time.
   a. true
   b. false

4. When a prescription is placed on hold, it can remain in that status for ____.
   a. 2 months
   b. 18 months
   c. an unspecified period of time
   d. 3 weeks

5. The color coding of prescription data in the patient prescription profile in a pharmacy software system is used to help pharmacy personnel quickly determine prescription status.
   a. true
   b. false

Thinking Like a Pharmacy Tech

1. Many pharmacies will fill prescriptions for *non*controlled substances early, without question. However, when asked to fill a prescription for a controlled substance early, nearly all will ask questions and deny early refills. Keep in mind that patient safety—as well as abuse and fraud prevention—plays a role in how pharmacy staff respond to early requests. Explain whether asking questions or denying early refills is an act of discrimination or a legitimate and acceptable action.

2. If a patient comes in to your pharmacy for a refill but has no information with her and you cannot find her name in the software system, what should you do?

3. How will you try to develop empathy for the patients and customers you will meet as a pharmacy technician? How important do you think this will be to the job?

Lab 10   *Processing a Refill*

Worksheet for Refill Request Processing

Sub-Lab Number	Refill Request Date	Patient Name, Birth Date	Rx Number, Prescription	Result (Circle one/Fill blank if needed)
10.1	03/15/2015	Donaldson, Vance, 05/15/1975	6001012, Accupril 10 mg	Refill Too Soon: Last fill ___days ago Invalid Prescription Refill Processed
10.2	03/03/2015	Gupta, Amala, 08/24/1949	Lorazepam 0.5 mg	Refill Too Soon: Last fill ___days ago Invalid Prescription Refill Processed
10.3	03/17/2015	Nguyen, Lily, 10/18/1978	4001009, Alprazolam 2 mg	Refill Too Soon: Last fill ___days ago Invalid Prescription Refill Processed
10.4	05/19/2015	Riley, Cas, 01/22/1998	6001020, Ciprofloxacin 250mg	Refill Too Soon: Last fill ___days ago Invalid Prescription Refill Processed
10.5	02/18/2015	Esparza, Miguel, 09/12/1953	Humalog Insulin	Refill Too Soon: Last fill ___days ago Invalid Prescription Refill Processed
10.6	07/24/2015	Jackson, Kimberly, 06/23/1988	Amoxicillin 250mg/5mL	Refill Too Soon: Last fill ___days ago Invalid Prescription Refill Processed
10.7	03/28/2015	Wilkins, Marquita, 02/29/1984	Patanol	Refill Too Soon: Last fill ___days ago Invalid Prescription Refill Processed
10.8	02/21/2015	Klein, Jeffrey, 10/18/1979	Fluoxetine 20 mg	Refill Too Soon: Last fill ___days ago Invalid Prescription Refill Processed

Obtaining Refill Authorization

Lab 11

Objectives

- Learn strategies for resolving problems associated with expired prescriptions.
- Demonstrate proficiency in using pharmacy management software for prescription refill authorization.
- Practice securing authorization for prescription refills via paper forms.
- Learn protocol for communicating refill authorizations through simulated telephone conversations with prescribers.

Supplies

- NRx-Based Training Software

Frequently, a patient will come into or telephone the pharmacy with a prescription that you cannot fill because the prescription has expired. A prescription expires when all refills have been exhausted or when the final date to fill the prescription has passed. Because state laws differ regarding prescription refills, you must be aware of your state's regulations. Federal regulations dictate that prescriptions may be refilled if authorized by the prescriber.

To secure authorization for further refills of an expired prescription, the pharmacy technician may—in many states—contact the prescriber. However, in some states, pharmacy technicians *are not permitted* to perform this duty and only the pharmacist may legally obtain authorization. Determine what the law is in your state. If your state allows pharmacy technicians to process refills, this lab is accurate as written. However, if your state prohibits pharmacy technicians from processing refills, replace the term "pharmacy technician" with "pharmacist" throughout the remainder of this lab. For the same prohibitive reason, your instructor may have you skip this lab.

Precise restrictions are in place at the federal level to regulate refilling the various prescription categories. Knowledge of these restrictions will eventually become second nature to you in your pharmacy work. Start to learn these rules and integrate them into your practice:

- Controlled Schedule II substances can *never be refilled* and require a new prescription (except in emergency situations, when a pharmacist must handle the situation).
- Substances controlled on Schedules III and IV may have *up to five refills* within a 6-month period.
- Noncontrolled prescriptions and controlled substances on Schedule V have *no limitation* on refills (stated as "PRN"), provided the prescription is not 365 days old and has not expired. Note that the prescriber can choose to prohibit refills or stipulate a maximum number of refills, on both controlled and noncontrolled prescriptions.

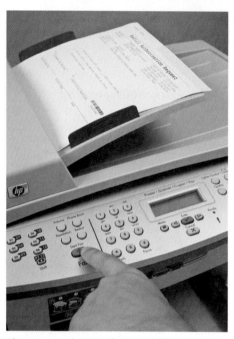

Pharmacy technician faxing a refill authorization request to prescriber's office.

Pharmacy technicians must follow a clear-cut process to refill an expired prescription. First, the technician generates a refill authorization request form by using the pharmacy's software program. Information on this form is then phoned in or faxed to the prescriber's office for authorization. Some prescriber offices will require you to send the request via fax so that they will possess a hard copy. However, in some cases the request can be phoned in by providing a specific series of patient and prescription information. You will be guided through the phoning-in process for refill requests during this lab.

Once the prescriber's office receives the refill request, it can either deny the request or approve it and designate a certain number of refills. When responding to the refill request, the prescriber may also communicate special instructions for the patient. For example, the patient may be required to obtain additional lab work or return for an office visit before receiving further refills. If the prescriber denies the request, a pharmacy technician must make a note of this decision and then notify the patient of the denial, relaying any special instructions given by the prescriber's office to the patient. If the prescriber approves the request, a pharmacy technician can generate a new prescription according to the prescriber's stipulations.

Procedure

In this lab, you will continue gaining skills with the NRx-based simulation by processing refill requests for prescriptions filled in earlier labs. At this time, however, those prescriptions will have expired. As in the previous lab,

Take Note

As you perform each of the NRx-based software simulation labs (Labs 8–14), be aware that you can choose "Print this screen" in the upper-right corner of any open screen. This printing option may be necessary under unusual circumstances, such as if you have to stop performing a lab in mid-stream due to closure of a campus computer lab, personal emergency, or similar circumstance. You may print the screen to demonstrate to your instructor just how far you progressed on the lab. Under ordinary circumstances, you will be printing only the final screen of the lab, the results screen that shows your numerical score and accuracy percentage. You will be clearly instructed when and how to print the results screen within the final steps of each lab.

some patients will present a prescription number, and others will not. Figures 11.1 through 11.5, located at the end of this lab, represent prescription labels brought in by patients and sticky notes jotted by pharmacy staff when patients have called in a refill request.

Because all of these prescriptions have expired, you must use the figure data to request and successfully obtain refill authorization before you can fill the patients' prescriptions. Following the steps below, you will practice generating a Refill Authorization Request form by using the NRx Simulation CD in Part I.

You will then spend class time off the computer to complete Parts II and III. In Part II you will communicate the authorization request to the prescriber by role-playing telephone conversations with a partner. Such role-play enables you to practice medical terminology, pronunciation, professionalism, and communication skills while guided by your instructor. In Part III, you will participate in a class discussion about procedures in your state regarding the roles of the pharmacy technician and the pharmacist when seeking refill authorization, the skills required to successfully perform those roles, and the varied state-based regulation of these roles.

Part I: Generating a Refill Authorization Request Form

You will perform this part of the procedure for each of the five patients requesting refills as presented in Figures 11.1 through 11.5 at the end of the lab. Once *all five* patient requests have been processed through Step 9, you will move on to procedure Part II, Step 10.

1 First install the NRx Simulation CD that accompanied your textbook by following the installation directions on page xii of the Preface. Begin this lab by clicking the PharmacyLabs icon that should now be on your desktop. When the sign-in fields appear, type in your First Name and Last Name and click OK.

2 When the menu for all available labs appears on the left, click the dark purple tab for Lab 11. When the list of sub-labs (for example, Lab 11.1, Lab 11.2, Lab 11.3, and so on) appears below the main lab tab, click the sub-lab you wish to perform, beginning with 11.1.

Tip: The sub-labs represent the different patients you will be processing through the lab procedures. Most labs present several sub-labs for processing; however, some labs have only one sub-lab.

3 When the NRx Security screen appears, log in to the NRx-based training software as the Primary User by typing "Student" as the Login ID and "Training" as the Password. Press Tab or click Log In.

Tip: After you have completed this log-in step for the first listed sub-lab (for example, Lab 10.1, Lab 11.1, Lab 12.1, and so on), you will not be prompted to log in again for the remaining sub-labs in that lab's listing and may then skip this log-in step.

4 From the Rx Processing Tasks menu, click Search or press F3. Begin with Miguel Esparza's refill request from Figure 11.1. If no prescription number was presented, type in the patient's name (in Lastname, Firstname format) or if the prescription number was presented, type it into the Search field and press Enter or click Find.

5 If you typed in the patient's name, follow Step 5a, or follow Step 5b if you typed in the prescription number.

5a *If you typed in the patient's name:* The Patient Information profile will display. Click the Rx Profile icon on the top toolbar. When the Patient Profile listing the patient's prescriptions appears, double click on the requested prescription or press the associated F-key. The Rx Summary screen will appear. Verify the patient name, medication name, and Last Filled date.

*Tip: The prescription profile is color coded for quicker reference. **Black:** Prescription is valid and has refills remaining; **Red:** No refills remain or the prescription has expired; **Purple:** Rx was placed into profile and has not been filled.*

5b *If you typed in the prescription number:* The Rx Summary screen will appear. Verify the patient name, medication name, and Last Filled date.

6 On the top toolbar, click the Print icon. From the drop-down menu, click Refill Request and the Refill Request Options dialog box will appear. Notice that the Print Call Physicians Form option is selected and click OK. A preview of the Refill Authorization Request form will be displayed. Click Print this screen in the upper-right corner of the screen. A small window associated with your printer options will appear. Make the necessary selections for the printer you wish to use and click as required to print the Refill Authorization Request form. Retrieve the printed form and set it aside to be used in Part II of the lab.

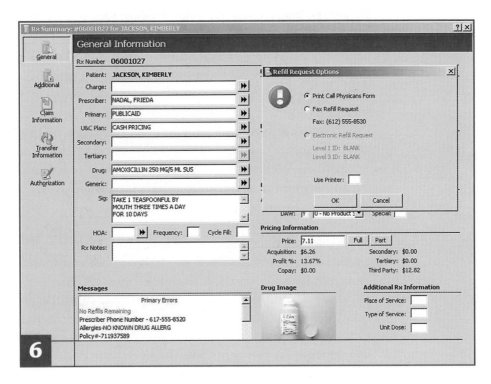

7 Click Next in the lower-right area of the screen. Within a few seconds, a results screen will appear, listing your name, the sub-lab number, your start and finish times, your numerical score and a maximum score, and your accuracy percentage. Print these results by clicking Print this screen in the upper-right corner. (Once again, a small window associated with your printer will appear and you should take the steps necessary to print the screen.) When you are sure the screen has printed, retrieve it and set it aside to be turned in at the end of the lab. Click Close this lab in the upper-right corner of the screen.

Tip: Do not close the lab until you are absolutely certain that your results screen has printed successfully. You will not be able to retrieve your results once you click Close this lab.

8 After printing Mr. Esparza's Refill Authorization Request form and your results screen for sub-Lab 11.1, you may process the refill requests for the four remaining patients. Repeat Steps 2 through 7 with the remaining refill requests, proceeding in numerical order as presented in Figures 11.2 through 11.5 in your textbook and represented as Labs 11.2 through 11.5 on screen in the sub-labs listing. When you have processed all five patients, proceed to Step 9.

9 Retrieve all five printed Refill Authorization Request forms and results screens and stack them separately. Set the results screens aside for turning in at the very end of the lab. You will use the Refill Authorization Request forms in the next step and should proceed now to Part II.

Part II: Phoning in the Refill Request

In this part of the procedure, you will seek authorization for the refills being requested. In practice, you may be required to fax the Refill Authorization Request form to the prescriber's office. However, refill requests are frequently communicated via telephone by following a specific procedure, as outlined in Steps 13–18.

To practice communicating refill requests, you will work with a partner, role-playing telephone conversations to simulate communication with a prescriber. Admittedly, because this is a practice scenario, there is no real telephone number to call and no actual prescriber to speak with. Nonetheless, you and your lab partner should do your best to role-play these pharmacy technician and prescriber conversations. The student pretending to be on the prescriber-end of the phone line should sometimes pretend to be a prescriber or prescriber's office staff member and sometimes pretend to be a recorded voice on the office's refill message line.

Keep in mind that you and your partner should each write on your own stack of Refill Authorization Request forms when directed to do so. Although your two sets of forms should be identical, each student should write on her or his own forms to have documents to turn in to your instructor at the end of the lab.

10 Review the medication names on the five Refill Authorization Request forms you have printed. If you are unsure how to correctly pronounce any of the names, ask your instructor or another student to model the pronunciations for you.

11 Select a partner and keep at hand each student's stack of five printed Refill Authorization Request forms. Keep one student's copy of *Pharmacy Labs for Technicians* open to these procedure steps and open the other student's copy to the patient refill requests (Figures 11.1–11.5).

12 Decide who will play which role initially: one of you will play the role of the pharmacy technician calling for authorization and the other will act as the prescriber or as a prescriber's office staff member and either deny or approve the refill request. If you deny the request, you must offer justification for the denial; if you approve the request, you must state how many additional refills are permitted.

Tip: You should switch roles partway through the procedure so that you each have a chance to role-play both sides of the conversation.

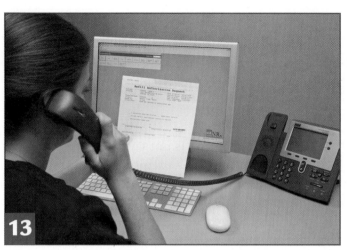

13

Pharmacy technician telephoning prescriber's office to request refill authorization.

13 Telephone the prescriber's office for the first authorization request.
Tip: Some offices will have you speak to a person and others will have pharmacy-specific refill message lines. In either case, remember to remain professional and courteous on the phone.

14 When the phone is answered, tell the person answering who you are, which pharmacy you are with, and that you have a refill authorization request. That person will either transfer you to the appropriate person or take the request immediately. If you get a recorded message, listen carefully to it before providing the information listed in Step 15.
Tip: For one or two of the refill requests, the student in the prescriber role should simulate a recorded message line at the prescriber's office.

15 Whether speaking to a person or on a message line, enunciate clearly and provide the following information, in this order:

1. Patient's last name (Say it and spell it out.)
2. Patient's first name (Say it and spell it out.)
3. Date of birth (This is important because you do not know how many John Smiths or Maria Garcias are seen at this office.)
4. Medication name (Say it and spell it out.)
5. Strength
6. Quantity
7. Signa (either in signa form or as it appears on the sticky note or label)
8. Date written
9. Last date refilled or dispensed
10. Prescriber name (Say it and spell it out.)
11. Your name, the name of the pharmacy you are with, and—most important—your call-back number
12. If you are on a message system, state the information again. If you are speaking to a person, repeat the information in the same order, or ask the person to repeat the information while you verify that it matches yours.

16 If you are speaking to a person, you could receive authorization right away or you might have to wait up to 48 hours. Ask for the person's name and note that name, the date, and the time in a blank area on the Refill Authorization Request form. Similarly, when leaving a recorded message, expect a return phone call within 48 hours and note on the form the date and time you left the message.

17 For the purposes of this lab, if authorization is not given right away or your request was left as a recorded message, all return phone calls should take place immediately during the role-play. Either during the initial call (if you receive authorization right away) or when the "prescriber" student calls back, the "pharmacy technician" student should record the prescriber's decision by checking off one of the three possible responses (refills are authorized, refills are denied, or prescriber asks the patient to make contact) located at the bottom of the Refill Authorization Request form. If refills are authorized, be sure also to write the quantity of additional refills in the blank.

*Tip: Take special care when filling in the number of "additional" refills because that number refers to fills authorized to take place **after** this one. For example, if the prescriber authorized only one refill, you must put a zero in the blank because **you are about to provide** that one additional refill.*

18 Follow Step 18a if the refill request was denied or Step 18b if the refill request was authorized.

18a *If authorization was denied*: Both students should write the reason for denial on the bottom of their own Refill Authorization Request form and set the forms aside for the moment. You will each have to submit these denied request forms to your instructor at the end of this lab. For now you may go on to process the next request, returning to Step 13. When you have received and recorded a response for all five requests, you may proceed to Part III.

Tip: At this point in pharmacy practice, the pharmacy technician would notify the patient—in person or over the telephone—of the denial and any special instructions given by the prescriber's office. If you wish to extend the role-play, you and your partner might play out such a conversation between the pharmacy technician and the patient.

18b *If authorization was granted*: You should temporarily put the approved Refill Authorization Request form aside and return to Step 13 to process the remaining requests. When you have received and recorded a response for all five requests, you may proceed to Part III.

Tip: At this point in pharmacy practice, the pharmacy technician would notify the patient—in person or over the telephone—of the approval and of when the refill will be ready. If you wish to extend the role-play, you and your partner might play out such a conversation between the pharmacy technician and the patient.

Part III: Further Discussion of the Refill Authorization Request Process—Roles, Skills, and Regulation

In this part of the lab, your class will meet as a whole and discuss three topics impacting the refill authorization request process: the evolving roles of pharmacy technicians and pharmacists in the process, the essential skills for professionally and successfully completing the process, and the variation in state-based regulation of the process.

Your instructor will facilitate the discussion and provide you with guidelines for participation. Keep those guidelines in mind as you work through the following steps as a class. The final step in this part instructs you in organizing your materials from Parts I and II and completing the lab.

19 Discuss the **evolving roles** of the pharmacist and the pharmacy technician in the process of *obtaining refill authorization* by considering the following questions, or others posed by your instructor: The pharmacist and the pharmacy technician play central roles as members of the pharmacy team providing quality care to patients, but how do these roles differ for this process? What are the limitations of both roles for this process? What opportunities for growth are inherent to these roles in this process?

20 Discuss the **essential skills** for professionally and successfully *obtaining refill authorization* as a pharmacy technician by considering the following questions, or others posed by your instructor: What does it mean to *act professionally* when seeking refill authorization? What are the rules for telephone etiquette when communicating with the prescriber's office staff? With the office's refill message line? What other communication skills might you have or seek to obtain for professionally and successfully *obtaining refill authorization*?

21 Discuss the **state-by-state variation in regulation** of the pharmacy technician's role in *obtaining refill authorization* by considering the following statements and questions, or additional questions posed by your instructor: The role of the pharmacy technician can differ greatly from state to state. (For example, pharmacy technicians in Texas are allowed to obtain refill authorization via telephone and fax and to electronically generate a new prescription from an older record in the computer software, provided they update only the number of allowed refills. In Iowa, pharmacy technicians, at the discretion of the pharmacist, may receive new orders via telephone and other means. At the time this text was written, some states—including Colorado, Hawaii, and New York—do not regulate pharmacy technicians at all.) What regulations does your state's pharmacy act impose regarding this job activity? For example, does your state consider what becomes authorized to be a new prescription, not a refill, even though the drug name, strength, and signa do not change?

22 **Conclusion:** Collect the five results screens that you set aside in Step 9 and the five approved or denied Refill Authorization Request forms that you set aside in Step 18. Because you are not identified on the Refill Authorization Request forms, sign and date them. Turn in all ten items to your instructor. On a separate sheet of paper, answer all questions in the following Lab Review section and turn in your answers to your instructor.

Lab Review

Check Your Understanding

1. To refill a prescription, you may search the pharmacy software by patient name and ____.
   a. NDC number
   b. prescription number
   c. last fill date
   d. DAW code

2. A prescription expires because the legal time limit passes or the ____.
   a. number of refills is exhausted.
   b. prescribed quantity is used.
   c. pharmacy runs out of stock.
   d. patient loses the prescription.

3. When communicating with a prescriber to seek authorization, you do not typically communicate which of the following pieces of information?
   a. signa
   b. last date refilled
   c. pharmacy address
   d. patient name

4. Refills for C-IIs may be authorized by phone and fax.
   a. true
   b. false

5. As the pharmacy profession evolves and each of the following skills becomes more important for pharmacy technicians, which *one* of these skills should rank the highest in your skills group?
   a. management
   b. billing
   c. communication
   d. hygiene

Thinking Like a Pharmacy Tech

1. Within the lab procedure, you read that it may take up to 48 hours for a refill to be authorized even if you phone in the request. Why does the authorization process take so long? Why can't the prescriber's office staff simply pull the patient's chart and speak to a nurse or physician to get approval right away?

2. Now that you've participated in a whole-class discussion of how regulation of the pharmacy technician's role in obtaining refill authorization varies from state to state, take a few moments to consider you own position on this topic. Write a paragraph or more first declaring whether you agree or disagree with the following statement and then explaining why or why not:

   The United States should have a single, federal-level regulation specifically outlining the role of the pharmacy technician in the process of obtaining refill authorization, and individual states should not be able to alter the regulation.

3. What are soft skills, and why are they important to your success on the job?

FIGURE 11.1 **Refill Request Noted from Phone Call**

Esparza, Miguel

09/12/1953

Humalog Insulin

FIGURE 11.2 **Refill Request from Previous Fill Label**

THE CORNER DRUG STORE
17 Main Street - Orlando, FL 32810
phone (407) 555-1212 fax (407) 555-1313

RX **6001020**

DATE FILLED: 02/17/2015
ORIGINAL DATE: FEB 17, 2015

RILEY, CAS
72650 Okade Court; Orlando, FL 32810 – DOB: Jan 22, 1998

**TAKE 1 TABLET BY MOUTH
2 TIMES A DAY FOR 14 DAYS**

CIPROFLOXACIN 250 MG TABLETS   **QTY: 28**

Prescriber: PHILIP MCCRACKEN, MD
REFILLS: 0   **JPS/LAM**

FIGURE 11.3 **Refill Request Noted from Phone Call**

Jackson, Kimberly

06/23/1988

Amoxicillin 250mg/5mL

FIGURE 11.4 **Refill Request Noted from Phone Call**

Wilkins, Marquita

02/29/1984

Patanol

FIGURE 11.5 **Refill Request from Previous Fill Label**

THE CORNER DRUG STORE
17 Main Street - Cedar Rapids, IA 52411
phone: (319) 555-1212 fax: (319) 555-1212

RX **6001019**

DATE FILLED: 02/20/2015
ORIGINAL DATE: FEB 20, 2015

KLEIN, JEFFREY
1157 North Plaza Avenue; Cedar Rapids, IA 52411 – DOB: Oct 18, 1979

**TAKE 1 CAPSULE BY MOUTH
FOUR TIMES DAILY.**

FLUOXETINE   **QTY: 30**

Prescriber: ETHEL JACOBSON, MD
REFILLS: PRN   **JPS/LAM**

Processing Third-Party Claims

Lab 12

Objectives

- Accurately process patient prescriptions with third-party, or insurance, claims.
- Understand how pharmacy management software processes third-party claims.
- Understand why third-party claims are rejected.
- Learn how to resolve common claim rejections using pharmacy management software.

Supplies

- NRx-Based Training Software

Third-party adjudication

An insurance company determination to pay the pharmacy an amount on behalf of the patient's account

Submitting insurance claims will be a regular part of your work processing prescriptions as a pharmacy technician. Because insurance companies act as a "third party" in the chain of events that moves payment from the first party—the patient—to the second party—the pharmacy—such processing is called "third-party adjudication," or "third-party processing." The word "adjudication" is related to "judging" and "judgment" and refers to someone in an outside position making a decision, or judgment, for those inside the situation.

In the case of **third-party adjudication**, the pharmacy submits an electronic claim to the third party, the insurance company. The insurance company then reviews the prescription claim and judges, based on the drug coverage plan a patient has already agreed to, whether and how much payment should be transmitted between those inside the situation: the patient and the pharmacy. Ultimately, the third party, the insurance company, pays the pharmacy on behalf of the patient for part of the patient's prescription cost.

A third-party adjudication will take place on nearly all of the prescriptions in a community pharmacy and will be a significant part of your daily work. In an institutional pharmacy, however, pharmacy technicians do not often process third-party claims. Instead, you would only begin the process by entering orders into the computer system, and the institution's billing or medical records department would bill the patient's insurance company.

While processing claims, you may come across unfamiliar terms, including adjudication, capture, BIN number, NDC, Group Code, and Person Code. You may have encountered these terms in previous labs, but take some time now to review and learn them better as you practice processing third-party claims. **Capturing** is particularly relevant to this lab, for as you resolve common insurance rejections, you will need to update claims and "capture" a paid claim. Capturing is your goal, and refers to the successful submission and payment of a claim.

Capturing

Successfully submitting and obtaining payment on an insurance claim

Once a claim is submitted, it will either be paid by the third party, or rejected. The most common rejections a pharmacy technician will encounter in community pharmacies are *NDC Not Covered*, *Patient Not Covered*, and *Refill Too Soon*. Most often, these errors occur because patients are unfamiliar with particular coverage rules under their insurance plans. Many patients have the impression that the prescriber or pharmacy will track their insurance plan and readily know which products are covered. While that would be ideal, it is not possible because of the wide variation in insurance plans. Therefore, additional communication must take place between the prescriber, the pharmacy, and the patient to resolve coverage questions. Most insurance issues may be resolved by a phone call to the insurance carrier or the prescriber's office. In fact, a good deal of your time as a pharmacy technician will be spent on the telephone resolving third-party issues.

As a consequence of this communication and verification process, patients may understandably become frustrated. By the time patients reach the pharmacy to have their prescriptions filled, they have often been through quite a lot: they may have been sick for a few days prior to seeking medical attention, then they may have had to wait at the prescriber's office for a length of time, and now, perhaps in considerable pain or discomfort, they must wait at the pharmacy to receive their prescription. You can see how this situation could contribute to impatience and cause patient–pharmacy misunderstandings. Remember that patients are not directly angry with you, but are frustrated with the process itself. Because you are involved in the process, you can become a target of their frustration. Please do not take any misunderstandings personally and try to remain calm and empathetic.

Procedure

Take Note

As you perform each of the NRx-based software simulation labs (Labs 8–14), be aware that you can choose "Print this screen" in the upper-right corner of any open screen. This printing option may be necessary under unusual circumstances, such as if you have to stop performing a lab in mid-stream due to closure of a campus computer lab, personal emergency, or similar circumstance. You may print the screen to demonstrate to your instructor just how far you progressed on the lab. Under ordinary circumstances, you will be printing only the final screen of the lab, the results screen that shows your numerical score and accuracy percentage. You will be clearly instructed when and how to print the results screen within the final steps of each lab.

At the end of this lab, you will find newly acquired insurance cards accompanying the associated prescriptions in Figures 12.1 through 12.5. You will use these figures through Parts I, II, and III of this lab to process a prescription claim for each patient. In Part I, you will enter the prescription claim data, using procedure Steps 1–14. Then either the prescription will process without incident or the software will notify you that the claim is rejected for one of three reasons: *"NDC Not Covered," "Patient Not Covered/Invalid,"* or *"Refill Too Soon."* To resolve each rejection in Part II, you will be advised to go through Steps 15 and 16 under the section matching the rejection reason. In Part III, the final section of the lab, Steps 17–20 will guide you through printing labels and results, and concluding the lab.

Admittedly, because this is a practice scenario, there is no patient present for you to speak with, should the described situations arise or should you have questions about the prescription or insurance card. Nonetheless, when a procedure step asks you to communicate with a patient, imagine the patient is in front of you and either whisper quietly to yourself as if having that conversation or silently imagine the patient's response. If your instructor permits it and time allows, you might also partner with another student to role-play these pharmacy technician and patient conversations.

Part I: Processing the Prescription Claim

1 First install the NRx Simulation CD that accompanied your textbook by following the installation directions on page xii of the Preface. Begin this lab by clicking the PharmacyLabs icon that should now be on your desktop. When the sign-in fields appear, type in your First Name and Last Name and click OK.

2 When the menu for all available labs appears on the left, click the dark purple tab for Lab 12 and when the list of sub-labs appears below the main lab tab, click sub-lab 12.1.

Tip: The sub-labs represent the different patients you will be processing through the lab procedures. Most labs present several sub-labs for processing; however, some labs have only one sub-lab.

3 When the NRx Security screen appears, log in to the NRx-based training software as the Primary User by typing "Student" as the Login ID and "Training" as the Password. Press Tab or click Log In.

Tip: After you have completed this log-in step for the first listed sub-lab (for example, Lab 10.1, Lab 11.1, Lab 12.1, and so on), you will not be prompted to log in again for the remaining sub-labs in that listing and may skip this log-in step.

4 On the Rx Processing Tasks menu, click Search or press F3.

5 When the Rx/Patient Search screen appears, type the patient's name in Lastname, Firstname format in the Search Criteria field (for the first profile, you will use Figure 12.1 and enter Donaldson, Vance). Click Find or press Enter.

Tip: Some pharmacy management software systems are case sensitive, and in your pharmacy work you will need to be careful about using upper case (capital) or lower case letters when typing in patient names and other data. However, for the purposes of these labs (Labs 8–14), you will not have to be concerned about case sensitivity.

6 When the Patient Information screen appears, click Payment Info at the bottom of the left menu bar. When the Patient Payment Information screen appears, click the New icon on the top toolbar.

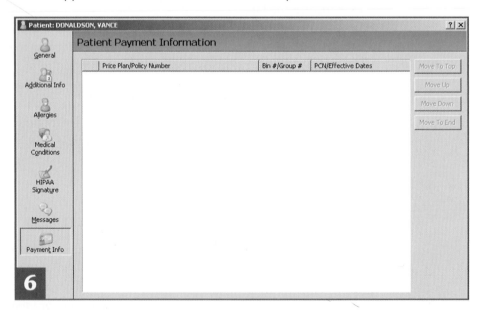

7 A blank Patient Insurance Record screen will appear. Click the Double Arrows to the right of the Payment Plan field.

8 When the Price Plan Scan screen appears, enter the name of the third-party plan (located under the words Insurance Card on the patient's card) into the search field and press Enter or click Find. Double-click the desired insurance plan or press the corresponding F-key.
Tip: If more than one plan shows the same name, match the BIN number on the insurance card to the BIN number on screen before selecting the plan name.

9 The blank Patient Insurance Record screen will reappear. Enter the patient's insurance plan information from the insurance card into the appropriate fields. First type in the Policy ID Number and press Tab. Then, for the Group Number you will have two options. If the insurance card indicates None, move on to the Relationship field; if a Group Number is given, type it in and then press Tab. If the card presents the Relationship category as Not Specified, leave the field as is and click Save or press CTRL+S; if another Relationship category is given, click on the Relationship drop-down menu and select the corresponding code number and name. Click Save or press CTRL+S.

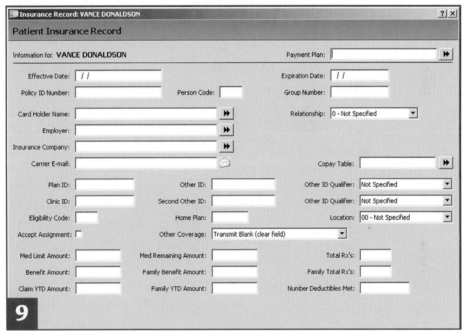

Take Note

Not all insurance carriers require the same information. All will require an ID number, but not all require a group number, person code, or relationship number. Note that you have relationship numbers on the insurance cards in this lab, but not person codes. Keep in mind that person codes are slightly different from relationship numbers. Person codes tend to be: 00—Cardholder; 01—Spouse; 02, 03, 04, etc.—Children, sequentially numbered in birth order. Take extra care at your pharmacy job to ensure that you enter the proper item— person code or relationship number— according to the information listed on the patient's insurance card.

10 Press Esc to return to the Patient Payment Information screen. Click the Update Profile icon on the top toolbar. A Payment Change Detected dialog box will appear displaying the message "The primary payment plan has changed for this patient. Do you wish to update the patient's prescription profile with the new payment plan?" Click Yes.

11 Press Esc again to return to the Rx Processing Tasks menu and process the prescription normally.

Tip: If you need help to process the prescription, review and follow the Procedure section of Lab 9.

12 When you have processed the prescription through the step of clicking the Fill icon and then clicking Fill in the Filling Options dialog box, one of two things will happen. Either a Clinical Checking dialog box or the prescription label preview screen will pop up and you should proceed to print the label (referring again, if needed, to Lab 9, Steps 17–18), or the Rx Summary/General Information screen will remain on screen, unchanged. You should proceed to one of the two "If" sections below, according to whether you were able to print the label or not (because the prescription requires additional attention to resolve a claim issue).

- ■ *If* *the prescription label printed, it was successfully filled on a third-party plan.* When you are sure the prescription label has printed and you have picked it up from the printer, set it aside for turning in at the end of the lab. Click Next in the lower-right area of the label preview screen.

  - • When the results screen appears, displaying your name, the lab number, your start and finish times, your numerical score and a maximum score, and your accuracy percentage, click Print this screen in the upper-right corner. A small window associated with your local printer options will appear. Make the necessary selections for the local printer you wish to use, and click as required to print the screen.

  - • When you are sure the results screen has printed, retrieve it and set it aside to be turned in at the end of the lab. Click Close this lab in the upper-right corner of the screen.

    Tip: Do not close the lab until you are absolutely certain that your results screen has printed successfully. You will not be able to retrieve your results once you click Close this lab.

  - • When the main screen listing all labs and sub-labs appears, you may process the next prescription by clicking on the next sub-lab (Labs 12.2–12.5), in numerical order, and referring to the corresponding Figure (Figures 12.2–12.5) for the associated patient data. Return to Step 4 to begin processing the next patient.

- *If, however, the Rx Summary/General Information screen remains on screen, unchanged, and you were thus unable to proceed with printing the prescription label,* a claim submission error has occurred. You should proceed to Step 13.

13 To view an explanation of the claim submission errors, press Esc and return to the Rx Processing Tasks menu. Click the Electronic Claims Log button or press F4. Find the patient name on the log and click it once to highlight it.

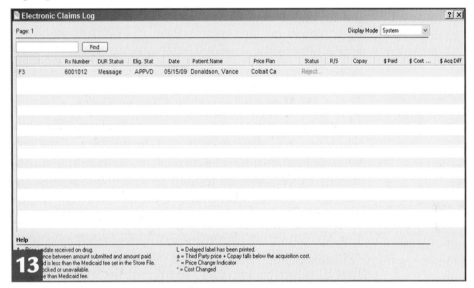

14 Click the DUR (Drug Utilization Review) button on the top toolbar and carefully review the information on the DUR screen. The data in the Conflict Description column determines which claim resolution section you should proceed to next, for Step 15 in Part II. Therefore, near the patient's prescription or insurance card, be sure to jot down all data appearing in the Conflict Description column, including the rejection reason (shown in red letters) and any additional free-text messages. Press Esc.

Take Note

Be sure to inform patients of the status of their prescriptions. In cases of rejection, patients may have helpful information to pass on to you or they may become upset. It is important, however, to keep them fully informed so they are not waiting in the pharmacy unnecessarily. Be prepared to answer additional patient questions in such situations.

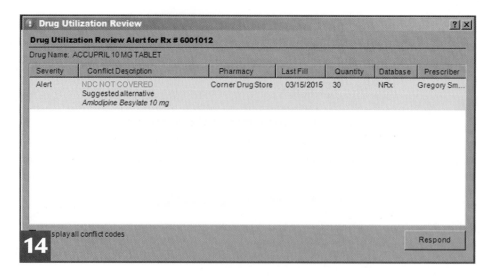

Part II: Resolving the Claim Rejection

In Part I you either processed a patient's claim without issue or were told why a patient's claim was rejected. In this part of the procedure, Part II, you will be shown how to correct the claim submission error based on rejection type. Move on to Step 15 within one of the three "If" sections below. Choose the section that corresponds to the claim rejection reason for the patient at hand. Take care to read the introductory paragraph for that section before proceeding. After you complete Steps 15 and 16 in the appropriate "If" section for a given patient, you will be clearly directed to Part III to perform Steps 17 or 18 to print labels and results screens, and, when you have completed all five sub-labs, to conclude the lab.

If "NDC Not Covered" causes the rejection:

On the DUR Screen you viewed in Step 14, the NDC Not Covered Conflict Description may have been accompanied by a free-text message offering additional explanations, limitation reminders, or alternate drugs. In practice, if the message lists an alternate drug, you would ask the pharmacist to contact the prescriber's office to request a new prescription for the alternate. For the purposes of this lab, proceed as instructed in the following scenario, Steps 15 and 16, to process this rejected patient claim.

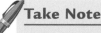

Take Note

If the drug is not covered, you should alert the patient to the situation and inform him or her that, unless he or she wishes to pay the retail, or cash, price for the prescription, the pharmacist will need to contact the prescriber to request a new prescription for a medication that may be covered.

15 You received a message in Step 14 that Vance Donaldson's prescription was rejected because the NDC is not covered. The pharmacist then contacted the prescriber for clarification and received orders to change the drug to amlodipine besylate 10 mg with the same directions (i po

QD), quantity (30), and refills (PRN). To take action on this patient's prescription, click the Correction icon on the top toolbar.

Take Note

In these "on hold" situations, patients will have to wait again for the pharmacist to reach the prescriber. Thus, you should inform patients that resolution could take some time and that, while they are welcomed to wait, going home is an option and the pharmacy will contact them when the prescription is ready. If patients become upset and begin to blame the pharmacy or the prescriber, explain that with so many insurance plans available, the prescriber or pharmacy cannot track each plan and drug formulary. Assure them that these situations are common, that you understand their frustration, and that they will be contacted as soon as the prescription is ready.

16 In the Rx Summary screen, update the drug name and strength by clicking atop the denied drug in the Drug field. When that field turns blank, type in Amlodipine Besylate 10 mg and press Enter. Click Fill on the top toolbar. When then Filling Options dialogue box appears, click your cursor in the small Resubmit box so that a check-mark appears and then click Fill. The prescription should now process and fill without rejection. Skip over the next two "If" sections to Step 17 in Part III, where you will print the prescription label and results screen and be directed how to continue with, or conclude, the lab.

Take Note

If, in a case similar to Vance Donaldson's, it had been later in the day and the pharmacist phoned the prescriber's office only to find it closed, you would ask the patient to contact the physician's office the next day for a new prescription. For the moment, you would place this prescription on hold in the patient's profile. The software would allow you to easily do so by clicking the Profile Only icon within the Correction process of the Electronic Claims Log. The prescription would then be on hold in the patient's profile and a label would print with the prescription information but without the drug monograph.

If "Patient (PT) Not Covered/Invalid" causes the rejection:

The DUR screen Conflict Description free-text message from the third party may have stated that the prescription was rejected because of data entry errors in the Patient Profile or Payment Info sections of the pharmacy software. It may also have been rejected because the patient has new insurance coverage or does not realize that the previous coverage has lapsed or been cancelled. In such cases, you would review the patient's profile and payment information to ensure that the data on screen matches the data on the insurance card, updating as necessary. You might also have to contact the insurance company to verify coverage, either receiving verification or filling the prescription on a cash payment basis if the patient agrees. For the purposes of this lab, proceed as instructed in the following scenario, Steps 15 and 16, to process this rejected patient claim.

15 Kimberly Jackson's prescription was rejected because she is no longer covered by her old insurance plan. After you ask her if she has new insurance, she reveals that she does not currently have any insurance. You would then ask if she agrees to cash payment for the prescription and when she agrees, you click the Correction icon on the top toolbar.

16 In the Rx Summary screen, you will need to update the Primary field from PublicAid to Retail Pricing to ensure that the prescription will not be billed to an insurance plan but be paid at the moment at the retail, or cash, pricing level. To do so, click atop the old insurance plan in the Primary field. When the field turns blank, type in Retail Pricing, and press Enter or click the Double Arrows to the right of the Primary field. Click the Fill icon on the top toolbar. When then Filling Options dialogue box appears, click your cursor in the small Resubmit box so that a check-mark appears and then click Fill. The prescription should now process and fill without rejection. Skip over the next "If" section to Step 17 in Part III, where you will print the prescription label and results screen and be clearly directed how to continue with, or conclude, the lab.

If "Refill Too Soon" causes the rejection:

The DUR screen Conflict Description free-text message from the third party may have indicated when the prescription was last filled—data that can help you discuss the rejection with the patient. For example, either you or the pharmacist could ask the patient whether he or she remembers the prescription's last fill date and, if not, remind the patient of that date. You would then seek further information about why the refill request is being made early. For the purposes of this lab, proceed as instructed in the following scenario, Steps 15 and 16, to process this rejected patient claim.

Take Note

When you engage patients in a conversation about refilling too soon, some will recall that they still have a supply of the prescription. The situation can then be easily resolved by canceling the request or placing it on hold. However, some patients may become upset or angry, in which case it is always best practice to have a pharmacist or experienced technician intervene to calm the situation. When patients become argumentative and demand a prescription be filled, the pharmacist may instruct you to change the primary price plan to Cash and fill the prescription.

15 Amala Gupta's prescription is for a controlled substance. It was last filled 16 days ago with a 20-day supply. Due to concerns in the pharmacy industry about potential abuse of controlled substances, it may not be prudent to fill the prescription early. In fact, the insurance company is not allowing an early refill, but is indicating the patient may refill in four days. You would remind the patient that she should have enough of the prescription remaining for four more days and ask her to return at that time to receive the fill when her insurance will cover the prescription. On the Electronic Claims Log screen, select the patient name and click it once to highlight it.

16 Click the DUR button to return to the DUR screen describing the rejection details. Click the Reversal icon on the top toolbar. When the Reverse Claim dialog box appears, notice that "Continue with reversal, only" is selected and click Submit. The dialog box Claim Reversal Results now advises you that this patient record is flagged for reversal. Click Ok. Because this fill has now been cancelled, a label will not be printed. Thus, as you move now into the final section of the lab, Part III, you should skip Step 17 (where a label would be printed) and proceed to Step 18, where you will print only your results screen and then be directed how to continue with, or conclude, the lab.

Part III: Printing Resolved Rejection Labels and Results Screens and Concluding the Lab

17 To print the prescription label, click Print this screen in the upper-right corner of the label preview screen. A small window associated with your local printer options will appear. Make the necessary selections for the local printer you wish to use, and click as required to print the screen. When you are certain that the prescription label has printed, set it aside for turning in at the end of the lab and click Next in the lower-right area of the label preview screen.

18 When the results screen appears, displaying your name, the lab number, your start and finish times, your numerical score and a maximum score, and your accuracy percentage, click Print this screen in the upper-right corner. (Once again, a small window associated with your local printer will appear and you should take the steps necessary to print the screen.) When you are sure the results screen has printed, retrieve it and set it aside to be turned in at the end of the lab. Click Close this lab in the upper-right corner of the screen.

Tip: Do not close the lab until you are absolutely certain that your results screen has printed successfully. You will not be able to retrieve your results once you click Close this lab.

19 When the main screen listing all labs and sub-labs appears, you may process the next prescription by clicking on the next sub-lab (12.2–12.5), in numerical order, and referring to the corresponding Figure (12.2–12.5) for the associated patient data. Return to Step 4 to begin processing the next patient.

20 **Conclusion:** When you have processed all the patient claims in Figures 12.1 through 12.5, resolving any rejections by following the associated procedure steps, you may conclude the lab as follows. Turn in to your instructor all labels and results screens that you have set aside during this lab. On a separate sheet of paper, answer all questions in the following Lab Review section and turn in your answers to your instructor.

Lab Review

Check Your Understanding

1. The act of judging, or making a ruling upon, a matter is known as _____.
   a. refilling
   b. capturing
   c. adjudicating
   d. submitting

2. The person code often assigned to a spouse is _____.
   a. 04
   b. 02
   c. 01
   d. 00

3. The most common cause of third-party rejection is _____.
   a. misprescribing
   b. mispronunciation
   c. technical error
   d. miscommunication

4. Patient–pharmacy misunderstandings are primarily due to _____.
   a. staff error at the pharmacy prompted by a too-heavy work load
   b. staff error at the prescriber's office because too many appointments are taken
   c. patients' frustration with the overall process and feeling especially ill by the time they reach the pharmacy
   d. patient error in telling the prescriber's office what is wrong or what doesn't feel well

5. A pharmacy is capable of tracking and automatically updating third-party information in each patient's profile.
   a. true
   b. false

Thinking Like a Pharmacy Tech

1. Processing third-party claims can be a multi-step task that takes up a lot of time. Make an argument that the pharmacy, nonetheless, should be responsible for filing these claims.

2. In contrast with your answer for #1, make an argument that patients should pay for their prescription(s) and then submit a claim for reimbursement on their own.

 3. After an interview, you should always send a thank you card. What does a typical thank you card include?

FIGURE 12.1
Patient Prescription and Insurance Card Data

Cobalt Care
Insurance card

VANCE DONALDSON
BIN: 00123
ID: ZVD996274638

GROUP: 11770
RELATIONSHIP: 01, CARDHOLDER

MEMBER SERVICES: 1-800-555-3232
CLAIMS/INQUIRIES: 1-800-555-6363

℞ John Ashfield, MD
Greta Zlatoski, FCNP
Gregory Smythe, MD
44 Medical Pkwy.
Austin, TX 78704
(512) 555-1212   fax: (512) 555-1313

DOB _May 15, 1975_ DEA# _____
Pt. name _Vance Donaldson_ Date _02/11/2015_
Address _12 Maple Leaf Trail_
Round Rock, TX 78664

Accupril
10 mg
30
i po QD

Refill __PRN__ times (no refill unless indicated)

Gregory Smythe _____ MD
_____ License #

FIGURE 12.2
Patient Prescription and Insurance Card Data

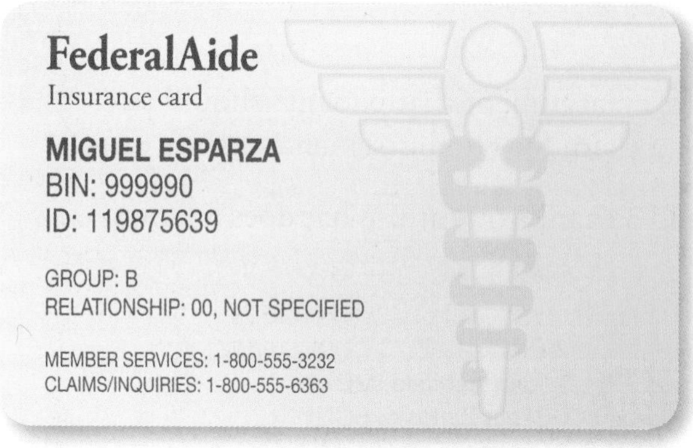

FederalAide
Insurance card

MIGUEL ESPARZA
BIN: 999990
ID: 119875639

GROUP: B
RELATIONSHIP: 00, NOT SPECIFIED

MEMBER SERVICES: 1-800-555-3232
CLAIMS/INQUIRIES: 1-800-555-6363

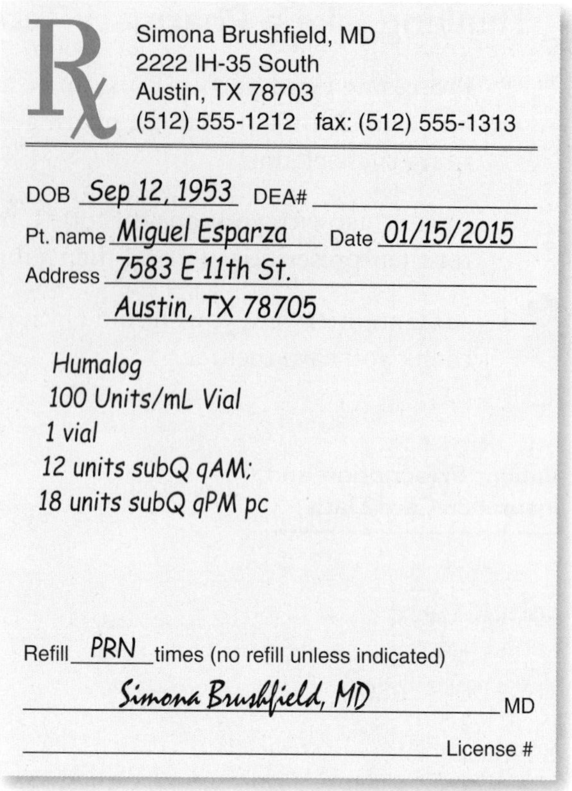

R_x Simona Brushfield, MD
2222 IH-35 South
Austin, TX 78703
(512) 555-1212   fax: (512) 555-1313

DOB _Sep 12, 1953_ DEA# _____

Pt. name _Miguel Esparza_ Date _01/15/2015_

Address _7583 E 11th St._
Austin, TX 78705

Humalog
100 Units/mL Vial
1 vial
12 units subQ qAM;
18 units subQ qPM pc

Refill _PRN_ times (no refill unless indicated)

Simona Brushfield, MD _____ MD

_____ License #

FIGURE 12.3
Patient Prescription and Insurance Card Data

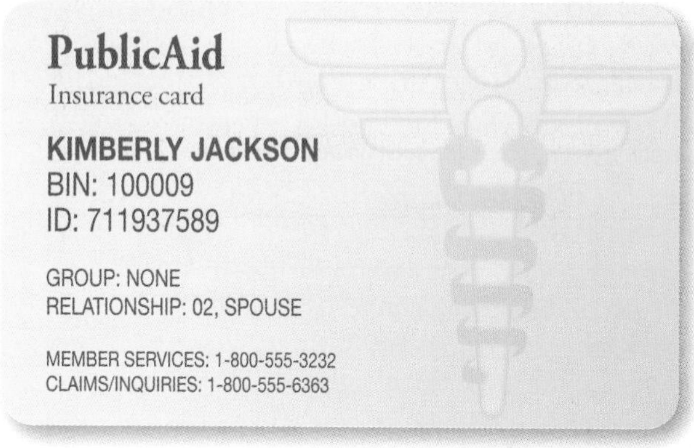

PublicAid
Insurance card

KIMBERLY JACKSON
BIN: 100009
ID: 711937589

GROUP: NONE
RELATIONSHIP: 02, SPOUSE

MEMBER SERVICES: 1-800-555-3232
CLAIMS/INQUIRIES: 1-800-555-6363

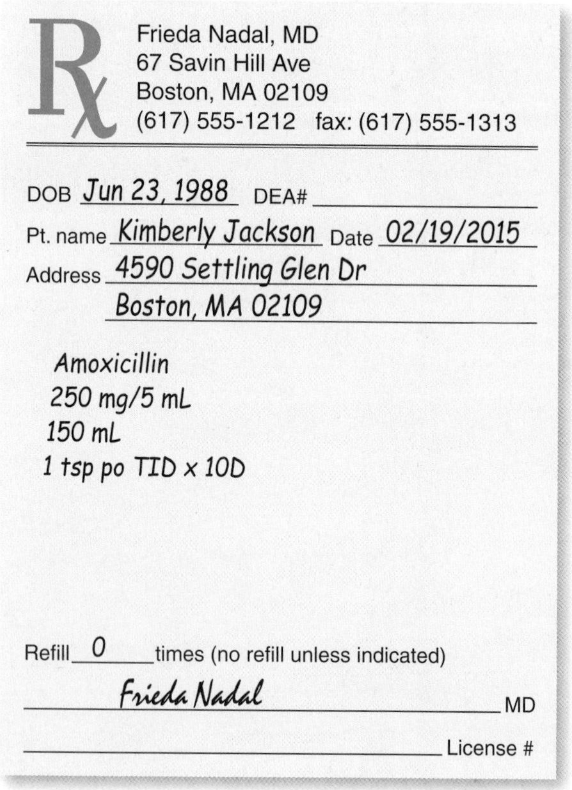

R_x Frieda Nadal, MD
67 Savin Hill Ave
Boston, MA 02109
(617) 555-1212   fax: (617) 555-1313

DOB _Jun 23, 1988_ DEA# _____

Pt. name _Kimberly Jackson_ Date _02/19/2015_

Address _4590 Settling Glen Dr_
Boston, MA 02109

Amoxicillin
250 mg/5 mL
150 mL
1 tsp po TID x 10D

Refill _0_ times (no refill unless indicated)

Frieda Nadal _____ MD

_____ License #

FIGURE 12.4
Patient Prescription and Insurance Card Data

```
------------------------------------------------------------------
!!! -- START SECURED ELECTRONIC PRESCRIPTION TRANSMISSION -- !!!
------------------------------------------------------------------
FROM THE OFFICES OF PHIL JACKSON, MD; ETHEL JACOBSON, MD;
                    PETER JARKOWSKI, PA; EUGENE JOHNSON, DO

OFFICE ADDRESS:          67 EAST ELM
                         CEDAR RAPIDS, IA 52411
OFFICE TELEPHONE:        (319) 555-1212   TRANSMIT DATE: 02/20/2015
OFFICE FAX:              (319) 555-1313   WRITTEN DATE:  02/20/2015
------------------------------------------------------------------
TRANSMITTED TO           THE CORNER DRUG STORE
PHARMACY ADDRESS:        875 PARADIGM WAY
                         CEDAR RAPIDS, IA 52410
PHARMACY TELEPHONE:      (319) 555-1414
------------------------------------------------------------------
PATIENT NAME:            JEFFREY KLEIN      D.O.B.: OCT 18, 1979
PATIENT ADDRESS:         1157 NORTH PLAZA AVE
                         CEDAR RAPIDS, IA 52411
------------------------------------------------------------------
PRESCRIBED MEDICATION:   FLUOXETINE 20 MG
SIGNA:                   i PO QD
DISPENSE QUANTITY:       30
REFILL(S):               PRN
------------------------------------------------------------------
PHYSICIAN SIGNATURE:     [[ ELECTRONIC SIGNATURE ON FILE ]]
                         [[ FOR DR. ETHEL JACOBSON ]]

------------------------------------------------------------------
!!! -- END SECURED ELECTRONIC PRESCRIPTION TRANSMISSION -- !!!
------------------------------------------------------------------
```

ApolloHealth
Insurance card

JEFFREY KLEIN
BIN: 459872
ID: 882646507

GROUP: NONE
RELATIONSHIP: 02, SPOUSE

MEMBER SERVICES: 1-800-555-3232
CLAIMS/INQUIRIES: 1-800-555-6363

FIGURE 12.5
Patient Prescription and Insurance Card Data

PublicAid
Insurance card

AMALA GUPTA
BIN: 100009
ID: 778342987

GROUP: NONE
RELATIONSHIP: 01, CARDHOLDER

MEMBER SERVICES: 1-800-555-3232
CLAIMS/INQUIRIES: 1-800-555-6363

R
Sunjita Patel, MD
7612 N. HWY 27
Cedar Rapids, IA 52404
(319) 555-1212   fax: (319) 555-1313

DOB _Aug 24, 1949_   DEA# _AP4756687_
Pt. name _Amala Gupta_   Date _02/16/2015_
Address _5473 W 10th Street_
Cedar Rapids, IA 52401

Lorazepam
0.5 mg
120 (one hundred twenty)
i po q4-6 h prn anxiety

Refill ___5___ times (no refill unless indicated)

Sunjita Patel, MD _____ MD

_____ License #

Verifying Cash Pricing

Lab 13

Objectives

- Understand the reasons for cash price payments in the community pharmacy.
- Demonstrate proficiency in the use of computer software for prescription pricing.

Supplies

- NRx-Based Training Software

Copay

The set price often paid by patients having third-party insurance coverage

Cash price

The price patients must pay when they do not have insurance coverage or their insurance plan is not accepted

Previous prescription-preparation labs in this book have focused on patients who have a third-party, or insurance, plan. When a patient has insurance, the third party covers part of the prescription cost and the patient often pays a set price—known as the **copay** amount, for the prescription. In copay situations, patients know that their cost will remain consistent. However, on some occasions, a pharmacy may not be able to accept a patient's insurance plan and the patient's payment amount will vary. As a pharmacy technician, you will then need to determine, or verify, how much the patient must pay for the prescription. This payment figure is known as the **cash price**.

Several factors can make cash price payment necessary. Sometimes a patient's insurance coverage is rejected because the patient is from another area of the country and the pharmacy is not named on the patient's insurance plan. At other times, the patient's insurance plan simply does not cover certain medications. When patients do not have a specific prescription benefit under the insurance coverage they do carry, they must pay the cash price for the prescription and then submit receipts to their insurance company for reimbursement under their medical benefits plan. In other cases, patients do not have any insurance coverage for prescriptions or have no health insurance at all and cash price payment is their only option.

The cash price for prescriptions, like the price on most products sold in more than one outlet, can vary from store to store and from pharmacy to pharmacy. Not all patients know this fact. Patients who must pay cash for their prescriptions and are aware of cash price variability will call many differ-

153

ent pharmacies in their area to search for the best prescription price. Patients save money when using this smart shopping strategy—particularly when they do not have prescription coverage. Thus, in your pharmacy technician work, you will need to know how to look up cash prices for patients.

When you initiate such an inquiry within a computer software program, the screen will display several categories of information, often including:

- **Description:** names the medication, whether brand or generic
- **NDC number:** is the National Drug Code
- **Price plan:** reveals the basis for the price, such as "cash pricing" or "retail pricing"
- **Cost:** displays what the pharmacy pays for the medication
- **Markup:** shows the amount of markup or the price increase to cover pharmacy operation costs
- **Discount:** notes any pricing discounts given to patients on this specific medication
- **The % Profit-AWP:** indicates the percentage of profit made from dispensing the medication compared to the average wholesale price, if available
- **Acquisition cost:** reveals how much it cost the pharmacy to purchase this amount of medication
- **The % Profit-Margin:** states the percentage of profit made above the cost of the medication
- **Price:** displays the price that should be quoted to the patient (notice that the size and prominence of the *Price* line make it easy for you to glance at the screen and quickly find this amount)

Procedure

Take Note

As you perform each of the NRx-based software simulation labs (Labs 8–14), be aware that you can choose "Print this screen" in the upper-right corner of any open screen. This printing option may be necessary under unusual circumstances, such as if you have to stop performing a lab in mid-stream due to closure of a campus computer lab, personal emergency, or similar circumstance. You may print the screen to demonstrate to your instructor just how far you progressed on the lab. Under ordinary circumstances, you will be printing only the final screen of the lab, the results screen that shows your numerical score and accuracy percentage. You will be clearly instructed when and how to print the results screen within the final steps of each lab.

In this lab, you will use the price quote feature of the NRx-based training software to verify cash pricing for the prescriptions listed on the worksheet at the end of the lab. As outlined above in the bulleted list, additional pieces of information will appear on screen for your reference.

1 First install the NRx Simulation CD that accompanied your textbook by following the installation directions on page xii of the Preface. Begin this lab by clicking the PharmacyLabs icon that should now be on your desktop. When the sign-in fields appear, type in your First Name and Last Name and click OK.

2 When the menu for all available labs appears on the left, click the dark purple tab for Lab 13 and when the list of sub-labs appears below the main lab tab, click sub-Lab 13.1.

Tip: Usually several sub-labs are listed, representing the different patients you are processing through the computer software procedures. This lab is one of the few with only one sub-lab, Lab 13.1. Because all patient prescriptions are grouped together on one "Verifying Cash Pricing" worksheet at the end of this lab, no additional sub-labs are required.

3 When the NRx Security screen appears, log in to the NRx-based training software as the Primary User by typing "Student" as the Login ID and "Training" as the Password. Press Tab or click Log In.

4 On the Rx Processing Tasks menu, click Price Quote.

5 In the Drug field, enter the *first word* of the drug name (not the additional words or initials; not the numerals or units) as found on the lab worksheet at the end of the lab. Press Tab.

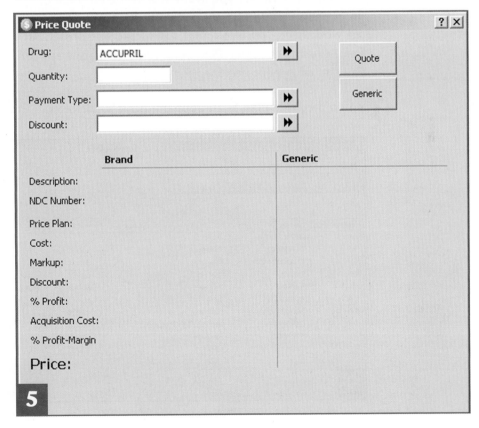

6 If the full drug name, strength, and form appear in the drug name field (because there is only one such drug to choose from and the software has populated the full details for you), you may proceed to Step 7. If the full drug description does not appear, the Drug Record Scan screen will appear instead (because the drug is manufactured in more than one strength or form and you will have to choose). Carefully review your options. When you find the exact match to the drug listed on the worksheet, double-click it or press the corresponding function key (or F-key, such as F3, F4, and so on, usually found along the top row of your keyboard) noted on screen to the left of the drug name, and proceed to Step 7.

Tip: *If multiple listings appear for the same drug description, be very careful to select the* **exact** *match by matching the strength (in mg, mL, concentration, and so on) and the form (as capsules, vials, tablets, and so on). In some cases you will need to go a step further to eliminate a duplicate option. In those cases you must check that the number in the on-screen NDC column exactly matches the NDC number listed on the worksheet.*

7 When the Price Quote screen appears, take care not to enter any data into the Discount field. If your cursor is not already there, click it in the Quantity field. Enter the quantity requested on the worksheet and press Tab.

Tip: *As you proceed down the list of drugs on your worksheet, if the number you need to enter is already present in the Quantity field, simply press Tab.*

8 If you are entering the first drug, your cursor should now be in the Payment Type field. Type in the words "retail pricing," press Tab, and proceed to Step 9. However, if you are entering the remaining drugs on the worksheet, "retail pricing" will already be present in the Payment Type field, causing the Price Plan Scan to immediately appear. In those cases, you should proceed to Step 9.

9 When the Price Plan Scan appears, double-click Retail Pricing or press F3.

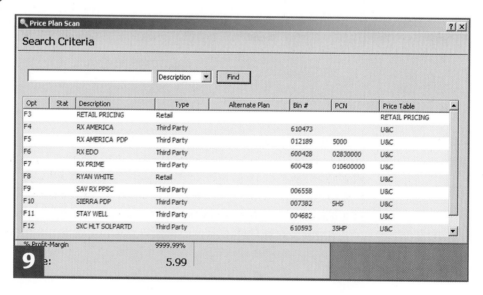

10 When the Price Quote screen returns, you will have the information you need to fill in the worksheet blanks. On the worksheet, record the requested data—the Acquisition Cost and the Cash Price—in the blanks on the right.

Tip: Do not use the first price, the Cost, for the Acquisition Cost. You will find the Acquisition Cost farther down the list of data on the Price Quote screen. You will find the cash price in large, bold type at the very bottom, listed simply as Price.

11 To determine the price for the next prescription listed on the worksheet, you may do one of the following:

a. If you need to change only the quantity and the drug name stays the same, click once atop the existing quantity, which will disappear. Type in the new quantity. Press Tab two times. Repeat Steps 9 and 10.

b. If you need to change the drug name *and* quantity, click once atop the existing drug name, which will disappear. Type in the next drug you wish to look up and press Tab. Repeat Steps 6 through 10.

12 When you have completed the worksheet for all 15 listed drugs and their quantity options, click the small black "X" that is next to the small black "?" in the upper-right corner of the Price Quote screen.

*Tip: Be careful! Do **not** click the large red "X" found in the upper-right corner of the lab window. Doing so will (always) close the entire lab and your work will be lost.*

13 The Rx Processing Tasks menu will appear briefly. Within a few seconds, a results screen will appear, listing your name, the sub-lab number, your start and finish times, your numerical score and a maximum score, and your accuracy percentage. Print these results by clicking Print this screen in the upper-right corner. (A small window associated with your local printer options will appear. Make the necessary selections for the local printer you wish to use and click as required to print the screen.) When you are sure the results screen has printed, retrieve it and set it aside to be turned in at the end of the lab. Click Close this lab in the upper-right corner of the screen.

Tip: Do not close the lab until you are absolutely certain that your results screen has printed successfully. You will not be able to retrieve your results once you click Close this lab.

14 **Conclusion:** Sign, date, and tear out both pages of your completed worksheet. Turn in your worksheet and the printed results screen to your instructor. On a separate sheet of paper, answer all questions in the following Lab Review section and turn in your answers (including your calculations and the costs per unit as requested in Question 1 of the "Thinking Like a Pharmacy Tech" section) to your instructor.

Lab Review

Check Your Understanding

1. Patients may need to pay the cash price for prescriptions because their health insurance does not have a pharmacy benefit.
   a. true
   b. false

2. A copay may be defined as the portion of the prescription cost that the _____ pays.
   a. pharmacy
   b. insurance company
   c. patient
   d. physician

3. The Markup line on the Price Quote screen shows the price _____ to cover _____.
   a. decrease; operation costs
   b. increase; operation costs
   c. decrease; inventory costs
   d. increase; inventory costs

4. The % Profit-Margin line states the percentage of profit that the pharmacy will make _____ the cost of the prescription.
   a. in comparison to
   b. in contrast to
   c. below
   d. above

5. The % Profit-AWP line indicates the percentage of profit that the pharmacy will make in relation to the average _____ of the prescription.
   a. windfall profits
   b. world pricing
   c. wholesale pricing
   d. wholesale profits

Thinking Like a Pharmacy Tech

1. On the same sheet of paper you will turn in to your instructor for these Lab Review exercises, perform your calculations and list the cost per unit (tablet, capsule, milliliter, etc.) for each prescription listed on the worksheet. *Note:* You will see that when a smaller quantity is requested, the cost per unit increases. Start to think about why cost levels are set up this way and whether you think the situation should remain as is.

   Discuss the advantages and disadvantages for the patient and the advantages and disadvantages for the pharmacy in the following two cases:
   a. The situation remains as is, with the unit price for the medication *decreasing* if the patient buys more.
   b. The pharmacy changes the pricing structure, keeping the price *at the same level* no matter how much the patient buys.

2. Looking at all the data provided by the Price Quote screen, think about how else this information might be used. For what additional purposes could an inventory pharmacy technician or pharmacy manager use this wealth of data?

3. Calculations are an important part of a pharmacy technician's duties. How comfortable are you performing calculations? What resources could you use to improve your skills?

Worksheet for Verifying Cash Pricing

Drug Description	NDC	QTY	Acquisition Cost ($)	Cash Price ($)
1. Accupril 10 mg tablets	00071-0530-23	30		
2. Lorazepam 0.5 mg tablets	00378-0321-05	120		
		60		
3. Cephalexin 500 mg capsules	00093-3147-05	40		
4. Alprazolam 2 mg tablets	00781-1089-05	120		
5. Ciprofloxacin ER 500 mg tablets	00378-1743-89	28		
		14		
6. Humalog 100 units/mL vial	00002-7510-01	20		
		10		
7. Zolpidem Tartrate 10 mg tablets	00054-0087-29	10		
		5		
8. Phenobarbital 64.8 mg tablets	00603-5167-32	90		
9. Propoxy-N/APAP 100-650 tablets	00172-4980-80	40		
10. Amoxil 250 mg per 5 mL suspension	00029-6009-22	150		
		75		
11. Gentamicin 3 mg per mL drops	00168-0178-03	10		
12. Zyprexa 15 mg tablets	00002-4415-30	30		

Name: _____ Date: _____

Drug Description	NDC	QTY	Acquisition Cost ($)	Cash Price ($)
13. Prednisone 2.5 mg tablets	00054-8740-25	32	_____	_____
		20	_____	_____
14. Fluoxetine HCL 20 mg capsules	00406-0663-01	30	_____	_____
15. Methylphenidate 20 mg tablets	00781-5754-01	60	_____	_____
		30	_____	_____

Producing an Audit Log

Lab 14

Objectives

- Demonstrate a basic understanding of using pharmacy management software for pharmacy audit log reporting.
- Become more informed about the evolving roles of the pharmacist and the pharmacy technician in pharmacy administration.

Supplies

- NRx-Based Training Software

Medication therapy management

Collaborative oversight of a patient's medications and their delivery to promote a safe, effective plan and encourage targeted outcomes

Pharmacy technicians play a central role in assisting the pharmacist with prescription preparation in the community pharmacy setting. Such assistance improves when you are familiar with a variety of hard-copy and online resources and confident about navigating within pharmacy software programs. When you take the initiative on a large number of daily responsibilities, both on the computer screen and at the counter, the pharmacist can focus on other duties, such as verifying prescriptions, counseling patients, administering immunizations, managing medication therapies, and overseeing the many components of pharmacy administration.

The vast majority of these administrative duties requires the education and professional judgment of a licensed pharmacist. However, because the role of the pharmacist continues to shift toward patient therapy management tasks, pharmacy technicians are increasingly assuming positions of greater administrative responsibility. Experienced pharmacy technicians, in particular, are moving up newly emerging and developing career ladders within independent and locally owned pharmacies and within hospital systems. Pharmacy technicians are also working as specialists, supervisors, and managers at all levels within the broader pharmaceutical industry. As the role of the pharmacist within direct patient care and **medication therapy management** continues to evolve, future pharmacy technicians will likely be asked to apply themselves to multiple pharmacy operations tasks.

One relatively new role that pharmacy technicians are taking on within pharmacy administration is report production. While several kinds of reports—including Inventory Management (a recommended order or listing of medications on hand), pricing, accounts receivable, accounts payable, billing, third-party receipts, DEA-prescribing, HIPAA-compliance, controlled-substance-compliance, prescriber, and drug reports—can be run with pharmacy management software, the audit log is a frequently produced and reviewed report. The audit log provides (for a designated time period programmed by the user) a list of pharmacists who logged in to the computer system, the total number of prescriptions filled under each person's user-ID, and a recap of every prescription filled. The log is often run at the end of the day for just that one-day period, as a daily summary of prescription sales. The log breaks down those sales into four categories: first, a line-by-line listing of prescriptions filled; second and third, newly filled prescriptions and refilled prescriptions broken down according to payment plan (cash price, Medicaid, and third party); and fourth, a cost-analysis breakdown by payment plan. Details for each category include:

- **Line-by-line breakdown of prescriptions filled:** provides prescription number, patient name, prescriber name, transaction number, drug name, quantity dispensed, dosage form unit (tablet, capsule, milliliter, etc.), original quantity prescribed, drug class, number of refills remaining, pharmacist logged in at the time, original date of prescription, date of last fill, price description, and price paid for the prescription.

- **Newly filled prescriptions by payment plan and refilled prescriptions by payment plan:** list number of prescriptions filled for each payment plan, cost of each prescription, amount charged or billed for the total quantity of prescriptions, and **profit margin** (the difference between prescription cost and amount charged) in dollars and also by percentage.

- **Cost-analysis breakdown by payment plan:** lists number of prescriptions filled for each payment plan (cash price, Medicaid, and third party), total cost of prescriptions filled for each payment plan, the total billed amount for all prescriptions, any discounts applied to the price, the amount of copays collected, any applicable sales tax, profit margin (in dollars and by percentage) for the total prescriptions, average price, and average dollar profit margin for each payment plan.

Pharmacy management staff rely on the large amount of information provided by the audit log to estimate total profits, losses, overhead costs, and future sales; and to schedule staff days and hours. You can contribute to pharmacy operations by using and understanding the audit log as part of your pharmacy work. Building your awareness level on the capabilities of the audit log and other pharmacy software reports increases your pharmacy management skills and adds value to your professional record, enhancing your ability to serve the pharmacy and its patients and, subsequently, to advance within the pharmacy profession.

Profit margin

The difference between the pharmacy's prescription cost and the amount charged to the patient or insurance provider

Procedure

In this lab, you will generate an audit log report and answer worksheet questions based upon on the report data.

1 First install the NRx Simulation CD that accompanied your textbook by following the installation directions on page xii of the Preface. Begin this lab by clicking the PharmacyLabs icon that should now be on your desktop. When the sign-in fields appear, type in your First Name and Last Name and click OK.

2 When the menu for all available labs appears on the left, click the dark purple tab for Lab 14 and when the list of sub-labs appears below the main lab tab, click sub-lab 14.1.

Tip: Usually several sub-labs are listed, representing the different patients you are processing through the computer software procedures. This lab is one of the few with only one sub-lab, Lab 14.1. Because all patient prescriptions are grouped together and printed on one Audit Log Report and examined further on the lab worksheet, no additional sub-labs are required.

3 When the NRx Security screen appears, log in to the NRx-based training software as the Primary User by typing "Student" as the Login ID and "Training" as the Password. Press Tab or click Log In.

4 Above the Rx Processing Tasks menu, click Reports on the topmost menu bar. On the menu that drops down, click Management and on the next drop-down menu, click Daily Audit.

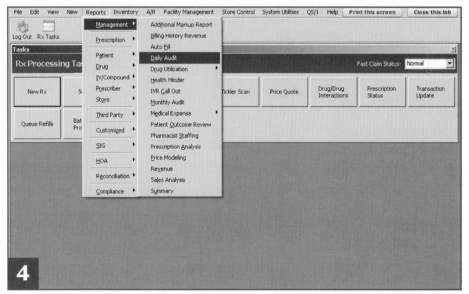

Take Note

As you perform each of the NRx-based software simulation labs (Labs 8–14), be aware that you can choose "Print this screen" in the upper-right corner of any open screen. This printing option may be necessary under unusual circumstances, such as if you have to stop performing a lab in mid-stream due to closure of a campus computer lab, personal emergency, or similar circumstance. You may print the screen to demonstrate to your instructor just how far you progressed on the lab. Under ordinary circumstances, you will be printing only the final screen of the lab, the results screen that shows your numerical score and accuracy percentage. You will be clearly instructed when and how to print the results screen within the final steps of each lab.

5 The Select Options screen will appear. Click your cursor under the Value column, on the line corresponding to the Field [RX Transaction].Date Filled *Dflt. When a blank field opens up under your cursor, type in the word All. Leave all other fields in their default, pre-set states, and click Next or press Enter.

Tip: In your pharmacy work, you will probably be asked to produce an audit log report for a single, specific date, and would enter the date in MM/DD/YY format. For example, if you wanted to process a report for December 21, 2015, you would enter the date as 12/21/15. At times you might also be asked to type in a range of dates or, as you do for this lab, to request a report for all available dates in the system.

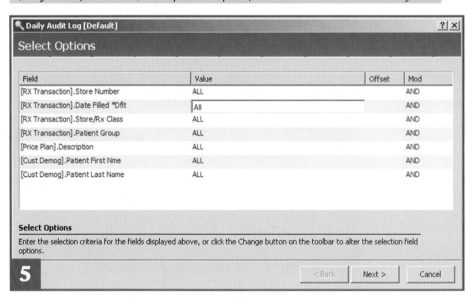

Take Note

The pre-set options are established for the purposes of this basic "Audit Log" lab. Since you are not yet trained to practice more detailed reports or more complex prescription processes, we are not discussing the advanced audit log report features in this lab. When you are at work in the field, you will be specifically trained to take advantage of additional pharmacy software capabilities in order to create the kinds of audit log reports (such as daily, monthly, drug-based, patient-outcome-based, and so on) that are useful to your individual pharmacy.

6 The Sort Options screen will appear. For the purposes of this lab, leave all values in their pre-set order and click Next.

Tip: In pharmacy practice, you would be able to adjust these fields so that your audit log report is organized to meet your pharmacy's needs. For example, you could sort the data by store (if you are part of a larger chain of stores), by date filled, by prescription drug class (Schedules II, III, etc.), or by prescription number.

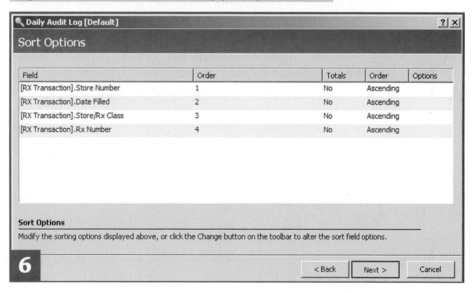

7 The Print Option Values screen will appear. Again, for the purposes of this lab, leave all values in their pre-set states and click Finish.

Tip: In pharmacy practice, you would be able to adjust these options so that your pharmacy's audit log report includes or excludes certain data, such as the prescription signa, new prescriptions, and summary report totals.

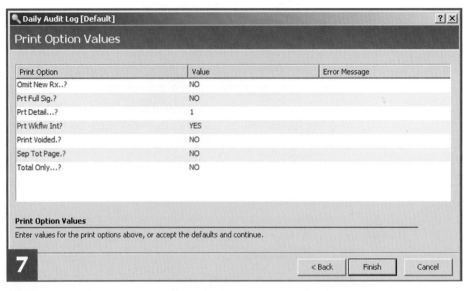

8 A preview of the Audit Log Report for your pharmacy, The Corner Drug Store, will appear. Click Print this screen in the upper-right corner of the report screen.

9 A small window associated with your local printer options will appear. For this report to print properly, you will need to go into the Properties area of your printer options dialog box and select a *landscape* orientation for the layout. Click as necessary to make the remaining selections for your local printer to print the screen. When you are certain that the Audit Log Report has printed, click Next at the bottom of the Audit Log Report preview screen.

10 A results screen will appear, listing your name, the sub-lab number, your start and finish times, your numerical score and a maximum score, and your accuracy percentage. Print these results by clicking Print this screen in the upper-right corner. (Once again, a small window associated with your local printer will appear and you should take the steps necessary to print the screen—landscape orientation is *not* required for this document.) When you are sure the results screen has printed, retrieve it and set it aside to be turned in at the end of the lab. Click Close this lab in the upper-right corner of the screen.

Tip: Do not close the lab until you are absolutely certain that your results screen has printed successfully. You will not be able to retrieve your results once you click Close this lab.

11 **Conclusion:** Pick up the Audit Log Report from the printer and use it to answer the questions on the worksheet at the end of the lab. Write your name and the date on the completed worksheet and the printed Audit Log Report and turn them in to your instructor along with the results screen you have set aside. On a separate sheet of paper, answer all questions in the following Lab Review section and turn in your answers to your instructor.

Lab Review

Check Your Understanding

1. A recap report of every prescription filled during a specific time period may be produced as _____.
   a. an audit analysis
   b. an audit log report
   c. a prescription analysis report
   d. a prescription audit

2. The daily audit log report breaks down pharmacy sales in four ways, but does *not* include a section on _____.
   a. newly filled prescriptions and refilled prescriptions broken down by payment plan
   b. cost-analysis broken down by payment plan
   c. prescriptions filled presented in a line-by-line listing
   d. average cost per pharmacist broken down by user-ID and controlled substance schedule number

3. The line-by-line breakdown on the audit log report includes all of the following information, *except* _____.
   a. dispensed quantity
   b. refills remaining
   c. DEA number
   d. price description

4. When setting the date of the audit log report, you must format it in this manner: _____.
   a. MM/DD/YYYY
   b. DD/MM/YYYY
   c. YY/MM/DD
   d. MM/DD/YY

5. Although the role of the pharmacist is changing, pharmacy technician duties still remain solely within the area of prescription preparation.
   a. true
   b. false

Thinking Like a Pharmacy Tech

1. As the profession of pharmacy continues to evolve, in what ways, aside from using software technology, might pharmacy technicians expand their role to better assist the pharmacist in providing pharmacy services, including duties based on pharmacy administration?

2. Many working in pharmacy believe it is crucial for pharmacy technicians to learn and master such complex packages of software as the NRx system. Think for a moment about possible future needs and changes within pharmacy practice. What do you envision as the next step for integrating technology into pharmacy services and administration?

3. Part of your duties as a pharmacy technician may include answering the phone in the pharmacy. How is communicating on the phone different from communicating in person? How important is it to develop a good phone demeanor?

Lab 14 *Producing an Audit Log*

Worksheet Based on Printed Audit Log Report

1. What prices did the following people pay for their prescriptions?

    a. Kimberly Jackson _____

    b. Miguel Esparza _____

    c. Marquita Wilkins _____

    d. Lily Nguyen _____

    e. Vance Donaldson _____

    f. Jeffrey Klein (his C-II) _____

    g. Amala Gupta _____

    h. Cas Riley _____

2. What is the total amount collected by the pharmacy on the report? _____

3. What is the total amount of copays collected on the report? _____

4. What was the total average price for all prescriptions on the report? _____

5. How many prescriptions did the pharmacist on duty fill? _____

6. How many prescriptions were paid via third party? _____

7. How many prescriptions were paid via cash pricing? _____

8. What is the control schedule of Ms. Nguyen's Alprazolam? _____

Unit

3

Institutional Pharmacy Practice

A day in the life of a pharmacy technician...

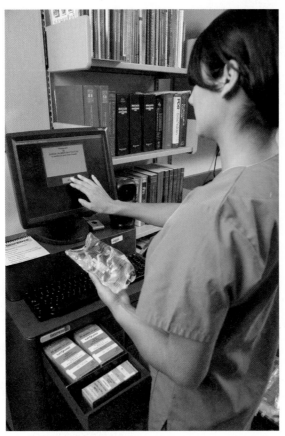

An ambulance pulls into the emergency room and doctors, nurses, and support staff throughout the hospital function as a team to care for the critically ill or injured patient. Multiple STAT medication orders arrive in the pharmacy for the newly admitted patient, along with a stack of urgent and routine orders for the hundreds of hospital patients who are undergoing treatment. The phone is ringing with doctors requesting drug information, and nurses needing medication refills or looking for a missing dose. The fax machine is whirring with new orders, the pneumatic tube system is dropping plastic tubes filled with more medication orders and refill requests. There is a backlog of crash carts to fill, floorstock is ready to be checked, there is a unit clerk at the pharmacy window waiting to pick up medicine for a patient in the intensive care unit.

What is your role? How do pharmacy technicians function seamlessly in what amounts to controlled chaos?

Pharmacy technicians are vital members of the hospital team. All members of the team—physicians, nurses, pharmacists, pharmacy technicians, and a multitude of other support staff must work together to care for patients who are recovering from injuries, disease, or surgical treatment. Each team member must know the role that they play in effective patient treatment. The pharmacy technician must perform numerous tasks with speed and accuracy. Timely treatment based on the accurate and precise delivery of pharmaceuticals is essential to the patient's recovery.

This unit will guide you in the essential tasks of the hospital pharmacy technician including 24-hour cart fill, floorstock, crash carts, narcotic record keeping, automated dispensing machine filling, and medication reconciliation.

Performing these important tasks with speed, and while maintaining 100% accuracy, will make you an indispensible member of the healthcare team.

Filling a Twenty-Four Hour Medication Cart

Lab 15

Objectives

- Demonstrate proficiency in accurately performing a 24 hour cart fill.
- Become familiar with the location, label information, class, general use, sigs, and abbreviations related to medications commonly used in a 24 hour cart fill.
- Discuss the procedures for, and the importance of, each step in the 24 hour cart fill process.

Supplies

- The Cart Fill Form
- Individual patient drawer, cassette, bin, or bag
- Access to a pharmacy lab stocked with common unit-dosed medications
- Access to standard pharmacy reference materials or the Internet

Unit dose

A medication packaged in a single dose, one-time-use container

The 24 hour cart fill is one of the most important basic functions that a pharmacy technician performs in institutional pharmacy practice. This process may be referred to as a cart fill, medication pick, medication fill, pick, or in similar terms as defined by the facility performing the procedure. Although cart fill specifics vary among institutions, the basic function is to quickly and accurately fill the required **unit-dosed** medications for one or more patients for a specified period of time. The variations you encounter might include slightly different terminology and procedures related to the process of filling a supply of medications for hospital patients.

For instance, some facilities might fill for a 24 hour supply, whereas others

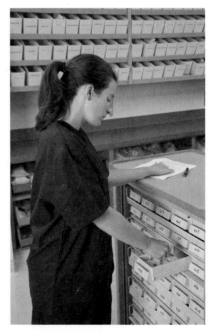

An important role of the pharmacy technician is to fill a medication cart.

175

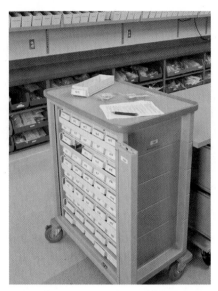
Medication cart.

might fill for a 12 hour, 48 hour, 72 hour, or even one week supply. In addition, the container into which a facility places a patient's pick medications might be a drawer, tray, bin, cart, cassette, or zip-lock type bag. Some larger facilities even have automated "robots" instead of pharmacy technicians performing the cart fill.

Despite these differences, it is crucial that you always check the expiration date of every dose you put into the drawer. Rules regarding expiration dating vary from state to state, but they generally require that all medications used for cart fill have a minimum of one month of "good" dating left. If the dose's dating is not acceptable, then it may not be used in the cart fill.

Standard procedure requires filling the cart by referring to a Cart Fill Form or pick list. The Form commonly presents several categories of information including:

- **Prescription # or Rx #:** A unique, computer-generated number that identifies a prescription and ties it to the patient information from the original medication order.
- **Drug name:** Most hospitals arrange medications by generic name within various sections such as fast movers, slow movers, topicals, injectables, etc. Exceptions include combination drugs with more than one active ingredient, in which case they are located under the brand name. However, such naming conventions may still vary between states and facilities.
- **Strength:** The individual tablet, capsule, ampule, or vial strength of the drug.
- **Directions:** The physician's directions for administration of the medication, including the route and the signa.
- **Number to dispense:** This number indicates the quantity of medication that you should place in the patient's drawer and is calculated based on the number of hours in the institution's fill period and the signa. Although in this lab you practice filling a medication cart based on a 24 hour fill period, the length of the fill period varies among institutions.

You will find an additional category on your Cart Fill Form: "Class or Primary Use," which is unique to this training lab. It has been added to help you learn the drug classification and primary uses of many common medications.

Procedure

For this lab, you will perform a 24 hour cart fill for one patient. You will find one version of a Cart Fill Form (version 15.1) at the end of this lab. Do not begin filling out that form until your instructor offers guidance. While you *may* be assigned to fill that particular form, you may also be given a completely different form by your instructor (numbered 15.2 and higher). He or she will probably have several different Cart Fill Forms to hand out, differing slightly in the quantities and items being requested. This form variety will prevent students from all having to be in the same part of the room at the same time. Your lab work can flow more smoothly and be completed within the allotted class time if you work on different forms. Thus, please do not begin performing the steps below until your instructor informs you which Cart Fill Form to use.

Tip: In practice, you will fill a 24 hour supply of medications for multiple patients. Be sure to verify the patient's name and room number; or make use of barcode technology to ensure that you place the patient's medications into the correct drawer.

1 Be sure to put your name and today's date on the Cart Fill Form.

2 Using the directions and signa, calculate how many doses you will need to fill a 24 hour supply of medications for the assigned patient. Write your answers for each medication in the "Number to Dispense" column on your Cart Fill Form.

3 Using pharmacy reference materials or the Internet, look up the class or primary use of each drug and record the information on your Cart Fill Form in the "Class or Primary Use" column. Write a few words describing the class or primary use of each drug (e.g., antihypertensive, analgesic, used to lower blood sugar, or used to treat upper respiratory infections).

Take Note

When performing an actual cart fill, you will not be required to look up or record the class or primary use of the medication. For the purposes of this lab, looking up the drug information will help you to familiarize yourself with various drugs and their use.

4 To help you locate where the medication is stored in the pharmacy, look up the brand/generic name of any drug that is unfamiliar to you on the Cart Fill Form.

5 Obtain the drugs you require from the appropriate pharmacy area. Be sure that each drug and its dose match *exactly* what is on the Cart Fill Form.

Tip: Watch out for abbreviations such as EC, ER, SR, or CR. Drug names followed by these abbreviations are different from drugs of the same name without them.

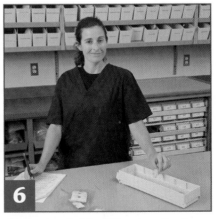

Pharmacy technician filling a medication cart drawer.

6 Place the appropriate amount of each drug into the patient's drawer (see "Number to Dispense" column).

7 **Conclusion:** Tear out and fold up the completed Cart Fill Form and place it in the drawer with the medications for your instructor to check. On a separate sheet of paper, answer all questions in the following Lab Review section and turn in your answers to your instructor.

Lab Review

Check Your Understanding

1. If the Cart Fill Form directions say "Give 1 tablet per tube TID," how many tablets would you put into the patient's drawer for a 24 hour cart fill?
   a. 2 tablets
   b. 3 tablets
   c. 4 tablets
   d. 5 tablets

2. The directions state "Give 1 tablet q8 h PRN pain." This signa indicates that the medication would be given how often?
   a. every 8 hours
   b. 3 times per day
   c. whenever the patient is in pain
   d. every 8 hours as needed to control the patient's pain

3. When filling a patient's drawer with medications, it is most important for the patient's health that you verify the correct _____.
   a. drug, strength, route, signa, and expiration date
   b. drug, strength, and route only
   c. strength, route, and signa only
   d. drug, route, and expiration date only

4. If a patient's medication was ordered to be given "1 tablet AC & HS," how many tablets would you place into the patient's drawer for a 24 hour cart fill?
   a. 2 tablets
   b. 3 tablets
   c. 4 tablets
   d. 5 tablets

5. If you look up a drug's primary use and discover that the drug is an antihypertensive, you might conclude that the patient has a condition of elevated _____.
   a. blood sugar
   b. liver enzymes
   c. blood pressure
   d. potassium levels

Thinking Like a Pharmacy Tech

1. Provide at least two reasons why it is valuable for a pharmacy technician to be familiar with a drug's class or general use.

2. Imagine that you are completing a Cart Fill Form and encounter a pharmacy abbreviation that is unfamiliar to you. Explain two ways that you could find the meaning of the abbreviation, other than by asking your instructor.

 3. Patient privacy is of utmost importance. With new technologies emerging in healthcare, such as e-prescriptions and electronic health records, how can you as a pharmacy technician ensure your patients' privacy? What are some ways the industry is working to protect patients' electronic information?

Name: _____   Date: _____

Lab 15   *Filling a Twenty-Four Hour Medication Cart*

Cart Fill Form (15.1)

Rx #	Drug Name	Strength	Directions/Sig	Number to Dispense	Class or Primary Use
11111	Acyclovir	200 mg	Give 1 capsule po BID	_____	_____
11112	Benazepril	10 mg	Give 1 capsule po q12 h	_____	_____
11113	Carbamazepine	200 mg	Give 1 tablet po QID	_____	_____
11114	Dicyclomine	20 mg	Give 1 capsule po q8 h	_____	_____
11115	Enalapril	5 mg	Give 1 tablet po BID	_____	_____
11116	Famotidine	20 mg	Give 1 tablet po AC & HS	_____	_____
11117	Gabapentin	100 mg	Give 2 capsules po TID	_____	_____
11118	Hydrochloro-thiazide	25 mg	Give 1 tablet po q6 h	_____	_____

Filling and Checking Floor Stock

Lab 16

Objectives

- Demonstrate skill and accuracy in filling and checking floor stock.
- Determine and discuss the rationale and procedures for filling and checking floor stock.

Supplies

- Floor Stock Request Form (FSRF)
- Access to a pharmacy lab stocked with floor stock items
- Access to a brand/generic handbook, pharmacy resource materials, or the Internet

Floor stock

A small supply of medications kept on each floor or unit

Most hospitals keep a small supply of certain medications on each floor or unit. This supply is commonly referred to as **floor stock** or unit stock. The number and types of medications kept in floor stock vary between facilities and even between floors or units of the same hospital. Floor stock medications generally include those items that need to be administered immediately, such as non-narcotic analgesics, antiemetics, antipyretics, and certain intravenous (IV) solutions.

When a pharmacy is very busy, the time it takes from the moment the physician writes an order until the pharmacy fills it and returns it to the nurse for administration—this is often referred to as the "turnaround time" of a pharmacy medication—can be quite long. The need to administer "STAT," "now," and initial doses quickly is the primary reason for having floor stock. Your timely and accurate filling and checking of floor stock items on the Floor Stock Request Form (FSRF) ensures that these medications are available to the nursing staff for immediate administration to patients.

Your role as a pharmacy technician requires familiarity with key terms used for filling and checking floor stock. Key terms include:

- **Unit:** The floor or nursing unit that placed the floor stock request. The unit may be identified by name, letter, abbreviation, or number (e.g., Obstetrics, ICU, or 4th floor).

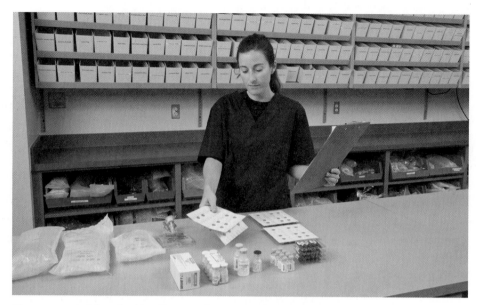

Pharmacy technician checking floor stock.

- **Fill #:** A number requested by designated nursing unit personnel to indicate the amount of each drug to be filled by the pharmacy in order to bring it up to par level. (par level minus the actual number on hand = the fill #).
- **Par Level:** The total number of a particular medication that the requesting unit keeps on hand when fully stocked.
- **Filled by:** The initials of the pharmacy staff member filling the FSRF.
- **Checked by:** The initials of the pharmacy staff member checking the FSRF.
- **The Double Check:** Takes place when pharmacy technicians do both floor stock procedures, filling and checking, rather than having a pharmacist, nurse, or other hospital staff member check a technician's fill work. The double check is allowed in many, but not all, states.

You should be aware that standard floor stock generally does *not* include the following:

- **Critical care medications:** Critical care items are commonly kept in a crash cart that is brought to the bedside for emergency administration to patients experiencing respiratory or cardiac arrest.
- **Medications requiring pharmacy compounding:** Some medications, such as creams, ointments, special oral solutions, and intravenous solutions with additives, require compounding in the pharmacy. The pharmacy sends such medications, whether prepared under nonsterile conditions or via strict aseptic technique, to the nursing unit as needed, based on physician's orders.
- **Narcotics:** Narcotics are kept in a separate, high-security area. Access to narcotics is restricted to authorized personnel, and special record keeping is required for their administration.

Procedure

This lab contains three procedure sections, Parts I, II, and III. You will learn the procedures for filling and checking a standard FSRF by practicing these two procedures separately, as "Part I: Filling Floor Stock" and "Part II: Checking Floor Stock," as outlined below. You will use the same FSRF for both parts, filling and checking. After you complete both of those procedures, you will turn in the single FSRF to your instructor as described in the final part, "Part III: Completing this Lab."

Part I: Filling Floor Stock

You will now fill a standard floor stock request using an FSRF. Note that one FSRF is included at the end of this lab. However, you *may* or *may not* be assigned to fill that particular form. Your instructor will probably choose to hand out several different FSRFs.

Therefore, it is important that you do not begin filling an FSRF until your instructor advises you which form to use. The forms differ slightly in the quantities and items being requested so that students will fill and check different requests, enabling the lab work to flow smoothly and be completed within the allotted class time. Once you have your designated FSRF in hand, you will begin with the first medication and proceed line by line, filling one medication at a time.

1 Because this lab will ask you to check the expiration date of each floor stock dose to be sure it is acceptable, you must first determine your state's expiration date requirements. Your instructor will have verified these state regulations so you should ask about them now.

2 Look up the brand and generic names of any medications on the FSRF that you are unfamiliar with. Note that you will fill *only* the medications and amounts written in the Fill # column. When the Fill # column is left blank, you will not fill that medication.

Tip: Once this medication is returned to the unit and added to that medication type kept in nursing unit floor stock, the total number of that medication will generally equal the par level. However, there are rare occasions when, based on temporarily increased usage, the nursing unit will request that a medication be refilled above the standard par level.

3 Find the first item to be filled. Make sure that what you are pulling from the pharmacy stock matches *exactly* what is ordered on the FSRF. The name, strength, form, and number of items must all exactly match the FSRF.

4 Pull out the correct number of that item (ie. the number in the "Fill #" column) and place it on an uncluttered section of counter or tabletop.

5 Check the expiration date of each dose to make sure it is acceptable.

6 Moving down the FSRF, continue pulling the correct number of each requested item (those with a quantity listed in the Fill # column).

7 Once you have pulled all of the items having a quantity in the Fill # column, arrange them so that the order of the items on the counter matches that on the FSRF. Organizing in this way makes the checking process more efficient.

8 Write your name and today's date in the blanks at the top of the Lab 16 worksheet, the FSRF. Near the bottom of the FSRF, write your name in the "Filled by" blank and the date in the "Today's date" blank.

Part II: Checking Floor Stock

While properly filling floor stock medications is crucial, it is also imperative that your checking process be thorough and accurate. Because many states now allow technicians to perform "the double check" (described in the background section of this lab) on standard floor stock items, you will now pair up with another student in the lab to do the double check.

Remember the importance of being thorough and accurate. When you receive the other student's completed FSRF, you will again begin with the first medication and proceed line by line, carefully checking one medication at a time.

As the "checker" you must check that the drug name, strength, form,

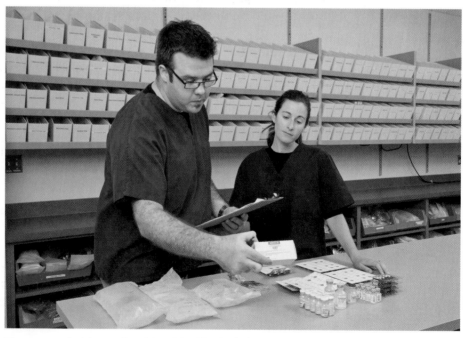

Pharmacy technician performing a "double check."

expiration date, and quantity match what is on the FSRF. Before you begin, have a pen or pencil ready to mark on the FSRF any errors you find while checking. When you are done checking the fill, you will be asked to point out the errors to the student who filled the FSRF and to count up the errors and write down the total number on the FSRF.

9 Find another student to perform a floor stock check on your work and have that student begin the check on the following step, Step 10.

10 On the completed FSRF, check the first item requested in the Fill # column. Verify that the name of the medication filled matches exactly what is ordered on the FSRF. If you find an error, circle the medication name.

11 Verify that the strength of the drug matches what is on the FSRF and circle any strength errors you find.

12 Verify that the route or formulation (form) of the drug matches what is on the FSRF and circle any route or form errors you find.

13 Verify that the technician filled the number that the nursing unit requested and circle any number errors you find.

14 Check the expiration date of each dose to make sure it is acceptable and note any dating problems near the medication line you are currently checking.

15 Repeat the entire procedure with the next medication on the FSRF, continuing until you have checked all items and noted any errors found.

16 Add up the total number of errors you have circled or noted on the FSRF. Write down this number at the bottom of the FSRF in the "Number of errors caught" blank and write your name in the "Checked by" blank.

Part III: Completing This Lab

17 Get together with the student who filled the stock for the FSRF you have just checked and exchange your FSRFs. Point out any errors to that student. He or she should now correct those errors. When your own FSRF is returned to you and your errors are pointed out, you should now correct any errors you made in your filling procedure.

18 **Conclusion:** Ask your instructor for a final check. The instructor will check what you have *filled* on your FSRF and also verify what you have *checked* by looking at the other student's FSRF. On a separate sheet of paper, answer all questions in the following Lab Review section and turn in your answers to your instructor.

Lab Review

Check Your Understanding

1. What is the primary reason for keeping some medications as floor stock?
   a. Nurses are impatient and need things right away.
   b. Some medications are not available from the pharmacy.
   c. Nurses on the floor can compound some medications.
   d. Long turnaround times necessitate that some initial doses, especially "now" or "STAT" doses, be given from floor stock.

2. The Fill # refers to the ____.
   a. amount of an item that a nursing unit requests to bring it up to par level
   b. total number of everything ordered on the FSRF
   c. total number of a medication that the unit keeps on hand when fully stocked
   d. number of the nursing unit or floor that ordered the drug

3. Which of the following items would *least* likely be kept in standard floor stock?
   a. ibuprofen tablets
   b. an IV bag with potassium chloride and multiple vitamins
   c. Benadryl capsules
   d. Pepto-Bismol tablets

4. Which of the following items would *most* likely be kept in standard floor stock?
   a. a prefilled narcotic injection
   b. penicillin intravenous piggyback
   c. acetaminophen tablets
   d. epinephrine injection

5. When filling and checking floor stock, it is important to verify accuracy. Which of the following lists items that *all* need verification for accuracy?
   a. medication name, strength, number of each item requested, expiration date
   b. medication name, room number, expiration date, number requested
   c. medication name, strength, room number, expiration date
   d. medication name, strength, number of each item requested, patient's name

Thinking Like a Pharmacy Tech

1. After a pharmacy technician has filled the floor stock, what are the advantages of having a second pharmacy technician, rather than a pharmacist, check the work?

2. How does the pharmacy technician's accurate and timely filling and checking of floor stock directly affect the nursing staff? How does it directly affect the patient?

 3. Punctuality is important in any job. Why might it be especially important to arrive to work on time as a pharmacy technician?

Name: _____   Date: _____

Floor Stock Request Form

Unit _____ Obstetrics _____

Fill #	Medication Being Requested (name, strength, form)	Par Level
8	Acetaminophen 325 mg tablets	10
5	Acetaminophen 500 mg caplets	10
	Amoxicillin 250 mg capsules	6
	Amoxicillin 500 mg capsules	6
3	Azithromycin 250 mg tablets	5
	Ciprofloxacin 500 mg tablets	2
	Dexamethasone 8 mg/2 mL injectable vial	4
2	Diphenhydramine 25 mg capsules	8
2	Dextrose 5% in Water 1000 mL for injection (IV bag)	6
1	Dextrose 5% in 0.45 Sodium chloride 1000 mL (IV bag)	4
	Dulcolax tablets	6
3	Furosemide 20 mg tablets	5
1	Furosemide 40 mg tablets	5
8	Ibuprofen 200 mg caplets	10
	Ibuprofen 600 mg caplets	10
	Maalox 30 mL oral liquid (unit-dose cups)	2
	Mylanta 30 mL oral liquid (unit-dose cups)	2
	Metoclopramide 10 mg tablets	4
	Promethazine 50 mg/2 mL for injection (ampule)	2
1	Sodium chloride 0.45% 1000 mL (IV bag)	4
6	Sodium choride 0.9% 30 mL vial (bacteriostatic)	10
5	Sodium chloride 0.9% 1000 mL (IV bag)	8
	Tobramycin 40 mg/1 mL for injection (multidose vial)	1
	Tucks Pads topical (jar)	1

Filled by _____ Today's date _____

Number of errors caught by checker (and corrected by filler) _____

Checked by _____

Instructor final check _____ Number of errors missed by checker _____

Filling and Recording Narcotic Floor Stock

Lab 17

Objectives

- Demonstrate proficiency in the counting and preparation of narcotic floor stock based on a narcotic floor stock refill form.
- Demonstrate accuracy in record keeping related to the filling of narcotic floor stock.
- Discuss the procedures and rationale for filling narcotic floor stock and for related record keeping and narcotic procedures.

Supplies

- Access to a narcotic cabinet, vault, or room stocked with common C-II through C-V narcotics for floor stock use
- Access to a brand/generic handbook or the Internet
- Access to a sample C-II perpetual log book
- Access to a sample C-III through C-V perpetual log book
- Narcotic Floor Stock Refill Form
- Counting tray and spatula
- Calculator
- Black pen
- Red pen

Narcotic cabinet

A double-locked location in the pharmacy where narcotic medications are securely stored

In an institutional setting, all narcotics are kept in the **narcotic cabinet** and are dispensed in a manner similar to standard floor stock dispensing. In larger institutions, a full-time pharmacy technician is often responsible for the operation of the narcotic cabinet (also referred to as the narcotic vault or room). Smaller institutions might require the pharmacy technician to work with narcotics only on an as-needed basis or in special situations, such as when compounding or delivering narcotics to the nursing unit. The technician responsible for handling narcotics will likely receive specialized on-the-job training.

Many institutional pharmacies now require pharmacy technicians to carry out all aspects of pharmaceutical narcotic duties. These duties are multiple and include ordering, pulling, counting, record keeping, filling, delivering, providing quality assurance, and placing the narcotic floor stock in a secure area on the unit. To order narcotic floor stock from

FIGURE 17.1 **Drug Enforcement Administration Form**

See Reverse of PURCHASER'S Copy for Instructions	No order form may be issued for Schedule I and II substances unless a completed form has been received (21 CFR 1305.04).	OMB Approval No. 1117-0010

TO (Name of Supplier) | STREET ADDRESS

CITY AND STATE | DATE | TO BE FILLED IN BY SUPPLIER

SUPPLIER'S DEA REGISTRATION NO.

TO BE FILLED IN BY PURCHASER

LINE No.	No. of Packages	Size of Package	Name of Item	National Drug Code	Packages Shipped	Date Shipped
1						
2						
3						
4						
5						
6						
7						
8						
9						
10						

SAMPLE

◀ LAST LINE COMPLETED (MUST BE 10 OR UNDER) | SIGNATURE OF PURCHASER OR ATTORNEY OR AGENT

Date Issued: **10302014** | DEA Registration No.: **AA4720581** | Name and Address of Registrant

Schedule: **2, 2N, 3, 3N, 4, 5**

Get Well Pharmacy
1000 Healthline Road
Wellness, TX 70000

Registered as a: **TRAINING ONLY** | No. Of this order Form: **002235985**

DEA FORM-222 (Oct. 1992) | **U.S. OFFICIAL ORDER FORMS - SCHEDULES I & II** | **DRUG ENFORCEMENT ADMINISTRATION** | **SUPPLIER'S Copy 1** | **75841302**

wholesalers and other suppliers, DEA Form 222 is used. An example of such a form is shown in Figure 17.1.

The technician is also responsible for record keeping: recording all narcotic withdrawals and additions in perpetual log books. The **perpetual log** book is an official, legal record with pages entitled "Perpetual Inventory Record" (Figure 17.2) or sometimes "Controlled Substance Record." Because there is one perpetual log book for C-II narcotics and a different perpetual log book for C-III through C-V narcotics, you should make sure you are using the correct book for each entry. Due to the importance of keeping an accurate narcotic record, you must become familiar with and practice these standard narcotic perpetual log book procedures:

Perpetual log

An official, legal record of all activity relating to medications in the narcotic cabinet; in some facilities, narcotic record keeping is maintained electronically using special narcotic tracking software

- Make all entries or additions into the perpetual log in black pen.
- Record withdrawals and negative balances in red pen. Note that only the number should be in red, not the entire line entry.
- Note errors by drawing a single line through the entire line entry. The initials of the person making the correction should be written next to the line-through, and circled.

FIGURE 17.2 Perpetual Inventory Record

Perpetual Inventory Record

Drug Name, Strength, and Dosage Form

NDC   Manufacturer

Date	Invoice #	Department/Floor/Unit #	Qty +/–	Balance	Initials	Verified by

- Errors in the narcotic records must remain traceable and legible. Therefore, never erase or scribble out errors, and note that it is *never acceptable* to use white-out or similar products.
- Always record information in the perpetual log on the next available line. There should never be an open or empty line in the perpetual log.
- Never write information on the bottom of a perpetual log sheet below the preprinted spaces. Rather, once you have filled the last available line on the page, you *must* start a new sheet.
- To start a new sheet, transfer the drug name, strength, manufacturer, and NDC number from the drug bottle onto the appropriate space at the top of the new sheet. Transfer the balance or actual count number into the first available balance space on this new sheet.

In order to provide the utmost security, be sure that narcotics, the keys to the narcotic cabinet, and all narcotic records are kept under your supervision while working in this area. These items should never be left unattended or unsecured. All narcotic records must be kept on hand in the pharmacy for a minimum of two years. The State Board of Pharmacy, the Drug Enforcement Administration (DEA), and other regulatory agencies may ask to review narcotic records, including the perpetual log books, so immediate access to these records is essential.

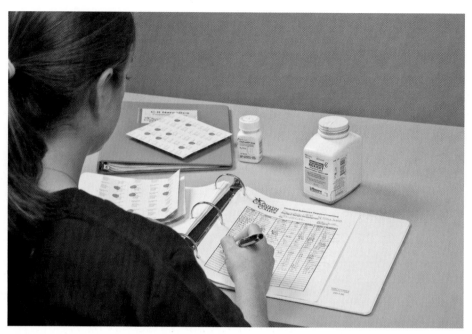

Pharmacy technician entering information into the Controlled Substance Perpetual Inventory Record.

Procedure

In this lab, you will fill a Narcotic Floor Stock Refill Form and record the dispensed narcotics in the appropriate perpetual log books.

1 Read through the Narcotic Floor Stock Refill Form completely. If necessary, look up the brand or generic medication names with which you are unfamiliar.

2 Open the appropriate (either C-II or C-III through C-V) perpetual log book and find the first medication listed on the Narcotic Floor Stock Refill Form. Verify that the drug name, strength, and form that are listed on the perpetual log match exactly what is ordered on the refill form.

3 Using a black pen, record today's date in the Date field on the first available line of the perpetual log for this medication. Under the Department or Unit # field, write the words "actual count." Record your initials under the Initials field. Leave the Invoice #, Qty +/−, and Balance fields blank for now.

4 Open the narcotic cabinet and locate the first item ordered on the Narcotic Floor Stock Refill Form. Pull out the bin or tray containing the first medication listed on the refill form. Verify that the drug name, strength, and form match exactly what is ordered and that all of the medications to be dispensed have acceptable expiration dating.

5 Count all tablets or capsules in the medication bin. Be sure to count everything in the bin, including unopened bottles, partial bottles, and unit-dosed medications. If necessary, use a counting tray and/or calculator.

6 Using a black pen, record the total number counted from this bin in the perpetual log book in the Balance field. Record your initials in the appropriate place on the same line.

7 Pull the requested number, as specified for the first Drug on your Narcotic Floor Stock Refill Form, out of the bin. The medication must be in unit-dose form. Consult your instructor if you do not have enough unit-dose medication to fill the entire order.

8 On the next available line for this medication (i.e., the line directly below the actual count), record today's date; the department, floor, or unit name and/or number as it appears on your Narcotic Floor Stock Refill Form; and your initials in the appropriate fields.

9 Using a red pen, record the amount that you pulled from the bin in the Qty +/– field. This number should match the number ordered by the department, floor, or unit.

> **Take Note**
>
> Be aware that in some facilities the recording of *both* entries and withdrawals are made in black pen. Refer to your facility policy and procedure manual for specific procedures for narcotic record keeping.

10 From the Balance (the actual count found in the first entry line), subtract the number to be dispensed (the number recorded under the Qty +/- field of the second entry line). This new count should be recorded, in black, under the Balance field of the second entry line and should be equal to the amount left in the bin.

Tip: Your formula is "Actual Count or Balance minus Amount Dispensed (or Qty +/–) = Amount Remaining in Bin."

11 Remember that when you are working with a perpetual log, the "actual count" must match the remaining balance that was written by the previous person recording entries for that medication. If you see a **discrepancy** during your work, report it immediately to your instructor.

Narcotic discrepancy

A disagreement between the actual count of a narcotic and the amount listed in the perpetual log or narcotic record

12 Move from the perpetual log to the Narcotic Floor Stock Refill Form. Fill in the "Balance," "# Dispensed," and "Remaining Balance" information that you determined for the first medication listed on the Narcotic Floor Stock Refill Form.

13 Place to the side, temporarily, the amount that was just filled for the first medication ordered.

14 Fill the other medications on the Narcotic Floor Stock Refill Form, following the same procedures listed above.

15 **Conclusion:** Once all of the medications on the Narcotic Floor Stock Refill Form have been filled and recorded in the perpetual log book(s), and you have filled in the necessary information on the Narcotic Floor Stock Refill Form, write your name and today's date on the Refill Form and ask for an instructor check. On a separate sheet of paper, answer all questions in the following Lab Review section and turn in your answers to your instructor.

Lab Review

Check Your Understanding

1. The actual count that has just been completed is 46 tablets of Dilaudid 2 mg. The balance that was previously recorded in the perpetual log for this medication is 47 tablets. How should you handle this discrepancy?
   a. Since the count is only off by one tablet, it may be ignored.
   b. Erase the previous record of 47 and write in the correct count of 46.
   c. Contact the State Board of Pharmacy and the DEA immediately.
   d. Double check to be sure the actual count is accurate. Double check the math from previous entries to see if errors were made. If unable to resolve the discrepancy by identifying a math or transcription error, notify the instructor (or pharmacist) immediately.

2. The term "actual count," as used in the lab above, refers to _____.
   a. a number that reflects the total amount of a specific narcotic currently in the narcotic cabinet
   b. the actual count of all narcotics in the narcotic cabinet
   c. the remaining count of a specific narcotic once the narcotic floor stock order has been dispensed
   d. a number that reflects the total amount of all narcotics in the perpetual log book

3. The term "perpetual log" refers to a _____.
   a. record book where all narcotic floor stock orders are kept
   b. method of recording the balance of, additions to, or withdrawals of medications from the narcotic cabinet
   c. method of recording the balance, additions to, or withdrawals of all medications in the pharmacy
   d. record book where all laws pertaining to narcotic records are kept

4. Suppose that you just made a transcription error in the perpetual log book. What procedure should you follow to correct the error?
   a. Use a white-out type product to cover up the error and then record the correct information over the entry where the error was made.
   b. Use a black pen to scribble out the entire line where the error was made and then write in the correct information on the next available line in the log book.
   c. Draw a single line through the entire entry in the log book where the error was made. Record your initials next to the error and circle it. Write in the correct information on the next available line in the log book.
   d. None of the above

5. According to federal law, how long must institutional pharmacy narcotic records be kept on hand?
   a. one year
   b. two years
   c. three years
   d. five years

Thinking Like a Pharmacy Tech

1. A Narcotic Floor Stock Refill Form states that the obstetrics unit needs meperidine 25 mg syringes × 10, and Vicodin 5 mg/325 mg tablets × 25. Should these drugs be recorded in the same perpetual log book? Why or why not?

2. *Scenario:* You have just completed an actual count of codeine 30 mg tablets and verified that there are 150 tablets on hand in the narcotic cabinet. You see that the perpetual log book containing the record for codeine 30 mg says there should be 155 tablets on hand. After verifying that the discrepancy is not a math or transcription error, you discuss the matter with the technician who recorded the most recent balance for this drug. This technician says, "Just erase the 155 count and write in the correct balance. That way there will not be a discrepancy." Discuss why this action is or is not an appropriate way to handle the situation.

3. While most employees are absent on occasion for uncontrollable circumstances such as illness, being absent frequently does not reflect well on your commitment to your job. What are some reasons why you might be absent, and how can you plan ahead to avoid missing work?

Lab 17   *Filling and Recording Narcotic Floor Stock*

Narcotic Floor Stock Refill Form (17.1)

Department/Floor/Unit Name or Number _____ Obstetrics _____

Floor Stock Narcotic Ordered by This Unit:

Tylenol #3 tablets x 50

Starting Balance_____ # Dispensed _____ Remaining Balance_____

Vicodin 5 mg/325 mg tablets x 25

Starting Balance_____ # Dispensed _____ Remaining Balance_____

Morphine 10 mg pre-filled syringes x 20

Starting Balance_____ # Dispensed _____ Remaining Balance_____

Instructor's initials _____   **Assignment grade** _____

Preparing Oral Syringes

Lab 18

Objectives

- Demonstrate competence in the preparation of oral syringes.
- Demonstrate accuracy in basic math calculations related to the preparation of oral syringes.
- Discuss the procedures and rationale for preparing oral syringes.

Supplies

- Ibuprofen oral suspension × 1 pint
- 10 mL oral syringe × 1
- 5 mL oral syringe × 1
- 3 mL oral syringe × 1
- Oral syringe caps × 3
- Rubber oral syringe bottle adaptor
- Paper and pencil for calculations
- Calculator

Enteral

A route of administration (oral, buccal, or rectal) delivering medication through a patient's gastrointestinal tract

Many **enteral** medications are available in an oral solid form. In some cases, the patient is unable or unwilling to swallow a capsule or tablet and the physician may request instead the oral liquid form of the medication. Some oral liquid medications are available prepackaged in unit-dosed cups. However, numerous oral liquid medications are supplied to hospital pharmacies in the original bulk bottle. In order to deliver the proper dosage to multiple patients in the most sanitary and cost-effective manner, the pharmacy technician will prepare individual doses in oral syringes by withdrawing them from the bulk bottle. This preparation process requires a special bottle adaptor that fits into the mouth of the bottle to facilitate easy withdrawal of the medication. A schematic illustration of oral syringe preparation is shown in Figure 18.1 on the next page.

Preparing oral syringes requires that you first perform precise calculations to determine the amount of liquid to draw into each syringe. You will use a basic formula called "ratio and proportion" to calculate how much liquid is needed for each individual dose. The calculation is based on the concentration of the liquid medication in the bulk bottle and the

FIGURE 18.1
Schematic illustration of oral syringe preparation

The syringe tip is seated inside the opening of a rubber bottle adaptor, which is seated inside the mouth of a bulk bottle of oral liquid.

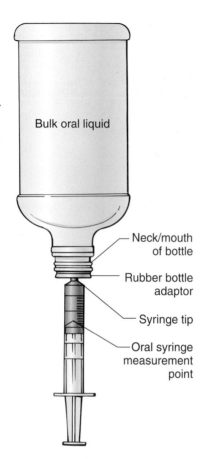

Bulk oral liquid

Neck/mouth of bottle

Rubber bottle adaptor

Syringe tip

Oral syringe measurement point

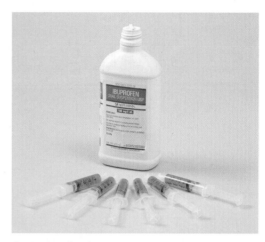

Capped oral syringes.

FIGURE 18.2
Enteral Feeding Tube Sites

Insertion sites for NG, G, and J tubes. Gastronomy tubes (G-tube), and jeujostomy tubes (J-tube) may also be used to administer medications via oral syringe.

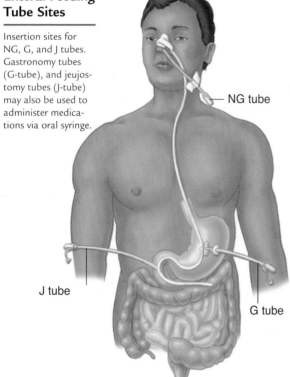

NG tube

J tube

G tube

dose you desire to prepare, and requires some familiarity with pharmaceutical math. An explanation of these basic calculations is provided on the next page. For more information on ratio and proportion, or other pharmacy calculation methods, refer to *Pharmacy Calculations for Technicians* by Don Ballington and Tova Wiegand Green.

Most oral syringes are administered by squirting them directly into the patient's mouth. Some oral syringes are administered by nurses who introduce them through a patient's nasogastric tube (NG tube or NGT). As illustrated in Figure 18.2, a NG tube is inserted into the patient's nose, continues past the throat, and ends in the stomach. Using an oral syringe with an NG tube eliminates the need to swallow, which may be difficult for some patients, and delivers medications and food directly to the patient's stomach. Remember that oral syringes are for one-time use only; they must be disposed of in the trash after the dose is administered to the patient.

General Explanation of Dose Calculation Process:

To determine the amount of liquid to draw into each syringe, you will use a basic "ratio and proportion" formula. Your calculation will provide you an answer to the question "How much liquid will I need to withdraw from the bulk bottle for an individual dose?"

First, look on the oral medication bottle label and find the concentration as provided in milligrams per milliliter. Write down the number in fraction form:

$$\frac{\text{Number of milligrams}}{\text{Number of milliliters}} \Bigg\} \text{ as stated on the medication label}$$

Tip: *To be accurate and clear when using ratios and proportions, always write down the abbreviation for the units (mg, mL, etc.) you are working with when you write down the numbers.*

Next to this concentration, or ratio, place an equals sign, and then write down the number of milligrams in the desired dose over x milliliters (the amount you are solving for).

$$\frac{\text{Number of milligrams (from medication label)}}{\text{Number of milliliters (from medication label)}} = \frac{\text{Number of milligrams in desired dose}}{x \text{ milliliters}}$$

You have created a proportion that communicates that one ratio is equal to another ratio. You can now cross multiply (work in a diagonal direction) and then divide, to calculate the missing x value in your ratio (to solve for x) and answer your dosage question:

- Multiply the Number of milligrams in desired dose by the Number of milliliters (from medication label).
- Take the result and divide it by the Number of milligrams (from medication label).
- Your answer is the missing value, x milliliters, the amount that you need to withdraw.

Specific Dose Calculation for This Lab:

In the following Procedure section, you will prepare three doses of ibuprofen. Below is the calculation process for one of those doses. Use this model to complete your calculations for the remaining two doses when you reach Step 4 of the Procedure.

For the ibuprofen 200 mg dose, your initial question is: "How many milliliters do I need to withdraw from the bulk bottle for the desired dose of ibuprofen 200 mg?"

Your bulk ibuprofen medication bottle label indicates a concentration of 100 mg/5 mL. Thus, your two ratios and the proportion between them (equality) result in this formula:

$$\frac{100 \text{ mg}}{5 \text{ mL}} = \frac{200 \text{ mg (in this desired dose)}}{x \text{ millilters (to be drawn up)}}$$

- First you cross multiply: 200 mg × 5 mL = 1000 mg/mL
- And then you divide: 1000 mg/mL ÷ 100 mg = 10 mL
- This final number, 10 mL, is your missing value for x and the answer to your question "How many milliliters do I need to withdraw from the bulk bottle for the desired dose of ibuprofen 200 mg?"

Procedure

In this lab, you will calculate three individual doses of oral liquid medication and prepare the doses using oral syringes and a bottle adaptor. The doses you will draw up are ibuprofen 200 mg, ibuprofen 100 mg, and ibuprofen 50 mg.

1 Wash hands thoroughly.

2 Gather the listed supplies. You may wish to wear gloves and scrubs or a lab coat when performing this lab.

3 Verify that the ibuprofen label indicates a concentration of 100 mg/5 mL.

4 On a separate sheet of paper, neatly perform your calculations to answer this question for each of the three desired ibuprofen doses: How many milliliters (mL) will I need to withdraw from the bulk bottle to prepare this dose? You will show your instructor your calculations sheet at the end of the lab.

Tip: Read the explanation and use the formula provided on the previous page to perform your dose calculations. Your instructor will guide you in practicing the calculations and you should ask for additional instruction as needed.

5 Remove the cap from the pint bottle of ibuprofen. Attach the bottle adaptor with a gentle twisting motion. The bottle adaptor should be firmly seated in the bottle top so that only the top one or two rings of the adaptor are visible. Do not push on the adaptor with too much force or it will fall directly into the liquid and render the bottle contents unusable.

6 Select an appropriate syringe for the dose you are preparing, choosing the size closest to the desired dose while ensuring that the entire dose fits. Also select an appropriate syringe cap, noting that they are available in different sizes and the cap should fit tightly and securely to the syringe tip.

7 Insert the tip of the first oral syringe into the hole on top of the bottle adaptor. Invert the bottle and syringe so that the syringe is now below the bottle.

Tip: If, upon inverting the bottle, you notice the medication leaking, then the syringe was not firmly seated in the bottle adaptor. To correct this problem, right the bottle and gently push and twist the syringe downward to attach it more firmly to the bottle adaptor.

8 Pull down on the plunger so fluid starts to flow into the syringe. Once the syringe is about one-third full, push up forcefully on the plunger to expel all the fluid and air bubbles back into the bottle.

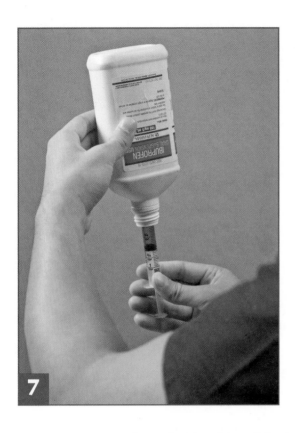

7

9 Pull down on the plunger again so fluid starts to flow into the syringe and then quickly push up on the plunger to expel the fluid and air bubbles. Repeat this process several times in quick succession. This technique is called "**crushing**." Crushing forces all of the air bubbles out of the syringe and allows only fluid to fill the syringe when you later draw up the full, prescribed volume. *Tip: Removing the bubbles when the syringe is only one-third full is important. You would find the crushing process very difficult if the syringe were more full or if you had drawn up the final proper volume.*

10 Once the air bubbles have been removed by using the crushing method, pull down on the plunger until you have the desired volume in the syringe. Take the measurement where the shoulder of the black stopper at the end of the syringe plunger meets the proper graduation on the syringe barrel.

Crushing

A method of removing air bubbles from a syringe

11 Invert the bottle and syringe duo again so that the bottle is right-side-up and the syringe is upside-down. Holding only the syringe barrel, remove the syringe in a twisting, pulling motion to break the suction that has been created. Once the suction is released, the syringe should easily detach from the bottle adaptor.

12 Place the properly fitting syringe cap firmly onto the syringe tip and set the syringe aside. Repeat the complete procedure for both remaining doses and place all three capped syringes on the work surface next to the ibuprofen bottle.

13 **Conclusion:** Write your name and today's date on the sheet where you performed the math calculations. Ask your instructor to check all three filled syringes, the medication bottle, and your calculations. Once the check has been done, on a separate sheet of paper, answer all questions in the following Lab Review section and turn in your answers to your instructor.

Lab Review

Check Your Understanding

1. Which of the following makes oral syringe dosing desirable?
   a. Doses from one bulk bottle can be easily dispensed to multiple patients.
   b. It is more sanitary to dispense a dose from an oral syringe than from a teaspoon.
   c. An oral syringe is a more accurate system of measure than is a dosing cup or spoon.
   d. All of the above

2. The area of the syringe where the measurement is made is the _____.
   a. hub of the syringe
   b. area where the shoulder of the plunger meets the barrel of the syringe
   c. area where the plunger enters the barrel of the syringe
   d. None of the above

3. The most appropriate size syringe for a 2.8 mL dose is a _____ syringe.
   a. 1 mL
   b. 3 mL
   c. 5 mL
   d. 10 mL

4. A common method used to remove air bubbles prior to filling the syringe to the desired final volume is often referred to as _____.
   a. squeezing
   b. pushing
   c. crushing
   d. withdrawing

5. How should you dispose of used oral syringes?
   a. Put them in the sharps container.
   b. Put them in a chemo waste container.
   c. Put them in a regular trash container.
   d. None of the above

Thinking Like a Pharmacy Tech

1. Compare oral syringes with syringes for parenteral use and describe some of the basic differences in procedures related to the use of these two products.

2. Describe two situations in which a patient would need to be given an oral liquid dose instead of an oral solid.

3. What does a pharmacy technician wear to work on a daily basis? Does this differ for techs working in a community pharmacy versus a hospital?

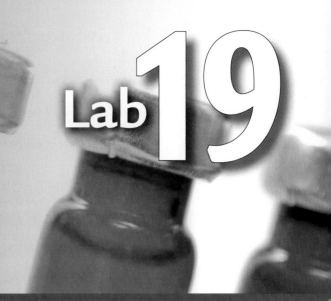

Charging and Refilling a Crash Cart

Lab 19

Objectives

- Identify and discuss the rationale for the preparation and use of a crash cart.
- Demonstrate proficiency in initiating patient charges for crash cart medications.
- Demonstrate skill and accuracy in filling a crash cart.

Supplies

- Access to a pharmacy lab stocked with standard emergency medications
- Access to a crash cart, tray, or tackle box
- Crash Cart Charge Form
- Crash Cart Refill Form
- Access to a brand/generic handbook

Parenteral

Any route of administration other than sublingual, enteral or topical, such as intravenous or intramuscular

Code

A life-threatening situation when a patient is in cardiac or respiratory arrest

Because hospitals care for people with potentially life-threatening conditions, it is vital to have a crash cart on hand for treating respiratory or cardiac arrest and other potentially fatal emergency conditions. Be aware that this cart may also be referred to as a crash tray, code cart, tackle box, or other names individual facilities may have developed. Many large facilities keep a crash cart on each floor or nursing unit, often in a specified location.

The arrangement and contents of crash carts vary widely among institutions. As a general rule, the crash cart is stocked with emergency medications, such as epinephrine, atropine, and nitroprusside. The cart may also contain standard IV base solutions, IV tubing, and a limited supply of syringes, needles, and other medication or supply items. Most of the items in the crash cart will be for **parenteral** use since a patient who is experiencing respiratory or cardiac arrest is generally unable to take oral medications.

When a hospital patient goes into cardiac or respiratory arrest, a "**code**" is called by hospital staff and usually announced on an overhead paging system. The code may also be referred to as a code blue, code zero, crash, zero, or other term preferred by the facility. A designated code team—a group of doctors and nurses trained in emergency medical care—commonly responds and assumes treatment of the patient. At that time, the charge nurse unlocks the crash cart, and the code team removes medications and

205

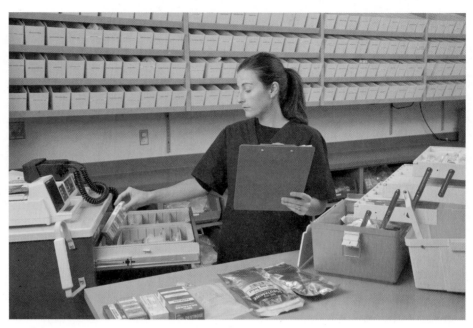

Pharmacy technician checking and refilling a crash cart.

supplies from the crash cart to treat the patient. Except for such code use, the crash cart must be kept locked at all times.

Once the code has ended, the crash cart is returned to the pharmacy to refill it and to determine which items should be charged to the patient. Accurate and timely initiation of patient charges and crash cart refilling are crucial tasks often performed by the pharmacy technician. As a technician, you must inventory the used crash cart and charge the patient for any items that were used during the code by recording the information on a crash cart charge form. You must also refill medications that were used to treat the patient and check expiration dates on all cart medications, replacing anything that does not have—within most states—a minimum of six months of acceptable dating. The number that is to be refilled on each item and recorded on a crash cart refill form will be determined by subtracting the number on hand in the cart from the par level (the number to be kept in the cart when it is full). The technician puts the resulting quantity, the refill number, into the cart.

Procedure

This lab requires you to practice two related procedures: initiating patient charges and refilling the crash cart. During the first procedure, you will use the Crash Cart Charge Form to charge the patient for medications and supply items used during the code. During the second part of the procedure, you will use the Crash Cart Refill Form to check medication expiration dates and refill the crash cart after the emergency has been addressed.

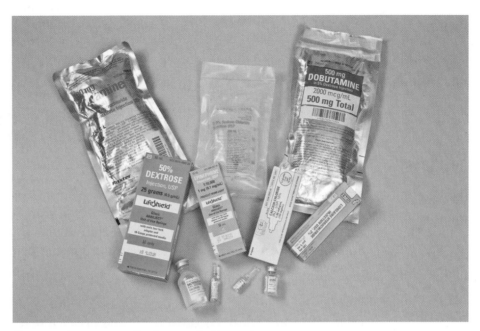
Common emergency medications stocked in crash carts.

Part I: Charging the Patient

You will first use a Crash Cart Charge Form to charge the patient for items used during the code. Your instructor will tell you, based on supplies available in your lab, whether to use the Charge Form provided at the end of the lab or wait for a different form to be handed out to you.

1 If necessary, look up the brand/generic names of any Crash Cart Charge Form medications with which you are unfamiliar.

2 Verify crash cart expiration dating with your instructor before beginning the lab. Six months is generally acceptable, but this may vary somewhat from state to state.

3 Open the top drawer of the crash cart (or the first section of the tray). Find the first item listed on the Charge Form. Note that the drawer may be divided into multiple sections and the first section (i.e., #1) should match the first item listed on the Charge Form.

4 Count the number of that item in the crash cart. This quantity should exactly match the item's par level as listed on the Charge Form. If it does not, the difference reflects the quantity of that item used to treat the patient and now to be replaced. Write the refill number on the corresponding line on the Charge Form.

Tip: Remember that Par Level — Number on Hand = Number to be Refilled.

5 Continue down the Charge Form, recording the refill number for each item listed. Once you have completed the Charge Form, write your name and today's date on the assignment. Temporarily set the Charge Form aside to await your instructor's check.

Tip: In an institutional setting, the Charge Form would now be used to enter patient charges into the facility's computerized billing system. For the purposes of this lab, however, the computer-based, data-entry portion of the charging process will be skipped.

Part II: Refilling the Crash Cart

You will now use a Crash Cart Refill Form to check expiration dates and refill the crash cart. Your instructor will tell you, based on supplies available in your lab, whether to use the Refill Form provided at the end of the lab or wait for a different form to be handed out to you.

6 Again locate, in the crash cart or tray, the first item in the crash cart, corresponding to the first item listed on the Refill Form. Find the expiration date for each dose of medication (which may be an ampule, vial, syringe, IV bag, or other supply) for this first item. Each dose must comply with your state's regulations regarding expiration dating. (Again, six months is generally acceptable, but this may vary somewhat from state to state.) If the dose does not comply (ie. it expires less than six months from today's date), remove it from the crash cart or tray.

7 If necessary, refill this item to bring it up to match the par level, replacing any missing (i.e., used) doses or doses you removed due to unacceptable expiration dating. Be sure that the replacement doses have at least six months of acceptable expiration dating. Place these items into the appropriate section of the crash cart, tray, or tackle box.

8 Write down the earliest expiration date—the one expiring first—for this item.
Tip: For example, if you are refilling six ampicillin 250 mg vials and each one has a different expiration date, you will write down only the earliest expiration date.

9 Repeat the entire procedure (checking expiration dates, removing, refilling, and recording the earliest expiration date) for each item listed on the Crash Cart Refill Form, until the entire cart has been refilled (brought up to par level) with items that have acceptable dating.

10 **Conclusion:** Write your name and today's date on the Crash Cart Refill Form. Retrieve the Charge Form that you set aside and then ask for an instructor check. The instructor will check both Crash Cart Forms—the Charge Form to verify that you have properly charged the patient, and the Refill Form to verify that you have refilled each item properly and recorded the correct expiration dates. On a separate sheet of paper, answer all questions in the following Lab Review section and turn in your answers to your instructor.

Lab Review

Check Your Understanding

1. The primary reason for keeping emergency medications in a crash cart is to supply ____.
   a. now and stat medications to the nursing staff
   b. medications and supplies that are not stored as floor stock
   c. medications that are used to treat chronic cardiac or respiratory conditions
   d. medications that are commonly used in a code situation

2. Of the following items, which would be least likely to be kept in a crash cart?
   a. nitroglycerin for IV use
   b. lactated Ringer's 1,000 mL IV bag
   c. epinephrine 1:10,000 injectable solution
   d. ibuprofen tablets

3. In reference to a crash cart, the term "par level" means the ____.
   a. quantity of a particular medication or supply item kept on hand within a filled crash cart
   b. total number of all medications or supply items kept on hand within the crash cart
   c. quantity of medications or supply items that must be refilled within the crash cart
   d. None of the above

4. Which of the following pairs of statements is most accurate?
   a. The Crash Cart Charge Form is used to charge the nursing unit. The Crash Cart Refill Form is used to record the earliest expiration date for each of the medications and supply items in the crash cart.
   b. The Crash Cart Charge Form is used to record the earliest expiration date for each of the medications or supply items in the crash cart. The Crash Cart Refill Form is used to charge the nursing unit.
   c. The Crash Cart Charge Form is used to record the earliest expiration date for each of the medications and supply items in the crash cart. The Crash Cart Refill Form is used to charge the patient.
   d. The Crash Cart Charge Form is used to charge the patient. The Crash Cart Refill Form is used to record the earliest expiration date for each of the medications or supply items within the crash cart to be returned to the nursing unit.

5. In most states, appropriate expiration dating for items stored in a crash cart is a minimum of ____.
   a. one month
   b. two months
   c. six months
   d. one year

Thinking Like a Pharmacy Tech

1. Describe the ways that the pharmacy technician might directly or indirectly affect the code team's response to a patient who is in cardiac or respiratory arrest.

2. What are three ways that you might verify your state's acceptable expiration dating for crash cart medications or supply items?

 3. A pharmacy technician must juggle many different tasks throughout his or her day. How can you practice good time management? What techniques do you use to manage your time as a student that may serve you well on the job?

Lab 19 *Charging and Refilling a Crash Cart*

Crash Cart Charge Form

Medication/Supply Item	Par Level	Number to Charge Patient
Vented IV tubing	2	
Bacteriostatic normal saline 30 mL vial	4	
Dextrose 50% 25 gram syringe	1	
Sodium bicarbonate 8.4% 50 mL syringe	2	
Heparin 5,000 units/mL syringe	4	
Naloxone 0.4 mg/mL syringe	2	
Lidocaine 2% pre-filled syringe	2	
Dexamethasone 4 mg/mL vial	1	
Atropine 0.1 mg/mL 10 mL syringe	3	
Furosemide 100 mg/10 mL vial	2	
Acyclovir 500 mg vial	1	
Adenosine 3 mg/mL vial	1	
Calcium chloride 10% pre-filled syringe	2	
Potassium chloride 2 mEq/mL 20 mL vial	2	
Theophylline 400 mg in 500 mL IV bag	2	
Dopamine 1,600 mcg in 250 mL IV bag	1	
0.9% Sodium chloride 1,000 mL IV bag	4	
Dextrose 5% in water 1,000 mL IV bag	4	

Lab 19

Charging and Refilling a Crash Cart

Crash Cart Refill Form

Medication/Supply Item	Par Level	Expiration Date
Vented IV tubing	2	_____
Bacteriostatic normal saline 30 mL vial	4	_____
Dextrose 50% 25 gram syringe	1	_____
Sodium bicarbonate 8.4% 50 mL syringe	2	_____
Heparin 5,000 units/mL syringe	4	_____
Naloxone 0.4 mg/mL syringe	2	_____
Lidocaine 2% pre-filled syringe	2	_____
Dexamethasone 4 mg/mL vial	1	_____
Atropine 0.1 mg/mL 10 mL syringe	3	_____
Furosemide 100 mg/10 mL vial	2	_____
Acyclovir 500 mg vial	1	_____
Adenosine 3 mg/mL vial	1	_____
Calcium chloride 10% pre-filled syringe	2	_____
Potassium chloride 2 mEq/mL 20 mL vial	2	_____
Theophylline 400 mg in 500 mL IV bag	2	_____
Dopamine 1,600 mcg in 250 mL IV bag	1	_____
0.9% Sodium chloride 1,000 mL IV bag	4	_____
Dextrose 5% in water 1,000 mL IV bag	4	_____

Filling an Automated Drug Storage and Dispensing System

Lab 20

Objectives

- Demonstrate skill and accuracy in the process of filling an automated drug storage and dispensing system.
- Determine and discuss the rationale and procedures for using an automated drug storage and dispensing system for pharmacy products.

Supplies

- An Automated Drug Storage and Dispensing System Refill Request Form
- Access to a pharmacy lab stocked with items commonly found in an automated drug storage and dispensing system cabinet or tower
- Access to an automated drug storage and dispensing system cabinet or tower and its networked computer
- Access to a brand/generic handbook

Many large hospitals use an automated drug storage and dispensing system (ADSDS) to assist with storing, dispensing, tracking, and charging some pharmaceuticals. The ADSDS generally consists of a cabinet or tower with an attached laptop computer that is networked to the pharmacy department. Each floor or unit of the hospital commonly has such a system.

Several different types or brands of ADSDSs are used in the institutional pharmacy setting. Some of the more common systems include Pyxis, Accudose, SureMed, MedDispense, and Omnicell. Although the systems have some procedural differences, they are all very similar in how they store, dispense, and track pharmaceuticals.

Hospitals invest in an ADSDS for speed, accuracy, cost savings, and security. In particular, the system provides nursing staff with immediate access to many medications and supply items, allowing the staff to avoid waiting for the pharmacy to fill the order. Because the system automatically prints out an accurate list for cabinet refills and patient charging, the chance for human error is reduced and labor costs are saved. Most

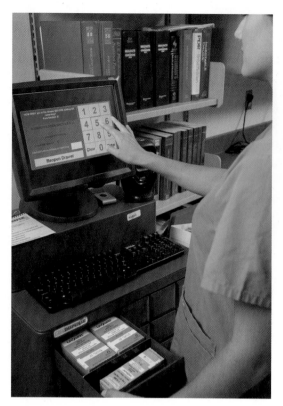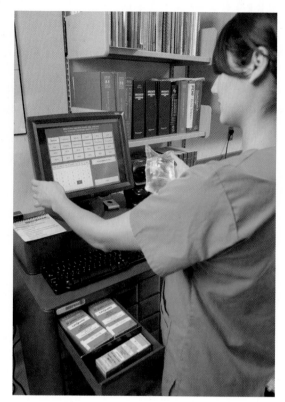

Pharmacy technician logging medications into the ADSDS (left) and placing drugs into specific drawers (right).

ADSDS discrepancy

A disagreement between the actual count of a medication in the ADSDS and the amount displayed on the verification screen

Drug diversion

Stealing or otherwise illegally taking or using drugs from the facility

importantly, the system offers a secure environment for pharmaceutical storage because each item is tracked along its path from the pharmacy to the nurse to the patient. Be careful to check and double-check your medication counts to avoid creating a count **discrepancy** and to prevent being suspected of the serious offense of **drug diversion**.

Your primary role in working with an ADSDS is to refill the system inventory according to the Refill Request Form. The ADSDS on each nursing unit automatically generates this Form. Each cabinet on each hospital unit or floor produces a separate Refill Form. Your job is to fill all the items on every Refill Form. In some institutions, you may also be responsible for delivering the medications to the unit and placing them into the individual ADSDS cabinets. In other settings, the nurse or unit assistant delivers and places the medications into the individual ADSDS.

Procedure

In this lab, you will refill medications for an automated drug storage and dispensing system (ADSDS). You will also properly enter the refilled items into the ADSDS cabinet. Your instructor may have you complete multiple repetitions of this lab to help you build speed and accuracy. It is vital that you pay close attention to accuracy with regard to the drug name, strength, number to refill, expiration date, computer entry, and proper placement within the ADSDS.

1 Verify acceptable expiration date requirements with your instructor before beginning this lab.

2 Look up the brand/generic names of any medications listed on the ADSDS Refill Request Form with which you are unfamiliar.

3 Find the first item to be filled. Make sure that what you are pulling from the pharmacy stock matches *exactly* what is ordered on the ADSDS Refill Request Form. The drug name, strength, dosage form, and amount ordered must all match those on the ADSDS Refill Request Form.

4 Pull out the correct number of that item and place it on an uncluttered section of counter or table top.

5 Check the expiration date of each dose to be sure it is acceptable. Remove expired doses or those with unacceptable dating, set them aside, and point them out to your instructor. Do not include these doses in your count for refilling the ADSDS.

6 Continue down the refill sheet, pulling the correct number of each requested item.
Tip: Your work with an ADSDS may require you to process Refill Request Forms for multiple nursing units. In such cases, be sure to keep the items from each Refill Request Form separate and clearly labeled so that you enter the correct items into each nursing unit's ADSDS.

7 Once you have pulled all of the items on the ADSDS Refill Request Form, arrange them in such a way that what is on the counter matches (from left to right) what is ordered on the ADSDS Refill Request Form (from top to bottom). This extra organizational step makes the checking process more efficient.

8 Write your name and today's date on the ADSDS Refill Request Form and ask for an instructor check.

9 Once your instructor has completed the check, take the ADSDS Refill Request Form and the medications to the ADSDS.

10 Enter your login and password, which have been provided by your instructor, into the computer. Enter the first medication name into the computer. The cabinet will automatically open the drawer (sometimes referred to as a cell) containing this medication.

Tip: Medications may be stored in the ADSDS by brand or generic name. Procedures may vary from state to state or between institutions.

11 Once the drawer opens, the computer will ask for verification of the medication count. Count the units (the exact number of pills, vials, bags, suppositories, etc.) in the drawer.

Tip: To avoid creating a count discrepancy, be sure to double-check the count in the drawer before verifying or denying the count in the computer.

12 If the count in the drawer matches the computer's count, answer "yes" or enter the matching quantity. If the count in the drawer does not match the computer's count, answer "no," or enter the correct quantity into the computer. The computer will generate a discrepancy, or error, report requiring later resolution by the nursing unit director and pharmacy quality assurance technician.

13 The computer will display the question "How many do you wish to add?" Enter the exact number of units (pills, vials, bags, suppositories, etc.) of the medication you are entering into the designated drawer.

14 The computer will ask you to verify the new count and close the drawer. Carefully follow the steps listed on the computer.

Tip: Again, to avoid creating a count discrepancy, be sure to double-check the count that you are adding before entering the number into the computer.

15 Repeat this process for each medication on the Refill Request Form.

16 Once you have entered all medications into the cabinet, log out of the computer. Logging out will cause the computer on the ADSDS to generate a receipt or printout. The receipt will list the actual count of everything in each drawer that you opened, track items added to the drawer, and highlight any discrepancies. Verify that the receipt contains your login name and the correct date.

17 **Conclusion:** Give the receipt and the completed ADSDS Refill Request Form to your instructor. On a separate sheet of paper, answer all questions in the following Lab Review section and turn in your answers to your instructor.

Lab Review

Check Your Understanding

1. What is/are the primary reason/reasons that a pharmacy might stock some medications in an automated drug storage and dispensing system?
   a. Nurses have immediate access to some necessary medications.
   b. The system helps prevent drug diversion or theft.
   c. The system reduces the need for manual charging for medications.
   d. All of the above

2. The proper procedure when filling an ADSDS Refill Request Form is to _____.
   a. pull out the correct medication, check to make sure it matches the Refill Request Form exactly, check the expiration date, and ask for an instructor check
   b. pull out the correct medication, check the expiration date, place it in the cabinet, and ask for an instructor check
   c. check the expiration date on the medication, place it in the cabinet, verify the count, and ask for an instructor check
   d. None of the above

3. The "receipt" refers to the _____.
   a. form that is used to refill medications for the ADSDS
   b. form that is used to refill medications for the 24 hr cart fill
   c. printout of what has been added to a specific cabinet or tower of an ADSDS and any discrepancies identified
   d. record of what has been added to the perpetual narcotic log of the ADSDS

4. In reference to adding medications to an ADSDS, the term "discrepancy" refers to _____.
   a. an error made in the process of filling the Refill Request Form
   b. a difference between the actual count of medication in a drawer within the automated drug storage and dispensing system cabinet and what the cabinet's computer states as being on hand
   c. a difference between the actual count of a narcotic in the perpetual log book and the remaining balance once the refill request has been filled
   d. an error made in the process of adding medications to the perpetual log book

5. As it relates to the process of filling an automated drug storage and dispensing system cabinet, the term "drug diversion" refers to a drug that is _____.
   a. diverted to the wrong nursing unit
   b. filled in error and diverted from the pharmacy
   c. removed from the cabinet by an unauthorized person, thereby creating an error in the drawer's medication count
   d. removed from the cabinet by a nurse or pharmacy technician for patient administration

Thinking Like a Pharmacy Tech

1. Consider the following scenario. What is the appropriate thing to do?

   Scenario: As you enter items into the automated drug storage and dispensing system cabinet on the nursing unit, a person wearing a scrub uniform approaches you and asks to use the cabinet to withdraw medications using your login and password.

2. What appropriate actions should you take if you have discovered a discrepancy or error that leads you to believe that someone may be diverting drugs?

 3. You may encounter patients working in the institutional pharmacy setting who are very ill. How can you provide compassionate care to these patients? How can you work through any misconceptions or fears you may have while maintaining professionalism?

Lab 20

Automated Drug Storage and
Dispensing System Refill Request Form

Medication Name and Strength	Number to Refill	Instructor Check
Acetaminophen 325 mg tablets	10	_____
Acetaminophen 500 mg caplets	8	_____
Ampicillin 125 mg vials	6	_____
Ampicillin 250 mg vials	3	_____
Ampicillin 500 mg vials	11	_____
Ampicillin 1,000 mg vials	2	_____
Bacteriostatic NS 30 mL vials	9	_____
Cimetidine 150 mg tablets	1	_____
Diphenhydramine 25 mg tablets	10	_____
Heparin lock flush 100 units/5 mL	6	_____
Furosemide 20 mg tablets	4	_____
Metoclopramide 5 mg/mL vial	3	_____
MOM 30 mL unit-dose cup	2	_____
Promethazine 25 mg/1 mL ampule	4	_____
D_5W 100 mL IVPB	2	_____
NS 50 mL IVPB	5	_____
D_5W 1,000 mL IV	2	_____

Medication Reconciliation

Lab 21

Objectives

- Describe the purpose of the medication reconciliation process.
- Describe the role of the pharmacy technician in the medication reconciliation process.
- Reconcile a patient-provided list of medications to a new or existing medical record.

Supplies

- *Pharmacy Labs for Technicians* textbook
- Drug reference book(s)

The Joint Commission

To learn more, search the web for The Joint Commission.

Institute for Safe Medication Practices

To learn more, search the web for Institute for Safe Medication Practices, or ISMP

Medication therapy and disease state management have grown increasingly complex. With steadily increasing options to effectively treat disease, the need for the healthcare team to maintain an accurate list of medications in the treatment of a hospital patient is very important. To ensure a patient's medication history is accurately maintained and updated in the continuum of care, The Joint Commission, has strongly emphasized the need for carefully documenting medication therapy throughout the treatment process within a hospital.

The weakest point for this communication, as identified by The Joint Commission and the Institute for Safe Medication Practices (ISMP), is when a patient is moved (transferred) from one care unit to another. During the transfer process, communication concerning the patient's treatment can break down due to the number of people involved, the lack of standardized procedures for moving a patient, potential for shift change, and other minor factors. When combined, all of these contributing factors—however small—can potentially lead to a medication error.

As a means to rectify and prevent further lapses in communication, The Joint Commission has included a reconciliation process in their medication management standards. The ISMP also strongly promotes this process as a means to eliminate medication errors. A pharmacy technician has a significant role in the medication reconciliation process.

One of the fastest growing areas of responsibility of a pharmacy tech-

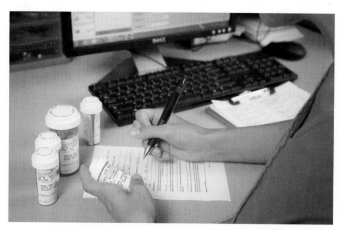

Pharmacy technician reviewing patient's prescription bottles.

nician lies in the medication reconciliation process. As a pharmacy technician, you may be asked to interview a patient and reconcile a list of medications at any point in the continuum of care. The most common points include admission and discharge, though pharmacy technicians may also help in the reconciliation process when patients present themselves to the emergency room or any other patient unit in the hospital. These units include Intensive Care, Intermediate Care, Labor and Delivery, Outpatient Surgery, and the Medical-Surgical Units.

Medication reconciliation may occur in many ways. Often a patient will bring his or her prescription bottles from home and the medication reconciliation technician must review each of the prescription bottles to determine if the prescriptions are still valid and currently being taken by the patient. Sometimes the technician will contact the prescriber or the pharmacy where the prescription was filled in order to get the most current medication information for the patient. However, often the first step is an initial interview with the patient, designated caregiver, or designated agent, followed by the review of a patient-provided list. The list is then transcribed to a document or a computer system for inclusion in the medical record as a reference for the physician or other healthcare providers to establish medication therapy while the patient is treated at the hospital.

A patient or their agent may not be able to provide accurate medication history due to injury, language barriers, being too young to communicate effectively, or a disability. In the event the patient cannot, or will not, communicate with the staff, does not know the details of their medication history, or is otherwise incapacitated, it may be necessary to call the patient's

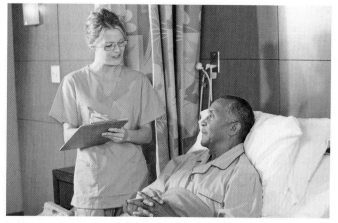

A pharmacy technician interviewing a patient about his medications.

local pharmacy (if identified), next of kin, pharmacy benefits provider, or insurance company to obtain the list of medications. This occurs more often than not, and while it is a potentially cumbersome process, it's important for you to work diligently to obtain the list and provide the highest level of care to each patient as you develop their medication history. The goal is to compile the best possible medication history during the reconciliation process.

The other equally important goal is to respect the dignity and privacy of the patient. You may be working in an area where many other people will be present, including patients, family members, healthcare providers, staff, and more. You will be speaking about protected health information under HIPAA, or the Health Information Portability and Accountability Act, and it is crucial you make a diligent effort to protect this information—even if it means asking other persons in the room to leave while you speak to the patient. Regardless of the reaction of the others, your duty is to protect the patient.

To properly obtain a patient's medication history through a direct interview of the patient or the patient's representative (family member, other healthcare provider, or insurance company), there are several steps to follow:

1. Identify yourself by full name, role, department, and the purpose for your visit.

2. Verify the identity of the patient to ensure you have the right patient and the right set of patient records. Each time you speak to a patient, even if it is the same patient, it is a best practice to verify the patient name, date of birth, and patient ID number. This may be accomplished by speaking to the patient and by looking at the patient identification bracelet.

3. If other persons are present in the room, ask the patient if they prefer other people leave the room while you discuss their personal and protected information.

4. Ask the patient to verify their height, weight, and allergies to ensure appropriate medication dosing. There are many medications used in a hospital that must be dosed according to this information.

5. Ask the patient to name each prescription medication they take, one at a time, providing the following information:
   a. Name
   b. Strength
   c. Route of administration
   d. Frequency of dosage
   e. Date/time of the most recent dose

6. Ask the patient to name each over-the-counter medication they take, one at a time, providing the following information:
   a. Name
   b. Strength
   c. Route of administration
   d. Frequency of dosage
   e. Date/time of the most recent dose

7. Ask the patient to name each herbal supplement or vitamin they take, one at a time, providing the following information:
   a. Name
   b. Strength
   c. Route of administration
   d. Frequency of dosage
   e. Date/time of the most recent dose

Take Note

While it may not seem important to obtain a list of over-the counter medications and herbal supplements, these items may interfere with prescription medications used in the hospital. Because of this, it is important for the medication history to be as accurate and complete as possible.

8. Once the list is completed, it may be necessary to transcribe it into a computer system or a fresh document, depending on the hospital's policies and procedures. Errors may have been made and changes may be needed to ensure accuracy.

Once completed, the list should be added to the patient chart by the healthcare staff as a point of reference for treatment and development of medication orders. In many cases, a patient may be able to provide you with their own list of medications and supplements. This will aid in the process, but it is still necessary to interview the patient or their representative for information on the last dose taken, if known. If this information is not known, it is important to note this on the completed document.

Once the process is finished, you may be asked to interview many more patients and complete their medication histories, or return to the pharmacy to assist in order preparation. Either way, the medication reconciliation process is crucial to medication safety, and should be treated with the utmost care.

Procedure

1 Using the information provided in the following patient medication lists (Figures 21.1, 21.2, and 21.3), complete the best possible medication reconciliation document.
Tip: Many times patient medication lists will contain spelling or other errors. You also have to read carefully to avoid misunderstanding a patient's handwriting.

2 If a piece of information is not known, make a note indicating as such—never guess. This could cause harm to the patient.

3 The use of signa abbreviations is accepted in many cases; however, there are many abbreviations prohibited in a hospital setting. When preparing the medication reconciliation document, be mindful to avoid these restricted abbreviations: www.paradigmcollege.net/pharmlabs2e/jointcommission

4 When you have finished the list, be sure to fill in the "Created by" line with your name, department (Rx), and the date.

5 Submit the completed forms to your instructor for review and grading.

Take Note

Medication reconciliation is a critical step in the continuum of care. Many medications sound alike and have similar dosing. When preparing a patient's medication history, a critical eye for detail is vital for the well-being and continued safety of the patient.

Lab Review

Check Your Understanding

1. When preparing to obtain medication history from a patient, the pharmacy technician identifies the patient by which of the following:
   a. Home phone number
   b. Social Security number
   c. Patient Identification Number
   d. Driver's license number

2. Which of the following organizations included medication reconciliation in the medication management standards?
   a. The Joint Commission
   b. Pharmacy Board
   c. ISMP
   d. ASHP

3. Medication reconciliation is conducted at which point of patient care?
   a. Admission
   b. Transfer
   c. Discharge
   d. All of the above

4. Medication reconciliation processes were developed to address a breakdown in:
   a. communication
   b. care
   c. transfer
   d. medications

5. Which of the following may be reasons which prevent a patient from giving a medication history to the technician?
   a. language barrier
   b. age
   c. disability
   d. all of the above

Thinking Like a Pharmacy Tech

1. Medication reconciliation can be a complex process involving many lines of communication between the patient, the patient's representatives, and other healthcare providers. What strategies can you use to ensure there is no breakdown or confusion when communicating with people involved in the process?

2. The Institute for Safe Medication Practices published an article entitled Building a Case for Medication Reconciliations (available at www.paradigmcollege.net/pharmlabs2e/ismp). Select three of the errors described in the article and identify a process to prevent each error from occurring with other patients.

3. Often a pharmacy technician performing medication reconciliation will have to ask people in the room to leave due to HIPAA considerations. How would you explain the importance of this action to them?

FIGURE 21.1 **A handwritten form with worn edges and multiple creases from having been folded and kept in a woman's wallet for an extended period.**

The patient is sitting in the ER in acute care after having an incident at a super market. She is in pleasant spirits since she arrived. She stated she took her medication through last night, but did not take anything today, April 17, 2015. She did take one Nitroglycerin tablet at the super market this morning around 7 a.m. She states she is allergic to shellfish and penicillin. In her interview, she states she is 5 feet 8 inches tall, and weighs approximately 250 pounds.

Prescription Medications	
Medication Name	**Dose/How often?**
Nitrogliserin	0.4 mg under the tongue for chest pain
Asperin	81mg in the morning
Alprazalam	1mg every 6 hours or as needed for my ~~sex~~ nerves
Glocotrol	5mg 2x/day
Xalatan Eye Drops	1 in left eye when I go to bed
Humulin 70/30	50 units in the morning
Lantis	22 units at bed time

Lab 21 **229**

FIGURE 21.2 **A handwritten list of medications and supplements provided to a pharmacy technician from a family member of an incapacitated patient.**

In an interview with the family member, Gloria, it was stated the patient, George Miller, was very relatively compliant. They were at the movies, when George collapsed around 2 p.m. George had taken his medications at 8 a.m. and through noon today, Saturday, February 28, 2015. He takes his evenings medications around 7 p.m. and nighttime medications around 10 p.m. George has no allergies. He was born on September 8, 1947, is 6 feet, 2 inches tall, and weighs 200 pounds.

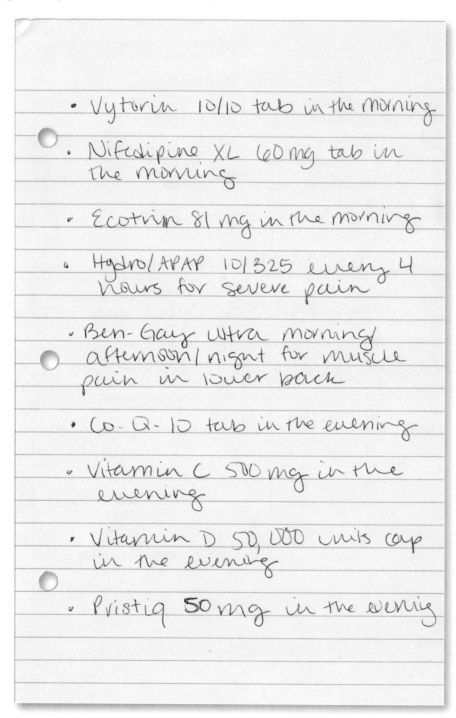

FIGURE 21.3 **A typed document from a local pharmacy faxed to the hospital emergency room at the request of a pharmacy technician.**

The patient arrived unconscious, but had an old prescription bottle in her purse.

The Corner Drug Store
875 Paradigm Way – Austin, Texas 78704
(512) 555-1212 – telephone

PATIENT PRESCRIPTION HISTORY REPORT

PATIENT INFORMATION

FELICIA JOHANSEN
1457 North Lamar Blvd
Austin, Texas 78738
(512) 555-1212

DOB: 04/27/1937
Height: 5ft 7in Weight: 115lbs

ALLERGIES: PCN, Codeine

Insurance
Apollo Health (115609)
ID: GT334918; Grp: RX12
PC: 00

Prescription	QTY	Directions	Prescriber	Date Written	Last Filled
PLAVIX 10MG TABLETS	30	TAKE 1 TABLET BY MOUTH DAILY	CARDOZA, FRANCISCO MD	01/12/15	02/13/15
LISINOPRIL 10MG TABLETS	30	TAKE 1 TABLET BY MOUTH DAILY	CARDOZA, FRANCISCO MD	01/12/15	02/13/15
SYNTHROID 0.05MG TABLETS	30	TAKE 1 TABLET BY MOUTH EACH MORNING BEFORE BREAKFAST	CARDOZA, FRANCISCO MD	01/12/15	02/13/15
LIPITOR 10MG TABLETS	30	TAKE 1 TABLET MY MOUTH AT BEDTIME	CARDOZA, FRANCISCO MD	01/12/15	02/13/15
PROTONIX 40MG TABLETS	30	TAKE 1 TABLET BY MOUTH EACH MORNING FOR GERD.	CARDOZA, FRANCISCO MD	01/12/15	02/13/15
ROZEREM 8MG TABLETS	10	TAKE 1 TABLET BY MOUTH AT BEDTIME AS NEEDED FOR SLEEP	CARDOZA, FRANCISCO MD	10/08/14	12/10/14

Lab 21   *Medication Reconciliation*

PARADIGM HOSPITAL MEDICATION RECONCILIATION DOCUMENT						
PATIENT INFORMATION NAME _____ D.O.B. _____ GENDER: ☐ MALE ☐ FEMALE			LIST OF ALLERGIES ____ Initial here for NO KNOWN ALLERGIES		Height (inches) _____ Weight (kg) _____	
Medication Name	Dose	Route	Frequency	Special Instructions	Last Dose	Status
Alprazolam	0.5mg	PO	Q 4 hours	PRN Anxiety	02/22/15 1645	EXAMPLE
						☐ ACTIVE ☐ D/C
						☐ ACTIVE ☐ D/C
						☐ ACTIVE ☐ D/C
						☐ ACTIVE ☐ D/C
						☐ ACTIVE ☐ D/C
						☐ ACTIVE ☐ D/C
						☐ ACTIVE ☐ D/C
						☐ ACTIVE ☐ D/C
						☐ ACTIVE ☐ D/C
						☐ ACTIVE ☐ D/C
Please provide the name, relationship, and phone number for the source of information contained on this document if other than patient:						

Created by Name/Credential: _____ Dept: _____ Date: _____

Reviewed by Name/Credential: _____ Dept: _____ Date: _____

Ordered by physician: _____ Date: _____

Lab 21   *Medication Reconciliation*

PARADIGM HOSPITAL MEDICATION RECONCILIATION DOCUMENT

PATIENT INFORMATION	LIST OF ALLERGIES	Height (inches) / Weight (kg)
NAME _____ D.O.B. _____ GENDER: ☐ MALE ☐ FEMALE	____ Initial here for NO KNOWN ALLERGIES	_____ _____

Medication Name	Dose	Route	Frequency	Special Instructions	Last Dose	Status
						☐ ACTIVE ☐ D/C
						☐ ACTIVE ☐ D/C
						☐ ACTIVE ☐ D/C
						☐ ACTIVE ☐ D/C
						☐ ACTIVE ☐ D/C
						☐ ACTIVE ☐ D/C
						☐ ACTIVE ☐ D/C
						☐ ACTIVE ☐ D/C
						☐ ACTIVE ☐ D/C
						☐ ACTIVE ☐ D/C
						☐ ACTIVE ☐ D/C

Please provide the name, relationship, and phone number for the source of information contained on this document if other than patient:

Created by Name/Credential: _____ Dept: _____ Date: _____

Reviewed by Name/Credential: _____ Dept: _____ Date: _____

Ordered by physician: _____ Date: _____

Lab 21   *Medication Reconciliation*

PARADIGM HOSPITAL MEDICATION RECONCILIATION DOCUMENT

PATIENT INFORMATION	LIST OF ALLERGIES	Height (inches)

NAME _____

D.O.B. _____

GENDER: ☐ MALE   ☐ FEMALE

____ Initial here for NO KNOWN ALLERGIES

Height (inches) _____

Weight (kg) _____

Medication Name	Dose	Route	Frequency	Special Instructions	Last Dose	Status
						☐ ACTIVE ☐ D/C
						☐ ACTIVE ☐ D/C
						☐ ACTIVE ☐ D/C
						☐ ACTIVE ☐ D/C
						☐ ACTIVE ☐ D/C
						☐ ACTIVE ☐ D/C
						☐ ACTIVE ☐ D/C
						☐ ACTIVE ☐ D/C
						☐ ACTIVE ☐ D/C
						☐ ACTIVE ☐ D/C
						☐ ACTIVE ☐ D/C

Please provide the name, relationship, and phone number for the source of information contained on this document if other than patient:

Created by Name/Credential: _____ Dept: _____ Date: _____

Reviewed by Name/Credential: _____ Dept: _____ Date: _____

Ordered by physician: _____ Date: _____

Unit

4

Extemporaneous Compounding

A day in the life of a pharmacy technician...

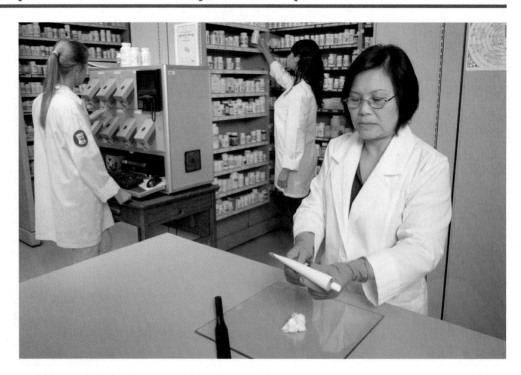

Grasshoppers Solution, Constanzi's Solution, testosterone cream, medicinal lollipops, pain capsules ... preparing compounded prescriptions such as these are all in a day's work for the pharmacy technician in the extemporaneous compounding environment.

Pharmacy technicians with special training in extemporaneous compounding prepare medications for patients who require a drug or dosage form that is not commercially available. Some patients require medications that are free of allergenic inactive ingredients such as dyes or preservatives; other patients require unique combinations or dosages of medication. Certain medications that may only be available as a pill might be ground into a powder and administered topically based on the patient's individual needs.

Pharmacy technicians who prepare extemporaneously compounded pharmaceuticals must have strict attention to detail in order to prepare the medication according to a specific recipe.

This unit will guide you through essential tasks related to extemporaneous compounding including use of a mortar and pestle, digital scale, weighing boat, and various graduated cylinders. You will learn how to prepare solutions, ointments, and creams, according to a pharmacy recipe. These tasks are the foundational aspects of extemporaneous compounding.

Reconstituting Powders

Lab 22

Objectives

- Demonstrate skill in measuring diluent and reconstituting powder medications for oral use.
- Demonstrate competence in calculations related to reconstituting powder medications for oral use.
- Discuss the rationale for and procedures related to reconstituting powder medication for oral use.
- Practice common pharmacy calculations related to the preparation of oral liquid medications.
- Become familiar with the compounding log as a means of recording the measurements, ingredients, and procedures used in compounding nonsterile products.

Supplies

- Augmentin 125 mg/5 mL (100 mL bottle)
- Reconstitube® (or similar device; 100 mL or larger attached to a water supply)
- Auxiliary labels
- Medication label
- Calculator

Introduction to Extemporaneous Compounding for Labs 22–27

Compounding

Preparing individualized medications per prescription order

Prior to the mass production of prepared pharmaceutical products in the 1940s and 1950s, pharmacies prepared individualized medications per a prescription order from a prescriber. This individualized preparation was termed **compounding** and included compressing tablets, creating suspensions, and filling capsules with a requested strength or amount of medication. Pharmacy technicians are still called upon to perform many types of extemporaneous, or nonsterile, compounding procedures, including preparing oral solutions, suppositories, capsules, troches, lozenges, creams, ointments, gels, and pastes. Today, compounding is required under several circumstances, including as a response to patients' unique needs, manufacturer-based difficulties, and physician-initiated requests. This type of compounding is often referred to as "extemporaneous compounding." Additionally, extemporaneous compounding is sometimes referred to as "non-sterile compounding."

While compounding in the pharmacy lab, safety, accuracy, and proper record keeping are essential. These safety precautions are used both in the lab setting, and also in practice. In most instances, you must wear gloves throughout all compounding procedures in order to protect (1) yourself from exposure to the medication, (2) the medication from degradation caused by skin cells and oils, and (3) the patient from potentially contaminated medications. Depending on the ingredients used to prepare the compound, you may also be required to wear safety glasses, a face mask, and/or a protective smock. Refer to the individual recipe for safety requirements. Accuracy is crucial in drug measurement and dose calculations. Some compounding lab procedures provide one or more **recipes**, which list the exact quantity of each ingredient. Other procedures provide dosage information and require your calculations to prepare the final product. Finally, you must keep careful and precise records each time you compound a prescription, by creating a **compounding log**, an official, detailed record of the processes and materials used. Because requirements for compounding-log recordkeeping may vary widely among states and individual facilities, you should check with your instructor about specific, local record-keeping procedures for compounded pharmaceutical products. An example of a compounding log is shown in Figure 22.1.

Recipe

A listing of the exact quantity of each ingredient and the processes required to compound a particular prescription

Compounding log

An official record of the processes and materials used to compound a prescription

Take Note

You must keep accurate records when preparing extemporaneous compounds. Each time you compound a prescription, even if it is a product you have previously prepared, you will create an entry in a compounding log. The compounding log contains detailed information and commonly includes: the name of the final compound; quantity prepared; a copy of the patient label, recipe, or instructions; the name, lot number, and quantity of all products and ingredients used; and a record of the steps followed to prepare the prescription. In addition, the compounding log will require you to create a unique lot number and expiration date to easily identify the compounded product. The process for recordkeeping in a compounding log may vary widely among states and individual facilities.

Reconstitute

To change into liquid form by adding water or other fluid to a powder

Many liquids and suspensions for oral use are supplied as commercially prepared powders that must first be **reconstituted**—changed into liquid form by having water or another fluid added to them—before they can be dispensed to the patient. When recon-

FIGURE 22.1   Pharmacy Compounding Log Sheet

Product Label

Date Prepared

Pharmacy Lot Number

Strength

AFFIX PHARMACY LABEL HERE

Quantity Prepared

Quantity Packaged

	Manufacturer's Lot Number	Ingredient Name	Amount Needed	Measured By	Verified By
1					
2					
3					
4					
5					
6					
7					
8					

Directions for Preparation:

Completion Time: _____

Prepared By

Auxiliary Labeling

Approved By

Date   Expiration Date

Diluent

The liquid added to a powder during reconstitution

stituting a powder medication, you should take special care to measure the proper amount of **diluent**—the liquid that is added to the powder—to ensure the correct concentration of medication. Facilities may vary in using distilled water, sterile water, or tap water for reconstitution.

Reconstituting powder medications requires particular equipment. Some facilities might have you use a graduated cylinder or similar product to measure diluent volumes. Easy and accurate diluent measurements can be made with a Reconstitube®, a modified graduated cylinder with two tubes attached. The upper tube connects the cylinder to a supply of water or other liquid, and the lower tube, which is open-ended, enters the medication bottle.

When you open a small clamp on the upper tube, diluent flows from the liquid source into the graduated cylinder of the Reconstitube®. Opening the lower tube allows the liquid to flow from the cylinder into the powder. You must add the diluent to the powder in two stages, shaking the solution at both stages to thoroughly mix the powder into an oral solution. To complete the reconstitution process, affix a medication label and appropriate auxiliary labels to the oral solution bottle.

In some instances, after preparing an amount of liquid medication, you will be asked to take the next step in getting the medication ready for patients: performing calculations to determine the volume of an individual dose. You will use a standard formula, as given below. Always start with the information that is provided on the label. In this case, Augmentin will have a concentration of 125 mg/5 mL once it has been diluted. Given that information, how many milliliters would you need to give a patient for the following doses: Augmentin 200 mg and Augmentin 250 mg?

Use the following formulas to calculate the doses:

$$\frac{125 \text{ mg}}{5 \text{ mL}} = \frac{200 \text{ mg}}{x \text{ mL}} \qquad \frac{125 \text{ mg}}{5 \text{ mL}} = \frac{250 \text{ mg}}{x \text{ mL}}$$

In order to solve for x, the unknown volume, you will cross multiply and then divide. (To review the cross multiplication process, refer to Lab 18, Preparing Oral Syringes.) In these two examples, your calculations will show you that a 200 mg dose of Augmentin is 8 mL and a 250 mg dose is 10 mL.

Procedure

In this lab, you will use a Reconstitube® (or similar device) to reconstitute a bottle of Augmentin suspension for oral use. You will measure an appropriate amount of diluent (in this case, water), add it to the powder medication, prepare the powder medication for dispensing, and practice related dose calculations. Prepare a compounding log, if and as directed by your instructor, to record the steps and ingredients that you use.

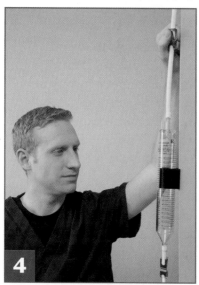

Pharmacy technician opening the upper clamp of a Reconstitube®.

1 Gather the supplies listed for this lab, set them on the workspace, and arrange them in an easily accessible and organized manner.

2 Wash your hands thoroughly, and, if directed to do so by your instructor, put on gloves, and wear them throughout the procedure.

3 Bring the Augmentin bottle to the area in the pharmacy where the Reconstitube® is located. Ensure that the lower clamp on the Reconstitube® is securely closed by pinching the clamp until it clicks shut.

4 Open the upper clamp on the Reconstitube® by pinching the clamp until it clicks open. You will see water from the storage container begin

flowing into the tube. Allow the water to flow freely into the Reconstitube® until it reaches approximately the 70 mL mark (You will ultimately be filling the Reconstitube® to the 90 mL mark).

5 Grasp the upper clamp on the Reconstitube® and squeeze softly such that the flow of water slows. While applying slight pressure to the upper clamp, allow water to continue slowly filling the Reconstitube®. When the tube is filled to the desired volume of 90 mL, close the upper clamp by pinching it shut until it clicks. See Figure 22.2 for an illustration of this technique.
Tip: *When reconstituting powder medications, read the accompanying package insert to verify the diluent amount prior to measuring it in the Reconstitube®. The diluent volume will be different with each medication.*

6 Ask for an instructor check of the diluent volume in the Reconstitube®.

7 Grasp the Augmentin bottle and carefully tap it against your palm or a countertop so that the powder is dislodged from the bottom of the bottle and moves freely within the container. Remove the cap from the Augmentin bottle.

FIGURE 22.2
Reconstitube® components

Illustration of a Reconstitube® containing 90 mL of diluent; notice that the lowest point of the meniscus rests on the 90 mL line.

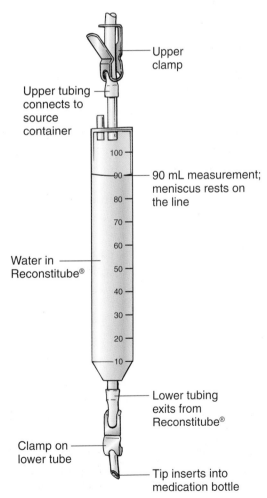

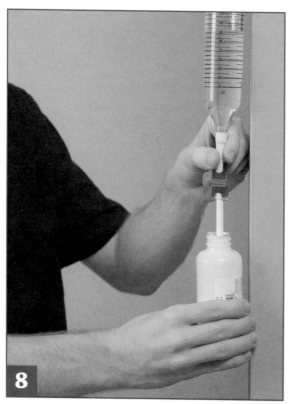

8 Place the tip of the lower tube of the Reconstitube® into the mouth of the Augmentin bottle and, while holding the medication bottle in place, open the lower clamp and allow water to flow into the bottle, maintaining slight pressure on the lower clamp to control the flow of diluent.

Tip: To prevent cross-contamination, take care not to get any powder on the lower tube.

Pharmacy technician opening the lower Reconstitube® clamp, which allows water to flow into the medication bottle.

9 When approximately one-third (or 30 milliliters) of the total volume of diluent has been added to the medication bottle, close the lower clamp.

Tip: You should add only a one-third portion of the diluent to the medication bottle at first, allowing the powder to dissolve gradually into the diluent. If you add all the liquid at once, the medication powder would likely stick to the bottom of the medication bottle and resist dilution. In addition, the water could overflow and you would end up with lost medication.

10 Recap the medication bottle and shake it vigorously.

11 Once again, remove the cap of the medication bottle and place the tip of the lower tube of the Reconstitube® into the mouth of the bottle. Open the lower clamp and allow all of the remaining diluent to flow freely into the medication bottle.

12 Tightly recap the medication bottle and again shake it vigorously. Verify that the powder has been fully incorporated into the diluent and that no powder remains stuck to the bottom of the Augmentin bottle. If you notice any undissolved powder, continue to shake the medication bottle until the drug is fully dissolved and the dilution is complete.

13 Affix the patient label to the medication bottle as directed by your instructor. Also affix Shake Well and Refrigerate labels to the medication bottle.

14 Prepare the compounding log, if and as directed by your instructor.

15 **Conclusion:** Present your log, if created, your calculations, and your final product to your instructor for a final check. On a separate sheet of paper, answer all questions in the following Lab Review section and turn in your answers to your instructor.

Lab Review

Check Your Understanding

1. If a Reconstitube® is unavailable, what other compounding equipment would be appropriate to use for measuring the diluent?
   a. mortar and pestle
   b. amber bottle
   c. graduated cylinder
   d. oral syringe

2. Once the diluent has been added to the powder medication, what is the final concentration in milligrams per milliliters?
   a. 25 mg/mL
   b. 50 mg/mL
   c. 100 mg/mL
   d. 250 mg/mL

3. Based on the concentration that was determined in question 2, how much of this medication would be needed for a 125 mg dose?
   a. 2 mL
   b. 3 mL
   c. 5 mL
   d. 10 mL

4. If the physician orders "Augmentin 125 mg po qid," how much of this solution would be needed for a 24-hour period?
   a. 5 mL
   b. 10 mL
   c. 15 mL
   d. 20 mL

5. When flowing from the source container through the Reconstitube®, diluent contacts the components in which order?
   a. source container, upper tube, upper clamp, graduated cylinder, lower tube, lower clamp, tip
   b. source container, graduated cylinder, upper clamp, lower clamp, tip
   c. source container, upper tube, upper clamp, lower clamp, lower tube, graduated cylinder, tip
   d. source container, lower tube, lower clamp, upper tube, upper clamp, graduated cylinder, tip

Thinking Like a Pharmacy Tech

1. Why is it important to add only one-third of the diluent at first, saving the remaining two-thirds until after the medication bottle has been vigorously shaken?

2. What are two ways that an oral liquid medication dose might be administered?

 3. Why is being a good listener an important skill for a pharmacy technician to possess? How important are good listening skills in the community pharmacy versus the institutional pharmacy?

Filling Capsules

Lab 23

Objectives

- Demonstrate proficiency in the process of compounding capsules from other dosage forms.
- Demonstrate skill in the punch method used to fill empty capsules.
- Demonstrate skill in use of laboratory equipment used in compounding.
- Become familiar with the compounding log as a means of recording the measurements, ingredients, and procedures used in compounding nonsterile products.

Supplies

- 10 placebo or metronidazole 500 mg tablets
- 6 empty gelatin capsules, size 0
- Counting tray and counting spatula
- Mortar and pestle
- Glass ointment slab
- 8- or 10-inch stainless steel spatula
- Digital balance that provides metric unit weights and displays three decimal spaces (e.g., 1.001 g)
- Clean, dry gauze pad or cloth
- Prescription vial for packaging the compounded capsules
- Weighing boat or paper

Introduction to Extemporaneous Compounding for Labs 22–27

Compounding

Preparing individualized medications per prescription order

Note: If you have completed Lab 22, you may skip the first two paragraphs.
Prior to the mass production of prepared pharmaceutical products in the 1940s and 1950s, pharmacies prepared individualized medications per a prescription order from a prescriber. This individualized preparation was termed **compounding** and included compressing tablets, creating suspensions, and filling capsules with a requested strength or amount of medication. Pharmacy technicians are still called upon to perform many types of extemporaneous, or nonsterile, compounding procedures, including

245

Recipe

A listing of the exact quantity of each ingredient and the processes required to compound a particular prescription

Compounding log

An official record of the processes and materials used to compound a prescription

Punch method

A technique for filling capsules from a leveled cake of drug powder

Triturate

To break up or grind into smaller pieces

Particulate

A powder or fine-textured material

preparing oral solutions, suppositories, capsules, troches, lozenges, creams, ointments, gels, and pastes. Today, compounding is required under several circumstances, including as a response to patients' unique needs, manufacturer-based difficulties, and physician requests. This type of compounding is often referred to as "extemporaneous compounding."

While compounding in the pharmacy lab, safety, accuracy, and proper record keeping are essential. These safety precautions are used both in the lab setting, and also in practice. In most instances, you must wear gloves throughout all compounding procedures in order to protect (1) yourself from exposure to the medication, (2) the medication from degradation caused by skin cells and oils, and (3) the patient from potentially contaminated medications. Depending on the ingredients used to prepare the compound, you may also be required to wear safety glasses. Refer to the individual recipe for safety requirements. Accuracy is crucial in drug measurement and dose calculations. Some compounding lab procedures provide one or more **recipes**, which list the exact quantity of each ingredient. Other procedures provide dosage information and require your calculations to prepare the final product. Finally, you must keep careful and precise records each time you compound a prescription, by creating a **compounding log**, an official, detailed record of the processes and materials used. Because requirements for compounding log record keeping may vary widely between states and individual facilities, you must check with your instructor about specific, local record-keeping procedures for compounded pharmaceutical products.

Although the practice of filling capsules in today's pharmacy is uncommon, it is still used. One method of filling capsules is known as the **punch method.** This method gets its name from the filling technique used—punching the capsules into a leveled cake of powder. Filling capsules using the punch method can be messy because you are dealing with large amounts of powder. Despite this challenge, you must maintain accuracy. When preparing the compounded prescription, work carefully and take your time. To create the powder, you will use a mortar and pestle to **triturate** tablets into a fine, uniform **particulate**. Adding and removing small amounts of powder from the capsules and weighing and reweighing them may be frustrating. However, you may also find it rewarding because you are preparing a specific product for a specific patient using essential ingredients.

Procedure

In this lab, you will practice using the punch method to prepare the number of capsules requested by prescription. Metronidazole is a manufactured product, but it is produced in tablet form. Because some patients have a difficult time swallowing tablets, a physician has asked your pharmacy to

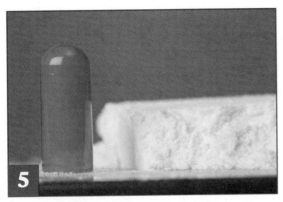

Powder leveled into a cake approximately one-half the height of the empty capsule body.

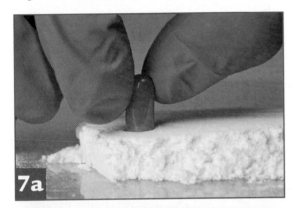

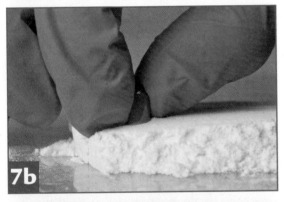

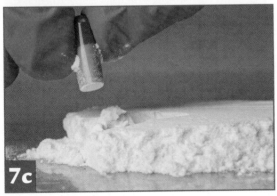

The punch method of capsule preparation.

compound tablets into capsules. You can help by filling five capsules to the requested weight (and preparing a compounding log, if and as directed by your instructor, to record the steps and ingredients that you use). In this case, a compounding formula is not needed; you will simply be given the recipe as the steps proceed.

1 Set your supplies on the workspace and arrange them in an easily accessible and organized manner. Visually inspect them to ensure that they are clean. If they are not, wash and dry them before use.

2 Wash your hands thoroughly, put on gloves, and wear them throughout the procedure.

3 Using the counting tray, count 10 tablets from the stock bottle and place them into the mortar. Use the pestle to triturate (break and grind) the tablets into a fine, uniform, particulate (powder).

4 Pour the contents of the mortar onto the ointment slab and with the spatula, scrape the sides of the mortar to get as much powder as possible out of the vessel and onto the slab.

5 Using the spatula, form the powder into a leveled cake approximately one-half the height of the empty capsule body.

6 Remove the capsule cap (the smaller section of the empty capsule) from five of the empty capsules and set them aside. Place the five capsule bodies (the larger sections of the empty capsules) on the ointment slab. Leave the sixth capsule intact.

7 Grasp the larger section of an empty capsule, open side down, with your thumb and forefinger. Punch the open capsule into the cake of powder (7a). When you reach the bottom of the powder, rotate the capsule slightly (7b), gently pinch the open end of the capsule, and withdraw the capsule from the powder (7c).

Tip: Do not use a scooping motion when removing the capsule body. Rather, be sure to pull it straight up and out of the powder cake.

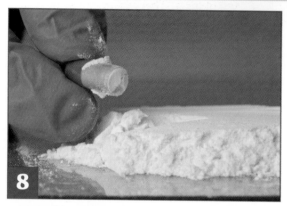

Filled capsule being withdrawn from powder.

8 Punch the capsule into the powder a second time, keeping the open end of the capsule pinched until you reach the top of the powder cake and then open the capsule just as you reach the cake, pushing into the powder. When you reach the bottom of the powder, rotate the capsule slightly, gently pinch the open end of the capsule, and withdraw the capsule from the powder.

9 Hold the capsule body with the open end upward, being careful not to spill any powder from the capsule. Place the cap of the capsule back onto the body of the capsule and set aside.

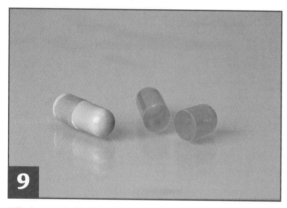

Filled capsule (left) and empty capsule (right). Both capsules will be weighed in the next several steps.

Tip: Some capsules have smooth bodies that allow for easy removal and application of the capsule top. Others, however, have a ridge in the middle of the capsule that acts as a locking mechanism. If you have ridged capsules, be careful not to reattach the capsule too tightly. You may not be able to reopen the capsule to adjust the weight of the capsule contents without damaging it. The pharmacy cannot dispense a damaged capsule.

10 Ensure that the digital scale is on a flat surface and set it level, following directions in the scale's user manual. Turn it on and allow it to zero.

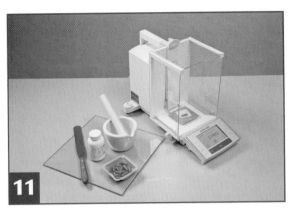

11

Empty capsule being weighed on a digital scale.

11 Place the intact, empty capsule (the sixth capsule) on the weighing pan and allow the scale to stabilize and provide a reading.

12 Press the "**tare**" or "re-zero" button. This resets the scale to zero and accounts for the weight of the capsule itself when weighing a capsule plus contents. The scale is now set to weigh only the capsule contents.

Tare

The container weight itself, or to allow for container weight when weighing an item or substance

13 Remove the empty capsule from the scale pan. Gently wipe the exterior of the filled capsule with the gauze pad to remove excess powder. Place the filled capsule on the pan and take the reading.

14 If this initial weight is *greater than* the required amount of 500 mg (the amount indicated by the prescription), open the capsule and gently tap out some powder onto the powder cake. Reseal, wipe, and reweigh the capsule, repeating the process until the desired weight is reached. However, if the initial weight of the capsule is *less than* the required amount, reshape the powder into a leveled cake as in Step 5, open the capsule, and repeat the punching process. Reseal, wipe, and reweigh the capsule. Repeat the process until the desired weight is reached. *Tip: You should do your best to fill the capsule to the exact amount of 500 mg. However, a margin of error of one or two milligrams is allowable for this lab.*

15 Reshape the powder into a leveled cake (Step 5), and perform the punching, weighing, and quantity-adjusting process (Steps 7–14) for the remaining four capsules.

16 Gently wipe the exterior of the five filled capsules with the gauze pad one more time to remove excess powder. Ask for an instructor check: he or she will verify the weight of each capsule. Once they are approved, place the five compounded capsules into a vial.

17 Wash, dry, and put away all supplies and clean up the work area. Prepare the compounding log, if and as directed by your instructor.

18 **Conclusion:** Present your log, if created, and your final product to your instructor for verification. On a separate sheet of paper, answer all questions in the following Lab Review section and turn in your answers to your instructor.

Lab Review

Check Your Understanding

1. The act of trituration _____ and _____ substances into _____ particles.
   a. compresses, binds, larger
   b. compresses, binds, smaller
   c. grinds, breaks, smaller
   d. grinds, breaks, larger

2. The tare button on a scale _____ the weight of the item on the weighing pan.
   a. adds/increases
   b. removes/zeroes out
   c. records/memorizes
   d. multiplies/increases

3. A ridge around the body of a capsule acts as _____.
   a. a locking mechanism
   b. a sanitary device
   c. a counter weight
   d. an opening mechanism

4. The powder cake used in punch-filling capsules is a leveled mound of triturated powder equal to the full height of the empty capsule.
   a. true
   b. false

5. The act of filling capsules in nonsterile compounding is commonly known as the _____ method.
   a. punch
   b. scoop
   c. push
   d. fill

Thinking Like a Pharmacy Tech

1. The act of compounding was once widely debated as an illegal practice. It was not until the FDA Modernization Act of 1997 that compounding was established as a legal practice. Why do you think this practice might have been considered illegal?

2. Since pharmaceutical companies invest so much time and expense in developing medications, it could be argued that these readily available manufactured products should be used for all patients instead of compounding separate preparations. Present your argument as to whether pharmacies should continue to compound.

3. What are good verbal communication skills? How are these important to the job of a pharmacy technician?

Creating Suspensions from Tablets

Lab 24

Objectives

- Demonstrate proficiency in the process of compounding an oral suspension from tablets.
- Demonstrate competence in mathematical calculations related to the preparation of an oral suspension from tablets.
- Discuss the procedure and rationale for compounding oral suspensions from tablets.
- Become familiar with the compounding log as a means of recording the measurements, ingredients, and procedures used in compounding nonsterile products.

Supplies

- A balance or scale (digital or otherwise)
- Two weighing boats
- Mortar and pestle
- Compounding spatula
- Beaker or Erlenmeyer flask (250 mL or larger)
- Stirring rod
- Gloves
- Metronidazole 500 mg tablets (bulk bottle) (or placebo)
- Syrpalta 200 mL (or similar)
- Amber bottle for liquid medications (8 ounce or larger)
- "Shake Well" auxiliary label
- Calculator

Introduction to Extemporaneous Compounding for Labs 22–27

Compounding

Preparing individualized medications per prescription order

Note: If you have completed Lab 22, you may skip the first two paragraphs.
Prior to the mass production of prepared pharmaceutical products in the 1940s and 1950s, pharmacies prepared individualized medications per a prescription order from a prescriber. This individualized preparation was termed **compounding** and included compressing tablets, creating suspensions, and filling capsules with a requested strength or amount of medication. Pharmacy technicians are still called upon to perform many types of

251

extemporaneous, or nonsterile, compounding procedures, including preparing oral solutions, suppositories, capsules, troches, lozenges, creams, ointments, gels, and pastes. Today, compounding is required under several circumstances, including as a response to patients' unique needs, manufacturer-based difficulties, and physician requests. This type of compounding is often referred to as "extemporaneous compounding."

While compounding in the pharmacy lab, safety, accuracy, and proper record keeping are essential These safety precautions are used both in the lab setting, and also in practice. In most instances, you must wear gloves throughout all compounding procedures in order to protect (1) yourself from exposure to the medication, (2) the medication from degradation caused by skin cells and oils, and (3) the patient from potentially contaminated medications. In addition, some compounding procedures will require you to wear safety glasses. Refer to the individual recipe for safety precautions. Accuracy is crucial in drug measurement and dose calculations. Some compounding lab procedures provide one or more **recipes**, which list the exact quantity of each ingredient. Other procedures provide dosage information and require your calculations to prepare the final product. Finally, you must keep careful and precise records each time you compound a prescription, by creating a **compounding log**, an official, detailed record of the processes and materials used. Because requirements for compounding log record keeping may vary widely between states and individual facilities, you must check with your instructor about specific, local record-keeping procedures for compounded pharmaceutical products.

Recipe

A listing of the exact quantity of each ingredient and the processes required to compound a particular prescription

Compounding log

An official record of the processes and materials used to compound a prescription

Many oral liquid medications are readily available as a **suspension**, a dispersion of fine solid particles in a liquid, which may be administered to the patient by using a spoon, oral syringe, or dosing cup. However, at times you may be required to compound such an oral suspension pursuant to a medication order or because a manufactured suspension may not be available.

Suspension

A dispersion of fine solid particles in a liquid

To compound a suspension, you will begin with a medication manufactured in either tablet or capsule form. (In this lab, you will use tablets as your starting material and in the next lab, Lab 25, you will use capsules as your starting material.) The original medication form is then reduced to a fine powder—either through tablet trituration or by releasing the medication from the capsules. The required amount of powder is weighed and then checked by the pharmacist. The liquid component, a suspending agent that is often a solution such as Syrpalta, is also measured as required and then checked by a pharmacist. Compounding oral solutions requires a digital balance for powder measurements and a beaker for solution measurement. In addition, oral solution compounded from tablets will require the use of a mortar and pestle. Once combined, the powder and solution must be shaken well to ensure that medication particles are thoroughly dispersed throughout the mixture.

Procedure

In this lab, you will prepare metronidazole oral suspension 500 mg/5 mL from tablets. You must prepare an amount that provides enough medication to supply the following prescription in its entirety: "Metronidazole 500 mg qid $\times$ 10 days."

You will need to perform calculations to determine how many tablets are required to prepare the final product. The tablets will be triturated, weighed, and then mixed with a suspending agent such as Syrpalta. If and as directed by your instructor, you will also prepare a compounding log to record the steps and ingredients that you use.

1 Set your supplies on the workspace and arrange them in an easily accessible and organized manner. Visually inspect them to ensure that they are clean. If they are not, wash and dry them before use.

2 Wash your hands thoroughly, put on gloves, and wear them throughout the procedure.

3 Complete the calculations provided below to determine the amount of metronidazole necessary to prepare the entire product ordered by the physician:

a. First, determine the **amount of medication** needed for **one day** of the prescription by setting up this statement:

500 mg *(number of milligrams per tablet)* $\times$ **4** *(number of doses per day)* = **2000 mg** *(needed per day)*

b. Second, determine the **number of tablets** needed to deliver that daily medication quantity **for one day of the prescription**. Do this by setting up a ratio and proportion problem.

Place the number of milligrams in one tablet over the words "1 tablet" (similar to writing down a fraction). Next to that item, place the number of milligrams in one day's prescription over the words "*x* tablets" (again, creating a fraction). Place an equals sign between the two fractions.

To solve this and all ratio and proportion problems, multiply across and then divide. In this case:

$$\frac{500 \text{ mg}}{1 \text{ tablet}} = \frac{2000 \text{ mg}}{x \text{ tablets}}$$

Solve by cross multiplying: **2000** mg $\times$ **1** tablet = **2000 mg-tablet**

And then dividing: **2000** mg-tablet divided by **500** mg = **4 tablets**

The answer to this problem is: **4 tablets** *(needed to compound **one day's** worth of prescription)*

c. Third, determine the **number of tablets** needed to compound the **entire prescription** by multiplying your answer from b (above) times the total number of days for the prescription.

In this case, the prescription is for 10 days, so:

4 tablets *(per day)* $\times$ **10** days *(duration of the entire prescription)* = **40 tablets** *(for the entire prescription)*

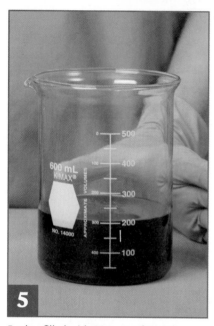

5

Beaker filled with 200 mL of Syrpalta

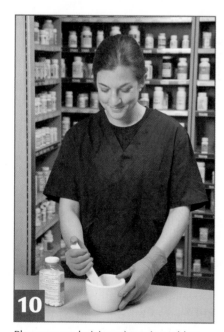

10

Pharmacy technician triturating tablets with a mortar and pestle.

4 Place the number of tablets needed for the entire prescription (calculated above) into a weighing boat and temporarily set the boat aside.

5 Pour 200 mL of Syrpalta into a beaker and temporarily set it aside.

6 If necessary, calibrate the balance according to standard procedures. Place an empty weighing boat on the balance and "tare" or "zero" it. If you have questions on this process, see Steps 10–12 in Lab 23 or ask your instructor for specific directions.

7 Remove the empty weighing boat and place the boat containing the metronidazole tablets onto the balance. Record the weight of the tablets here: _____ . This is the amount you will need for the final product that you are going to compound.

8 Ask for an instructor check on the quantity of tablets and the volume of Syrpalta.

9 Place the metronidazole tablets into the mortar. Add an additional three tablets of metronidazole to the mortar.
Tip: Adding this extra amount will allow for the powder loss that results from the medication adhering to the mortar and pestle and will ensure that you have adequate powder to measure for the final product.

10 Triturate to a fine powder, approximately the consistency of flour.
Tip: In this and other situations where you want to reduce the product to a very fine powder with the mortar and pestle, it is most effective to use a forceful, back and forth, grinding motion, not a stirring or pounding motion.

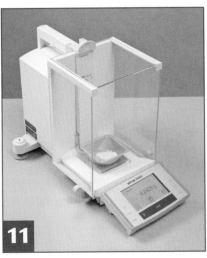

Drug powder being weighed on a digital scale.

11 Place an empty weighing boat onto the scale and tare it. Using the spatula, transfer an amount of powder from the mortar into the weighing boat equal to the "weight of the tablets" you recorded above, in Step 7. This amount must be no more than ± 5% of that amount.

Tip: While the standard margin of error is ± 5%, the allowed margin may vary in the case of medications used in chemotherapy treatments, neonate or geriatric medications, and other unique-needs situations.

12 Ask the instructor to verify the weight of the triturated metronidazole.

Tip: Always get an instructor to check your ingredient quantities (weights, volumes, or other measurements) before you begin mixing.

13 After a check of both ingredients, use a spatula to transfer a small amount of powder from the weighing boat into the beaker that contains the Syrpalta. Stir the suspension until that small amount of powder is dissolved in the Syrpalta.

14 Gradually add more metronidazole until it has all been incorporated into the Syrpalta.

Tip: Stir continuously as you add the rest of the powder, to promote uniform consistency. Be sure to scrape the metronidazole completely from the weighing boat into the Syrpalta so that the proper concentration of drug is contained in the final product.

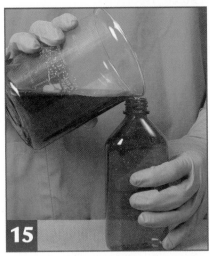

Syrpaltra being poured into the amber bottle.

15 Carefully pour the suspension from the beaker into the amber bottle.

Tip: To ensure that all of the medication is transferred into the final container, swirl the final product in the beaker as you gradually pour it into the amber bottle.

16 Label the product according to your instructor's directions, place a Shake Well auxiliary label on the bottle, and ask your instructor for a final check.

17 Wash, dry, and put away all supplies and clean up the work area. Prepare the compounding log, if and as directed by your instructor.

18 **Conclusion:** Present your log, if created, and your final product to your instructor for verification. On a separate sheet of paper, answer all questions in the following Lab Review section and turn in your answers to your instructor.

Lab Review

Check Your Understanding

1. Why is it important to add three extra tablets of metronidazole to the mortar prior to triturating the tablets?
   a. The actual amount required for the entire prescription is three tablets more than the weighed amount.
   b. That is the amount the physician ordered.
   c. To make up for the amount that sticks to and is "lost" in the weighing boat.
   d. To make up for the amount that sticks to and is "lost" in the mortar and pestle.

2. Why is it important to weigh out the tablets needed for the final prescription prior to trituration?
   a. It is important to know the weight of the powdered metronidazole that will be needed for the final prescription.
   b. It is not important when the medication gets weighed, as long as it is weighed prior to putting it in the beaker.
   c. It is not important when the medication gets weighed, as long as it is weighed prior to putting it in the amber bottle.
   d. None of the above

3. The most appropriate way to mix a powder into Syrpalta is to _____.
   a. pour all of the powder into the Syrpalta and stir continuously
   b. pour all of the powder into the Syrpalta and shake vigorously
   c. gradually add the powder into the Syrpalta and stir continuously
   d. gradually add the powder into the Syrpalta and shake vigorously

4. Once the final prescription has been compounded, the amber bottle will contain 20,000 mg of metronidazole in 200 mL of Syrpalta. What is the concentration in milligrams/milliliter?
   a. 50 mg/mL
   b. 100 mg/mL
   c. 250 mg/mL
   d. 250 mg/5 mL

5. The proper procedure used for trituration includes which of the following?
   a. stirring the powder with a stirring rod
   b. grinding the tablets in a mortar and pestle
   c. swirling the suspension in a beaker
   d. All of the above

Thinking Like a Pharmacy Tech

1. Think about why it matters that you "tare" or "zero out" the balance with an empty weighing boat on the scale prior to compounding. How would the concentration of your final product be affected if you failed to do this?

2. Surely it is important to make certain that your compounding supplies are clean prior to using them. What are two ways that patients might be negatively impacted if dirty compounding supplies are used to prepare their medications?

3. Working in the pharmacy can be hectic at times—there might be patients waiting for prescriptions, e-prescriptions to fill, and phone calls coming in. How can you juggle everyone's needs? How can you maintain composure and good customer service to the patients who are waiting?

Creating Suspensions from Capsules   Lab 25

Objectives

- Demonstrate proficiency in the process of compounding an oral suspension from capsules.
- Demonstrate competence in calculations related to the preparation of an oral suspension from capsules.
- Discuss the procedure and rationale for compounding oral suspensions from capsules.
- Become familiar with the compounding log as a means of recording the measurements, ingredients, and procedures used in compounding nonsterile products.

Supplies

- Weighing boat
- Beaker or Erlenmeyer flask (250 mL or larger)
- Stirring rod
- Gloves
- Amoxicillin 250 mg capsules (bulk bottle)
- Syrpalta 200 mL (or similar)
- Amber bottle for liquid medications (8 ounce or larger)
- Calculator

Introduction to Extemporaneous Compounding for Labs 22–27

Compounding

Preparing individualized medications per prescription order

Note: If you have completed Lab 22, you may skip the first two paragraphs.
Prior to the mass production of prepared pharmaceutical products in the 1940s and 1950s, pharmacies prepared individualized medications per a prescription order from a prescriber. This individualized preparation was termed **compounding** and included compressing tablets, creating suspensions, and filling capsules with a requested strength or amount of medication. Pharmacy technicians are still called upon to perform many types of extemporaneous, or nonsterile, compounding procedures, including preparing oral solutions, suppositories, capsules, troches, lozenges, creams, ointments, gels, and pastes. Today, compounding is required under several

circumstances, including as a response to patients' unique needs, manufacturer-based difficulties, and physician requests.

While compounding in the pharmacy lab, safety, accuracy, and proper record keeping are essential. These safety precautions are used both in the lab setting, and also in practice. In most instances, you must wear gloves throughout all compounding procedures to protect (1) yourself from exposure to the medication, (2) the medication from degradation caused by skin cells and oils, and (3) the patient from potentially contaminated medications. In addition, some compounding procedures will require you to wear safety glasses. Refer to the individual recipe for safety precautions. Accuracy is crucial in drug measurement and dose calculations. Some compounding lab procedures provide one or more **recipes**, which list the exact quantity of each ingredient. Other procedures provide dosage information and require your calculations to prepare the final product. Finally, you must keep careful and precise records each time you compound a prescription, by creating a **compounding log**, an official, detailed record of the processes and materials used. Because requirements for compounding log record-keeping may vary widely between states and individual facilities, you must check with your instructor about specific, local record-keeping procedures for compounded pharmaceutical products.

Recipe

A listing of the exact quantity of each ingredient and the processes required to compound a particular prescription

Compounding log

An official record of the processes and materials used to compound a prescription

Suspension

A dispersion of fine solid particles in a liquid

Many oral liquid medications are readily available as a **suspension**, a dispersion of fine solid particles in a liquid, which may be administered to the patient by using a spoon, oral syringe, or dosing cup. However, at times you may be required to compound such an oral suspension pursuant to a medication order or because a manufactured suspension may not be available.

To compound a suspension, you will begin with a medication manufactured in either tablet or capsule form. (In this lab, you will use capsules as your starting material, whereas in the previous lab, Lab 24, tablets are your starting material.) The original medication form is then reduced to a fine powder—either through tablet trituration or by releasing the medication from the capsules. The required amount of powder is weighed and then checked by the pharmacist. The liquid component, a suspending agent that is often a solution such as Syrpalta, is also measured as required and then checked by a pharmacist. Compounding oral solutions from capsules requires a weighing boat to provide a temporary receptacle for the capsules, and a beaker for solution measurement. Once combined, the powder and solution must be shaken well to ensure that medication particles are thoroughly dispersed throughout the mixture.

Procedure

In this lab, you will compound an oral suspension from capsules in order to prepare amoxicillin 250 mg/5 mL, an oral liquid medication. You must prepare enough medication to supply the following prescription in its entirety: "Amoxicillin 250 mg qid × 10 days."

You will need to perform calculations to determine how many capsules are required to prepare the final product. Before mixing the medication with a suspending agent such as Syrpalta, you will open the capsules and remove the powder from within the capsule shell. If and as directed by your instructor, you will also prepare a compounding log to record the steps and ingredients that you use.

1 Set your supplies on the workspace and arrange them in an easily accessible and organized manner. Visually inspect them to ensure that they are clean. If they are not, wash and dry them before use.

2 Wash your hands thoroughly, put on gloves, and wear them throughout the procedure.

3 Use the following calculations to determine the amount of amoxicillin necessary to prepare the entire product ordered by the physician:

a. First, determine the **amount of medication** needed for **one day** of the prescription by setting up this statement:

250 mg *(number of milligrams per capsule)* × **4** *(number of doses per day)* = **1000 mg** *(needed per day)*

b. Second, determine the **number of capsules** needed to deliver that daily medication quantity **for one day of the prescription**. Do this by setting up a ratio and proportion problem.

Place the number of milligrams in one capsule over the words "1 capsule" (similar to writing down a fraction). Next to that item, place the number of milligrams in one day's prescription over the words "x capsules" (again, creating a fraction). Place an equals sign between the two fractions.

To solve this and all ratio and proportion problems, multiply across and then divide. In this case:

$$\frac{250 \text{ mg}}{1 \text{ capsule}} = \frac{1000 \text{ mg}}{x \text{ capsules}}$$

Solve by cross multiplying: **1000** mg × **1** capsule = **1000 mg-capsule**

And then dividing: **1000** mg-capsule divided by **250** mg = **4 capsules**

The answer to this problem is: **4 capsules** *(needed to compound **one day's** worth of prescription)*

c. Third, determine the **number of capsules** needed to compound the **entire prescription** by multiplying your answer from b (above) times the total number of days for the prescription.

In this case, the prescription is for 10 days, so:

4 capsules *(per day)* $\times$ **10** days *(duration of the entire prescription)* = **40 capsules** *(for the entire prescription)*

4 Pour 200 mL of Syrpalta into a beaker or Erlenmeyer flask and temporarily set it aside.

5 Place the number of capsules (calculated above) needed for the entire prescription into a weighing boat and temporarily set aside.

6 Ask your instructor to check the number of capsules and the volume of Syrpalta. *Tip: Always have your instructor check your ingredients (capsules, volumes, other measured quantities) before you begin mixing.*

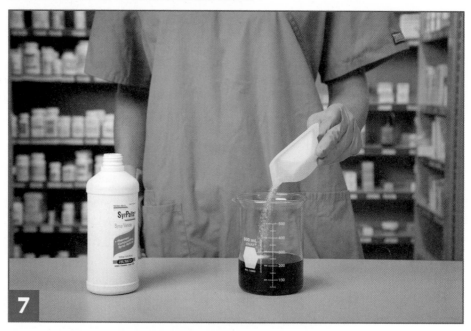

Pharmacy technician emptying capsule into a beaker of Syrpalta

7 Carefully open a capsule and empty it into the beaker containing the Syrpalta. All of the powder must be transferred into the Syrpalta, so examine the inside of both capsule halves and if any powder remains, tap the capsule shell gently against the inside of the beaker so the powder is dislodged and enters the Syrpalta.

8 Continue the process until all of the contents of all of the capsules have been emptied into the Syrpalta. Stir the suspension until the powder is thoroughly incorporated into the Syrpalta.

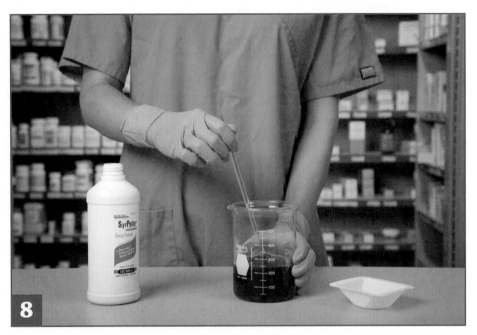
8

Pharmacy technician mixing powder and Syrpalta in a beaker.

9 Carefully and gradually pour the suspension from the beaker into the amber bottle.
Tip: While you are pouring, swirl the final product in the beaker to ensure that all of the medication remains in suspension and is transferred into the final container.

10 Consult your instructor for labeling instructions and also place a Shake Well auxiliary label on the bottle. Ask your instructor for a final check of the finished product.

11 Wash, dry, and put away all supplies and clean up the work area. Prepare the compounding log, if and as directed by your instructor.

12 **Conclusion:** Present your log, if created, and your final product to your instructor for verification. On a separate sheet of paper, answer all questions in the following Lab Review section and turn in your answers to your instructor.

Lab Review

Check Your Understanding

1. Why must gloves be worn when performing extemporaneous compounding?
   a. to protect the worker from potential exposure to the medication
   b. to protect the medication from degradation caused by contact with oil from the preparer's skin
   c. to protect the patient from potentially contaminated medication
   d. All of the above

2. During extemporaneous compounding procedures, at what point must the instructor/pharmacist check the technician's work?
   a. The instructor/pharmacist must check all the supplies once they have been gathered, prior to measuring the ingredients.
   b. The instructor/pharmacist must only check the ingredients once they have been measured, counted, or weighed.
   c. The instructor/pharmacist must only check the final product, just prior to labeling.
   d. The instructor/pharmacist must check all measured ingredients prior to mixing and must also check the final product.

3. The most appropriate way to remove any powder remaining in the opened capsule is to _____.
   a. tap the open capsule against the inside of the beaker
   b. scrape the powder out of the capsule with a stirring rod
   c. scrape the powder out of the capsule with a compounding spatula
   d. blow air into the capsule to dislodge the powder

4. Once the final prescription has been compounded, the amber bottle will contain 10,000 mg of amoxicillin in 200 mL of Syrpalta. What is the concentration of this product in milligrams/milliliter?
   a. 50 mg/mL
   b. 100 mg/mL
   c. 250 mg/mL
   d. 250 mg/5 mL

5. Oral suspensions may be administered by the following delivery methods: _____.
   a. spoon, oral dosing cup, oral syringe
   b. spoon, oral dosing cup, syringe for injectable use
   c. spoon, Erlenmeyer flask, oral syringe
   d. None of the above

Thinking Like a Pharmacy Tech

1. You are advised to have your instructor/pharmacist check each of the ingredients prior to mixing them. Why is it insufficient to simply have the instructor/pharmacist check only the final product?

2. Discuss whether extemporaneous compounding would be appropriate for a patient who is allergic to amoxicillin.

 3. Most employers will frown upon using the workplace to conduct personal business. What activities at work should you avoid?

Preparing Creams, Ointments, Gels, and Pastes
Lab 26

Objectives

- Demonstrate proficiency in the process of nonsterile compounding, specifically in the preparation of a topical gel.
- Discuss the procedure and rationale for compounding nonsterile creams, ointments, gels, and pastes.
- Become familiar with the compounding log as a means of recording the measurements, ingredients, and procedures used in compounding nonsterile products.

Supplies

- A balance or scale (digital or otherwise)
- Two weighing boats
- Mortar and pestle
- Two compounding spatulas
- Ointment slab
- Small ointment jar
- Gloves
- Thirteen aspirin 325 mg tablets (without film coating)
- One tube of surgical lubricant (minimum 15 grams)

Introduction to Extemporaneous Compounding for Labs 22–27

Compounding

Preparing individualized medications per prescription order

Note: If you have completed Lab 22, you may skip the first two paragraphs.
Prior to the mass production of prepared pharmaceutical products in the 1940s and 1950s, pharmacies prepared individualized medications per a prescription order from a prescriber. This individualized preparation was termed **compounding** and included compressing tablets, creating suspensions, and filling capsules with a requested strength or amount of medication. Pharmacy technicians are still called upon to perform many types of extemporaneous, or nonsterile, compounding procedures, including preparing oral solutions, suppositories, capsules, troches, lozenges, creams, ointments, gels, and pastes. Today, compounding is required under several

circumstances, including as a response to patients' unique needs, manufacturer-based difficulties, and physician requests. This type of compounding is often referred to as "extemporaneous compounding."

While compounding in the pharmacy lab, safety, accuracy, and proper recordkeeping are essential. These safety precautions are used both in the lab setting, and also in practice. In most instances, you must wear gloves throughout all compounding procedures in order to protect (1) yourself from exposure to the medication, (2) the medication from degradation caused by skin cells and oils, and (3) the patient from potentially contaminated medications. In addition, some compounding procedures will require you to wear safety glasses. Refer to the individual recipe for safety precautions. Accuracy is crucial in drug measurement and dose calculations. Some compounding lab procedures provide one or more **recipes**, which list the exact quantity of each ingredient. Other procedures provide dosage information and require your calculations to prepare the final product. Finally, you must keep careful and precise records each time you compound a prescription, by creating a **compounding log**, an official, detailed record of the processes and materials used. Because requirements for compounding log recordkeeping may vary widely among states and individual facilities, you must check with your instructor about specific, local record-keeping procedures for compounded pharmaceutical products.

Most topical preparations are readily available as pre-made creams, ointments, gels, or pastes. However, there are times when you may be required to compound nonsterile topical products pursuant to a prescription or medication order. In such compounding, a **base ingredient** is combined with an **active ingredient**. The base ingredient is an inert delivery vehicle such as a cream, ointment, gel, or paste. The required amount of base is carefully weighed and then verified by a pharmacist. The active ingredient, or medication, is commonly provided in either tablet or capsule form by the manufacturer. For the process of compounding topical products, the original form is then reduced to a fine powder, either through tablet trituration or by releasing the medication from the capsules. The required amount of powder is also carefully weighed and then checked by the pharmacist.

Compounding of a topical preparation is performed on an ointment slab, using compounding spatulas to mix the preparation. With this compounding method—often referred to as **spatulation**—the powder should slowly be incorporated into the base to ensure that the final product is prepared to a uniform consistency and concentration. While there are some differences in the consistency and uses of creams, ointments, gels, and pastes, the basic compounding process, as you will practice in this lab, is the same.

Recipe

A listing of the exact quantity of each ingredient and the processes required to compound a particular prescription

Compounding log

An official record of the processes and materials used to compound a prescription

Base ingredient

An inert substance, such as a cream, ointment, gel, or paste, to which an active ingredient is added during compounding

Active ingredient

The medication that is added to the base ingredient during compounding

Spatulation

A method of mixing ingredients together into a homogeneous mixture by combining and smoothing them on a slab with a spatula

Procedure

In this lab, you will compound a gel for topical application, using aspirin tablets as the active ingredient and surgical lubricant as the base gel (and prepare a compounding log, if and as directed by your instructor, to record the steps and ingredients that you use). In this case, a compounding formula is not needed; you will simply be given the recipe as the steps proceed.

1 Set your supplies on the workspace and arrange them in an easily accessible and organized manner. Visually inspect them to ensure that they are clean. If they are not, wash and dry them before use.

2 Wash your hands thoroughly, put on gloves, and wear them throughout the procedure.

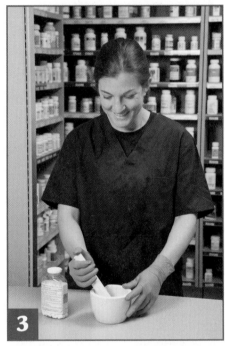

3

Pharmacy technician triturating tablets with a mortar and pestle.

3 Crush 13 (10 for the compound, plus three additional tablets to allow for some extra powder as some of the product may be lost during trituration and the pouring processes) aspirin 325 mg tablets with a mortar and pestle. Triturate to a fine powder, approximately the consistency of flour.
Tip: *It is most effective to use a forceful, back and forth, grinding motion when using a mortar and pestle, and not a stirring or pounding motion.*

4 If necessary, calibrate the balance according to standard procedures, and then place an empty weighing boat on the balance and tare ("zero") it.

5 Weigh out 2.5 grams of the finely ground aspirin powder into the empty boat. Set the boat filled with powder to the side.

6 Repeat the process with a second, empty weighing boat: place it on the scale, tare the scale, and weigh out your quantity— here, 10 grams of the surgical lubricant.

7 Ask the instructor to verify the weight of the aspirin and the surgical lubricant.
Tip: *Always get an instructor to check your ingredient quantities (weights, volumes, or other measurements) before you begin mixing.*

8 Once the two ingredients have been checked, you will put them onto different parts of a single ointment slab. First, carefully scrape the

powdery contents of the first boat into a small pile at one upper corner of the ointment slab, using the spatula to scrape the remnants from the boat onto the slab.

9 Second, carefully scrape the contents of the second boat into a small pile at the upper corner of the *opposite side* of the slab, using the spatula to scrape out the remnants.

10 To begin the mixing process, use the spatula to drag a small amount (approximately one-fifth of the total amount) of powder to the center of the slab.

11 Using the same spatula, drag a small amount (again, approximately one-fifth of the total amount) of surgical lubricant to the center of the slab.

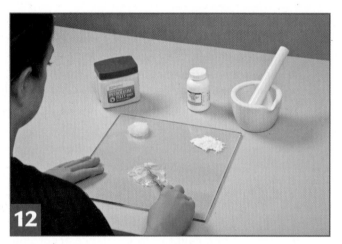

Technician mixing a small amount of powder and base on an ointment slab.

12 Mix the two ingredients together by using the flat surface of the spatula against the flat surface of the slab. You should apply a downward force and move the spatula back and forth in a sideways "S" pattern, as illustrated in Figure 26.1. The motion is similar to the hand motion you might use to frost a cake.

FIGURE 26.1
The "S" method of spatulation

Powder and gel are mixed together in an "S" motion against the slab, similar to the motion used to frost a cake.

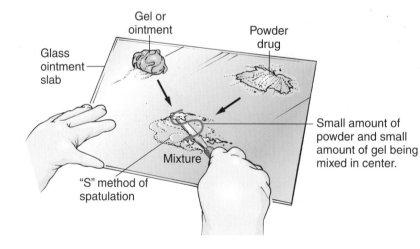

13 Gradually mix the small amounts of the two ingredients together by continuing to apply downward pressure as the mixture takes on a smooth, uniform texture.

14 Now use the spatula to drag an additional, similarly small, amount of both ingredients into the center of the slab. Using the same process, blend the ingredients together while incorporating them into the portion that you have already mixed.

15 Continue this process, gradually adding more of each ingredient until both piles of ingredients have been moved from the corners to the center of the slab and the entire product is of a smooth and uniform texture.

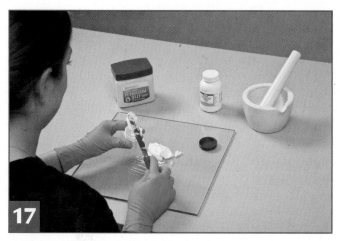

Pharmacy technician placing finished topical preparation into an ointment jar.

16 Ask your instructor to check the consistency of your product.

17 Once your product is approved, scrape everything off the slab and into an ointment jar.

18 Wash, dry and put away all supplies and clean up the work area. Prepare the compounding log, if and as directed by your instructor.

19 **Conclusion:** Present your log, if created, and your final product to your instructor for verification. On a separate sheet of paper, answer all questions in the following Lab Review section and turn in your answers to your instructor.

Lab Review

Check Your Understanding

1. The types of situations that might require extemporaneous compounding include _____.
   a. the prescribed dose is unavailable from the wholesaler or manufacturer
   b. the patient is allergic to the fragrance in the pre-made product
   c. the physician prefers to use a special mixture of ingredients that is not available in a pre-made product
   d. All of these situations might require extemporaneous compounding.

2. In reference to the material in this chapter, the word "base" means _____.
   a. the foundation upon which all extemporaneous compounding is completed
   b. an active ingredient that is mixed with a gel
   c. a sterile cream to which aspirin is added
   d. an inert delivery vehicle for the active ingredient

3. The most appropriate way to mix a powder ingredient with a gel ingredient is to mix _____.
   a. a small amount at a time in the center of the slab
   b. all of the ingredients together at the same time
   c. all the powder with a little bit of the gel
   d. all the gel with a little bit of the powder

4. Why is it important to "zero" or "tare" the scale while the boat is on, before weighing anything?
   a. To make sure it is calibrated properly.
   b. So that the weight of the boat does not affect the weight or amount of the ingredient you are measuring.
   c. Because you should always start at zero and work your way up.
   d. It is not important to "zero" the scale with the boat on it.

5. Why is it important to be sure that all of your supplies are clean prior to performing extemporaneous compounding?
   a. To make sure that the final product is not discolored.
   b. Since it is not sterile compounding, it is not important that the supplies are clean.
   c. So that the final volume is accurate.
   d. To make sure that the final product is safe, prepared as ordered, and free of contaminants.

Thinking Like a Pharmacy Tech

1. When performing extemporaneous compounding, why is it important to do so with attention to accuracy and to maintain a focus on creating a final product of a smooth and uniform consistency?

2. There are advantages to having some medications used topically. In what types of situations might a topical preparation be preferred over an oral medication?

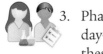

3. Pharmacy technicians work with many different people throughout their work day—patients, other technicians, and pharmacists. How can you get along with these many different types of people? How will you deal with difficult people you may end up working with?

Making Lozenges

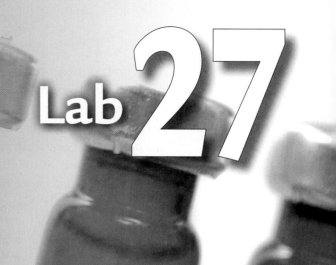

Lab 27

Objectives

- Demonstrate proficiency in the preparation of compounded, custom-made lozenges.
- Demonstrate skill in the use of laboratory equipment required for compounding.
- Become familiar with the compounding log as a means of recording the measurements, ingredients, and procedures used in compounding nonsterile products.

Supplies

- Saucepan
- Thermometer capable of reaching 155 °C (311 °F)—a candy thermometer is best
- Hot plate capable of generating temperatures of 155 °C (311 °F)
- 10 fl. oz tap water (for hot water bath)
- Can of cooking spray (canola or olive oil)
- Glass stirring rod

- Two 100 mL or 125 mL beakers
- Beaker tongs or one pair of heat-resistant gloves
- Set of protective eyewear
- 0.25 oz lozenge mold (20 lozenges per mold)
- Twenty individual aluminum wrappers or aluminum foil pieces cut into 3 × 3 in. squares
- Access to a freezer
- Lozenge ingredients:
  - 2.5 oz (70 g) granular sugar, powdered sugar, or Splenda® or equivalent of other sugar substitute (for diabetic patients)
  - 1.5 oz (45 g) light corn syrup
  - 1 oz (30 mL) distilled water
  - Bottle of food flavoring (per customer/prescriber request)
  - Bottle of food coloring
  - 9 g benzocaine powder, USP

Introduction to Extemporaneous Compounding for Labs 22–27

Note: If you have completed Lab 22, you may skip the first two paragraphs.
Prior to the mass production of prepared pharmaceutical products in the 1940s and 1950s, pharmacies prepared individualized medications per a

Compounding

Preparing individualized medications per prescription order

Recipe

A listing of the exact quantity of each ingredient and the processes required to compound a particular prescription

Compounding log

An official record of the processes and materials used to compound a prescription

Lozenge

A dosage form that resembles hard candy and is administered orally; also known as a troche or pastille

prescription order from a prescriber. This individualized preparation was termed **compounding** and included compressing tablets, creating suspensions, and filling capsules with a requested strength or amount of medication. Pharmacy technicians are still called upon to perform many types of extemporaneous, or nonsterile, compounding procedures, including preparing oral solutions, suppositories, capsules, troches, lozenges, creams, ointments, gels, and pastes. Today, compounding is required under several circumstances, including as a response to patients' unique needs, manufacturer-based difficulties, and physician requests. This type of compounding is often referred to as "extemporaneous compounding."

While compounding in the pharmacy lab, safety, accuracy, and proper record keeping are essential. These safety precautions are used both in the lab setting, and also in practice. In most instances, you must wear gloves throughout all compounding procedures in order to protect (1) yourself from exposure to the medication, (2) the medication from degradation caused by skin cells and oils, and (3) the patient from potentially contaminated medications. In addition, some compounding procedures will require you to wear safety glasses. Refer to the individual recipe for safety precautions. Accuracy is crucial in drug measurement and dose calculations. Some compounding lab procedures provide one or more **recipes**, which list the exact quantity of each ingredient. Other procedures provide dosage information and require your calculations to prepare the final product. Finally, you must keep careful and precise records each time you compound a prescription, by creating a **compounding log**, an official, detailed record of the processes and materials used. Because requirements for compounding log recordkeeping may vary widely among states and individual facilities, you must check with your instructor about specific, local record-keeping procedures for compounded pharmaceutical products.

The hard **lozenge** is another common dosage form created by compounding. Also known as a **troche** (pronounced tro-shay or tro-kee) or **pastille** (pas-teel), a lozenge is a hard candy-like dosage form that contains an active ingredient and may contain flavoring, sugar, or another form of sweetener. Hard lozenges are administered orally (by mouth), and patients suck on the lozenge until it dissolves, like hard candy; patients are not to swallow the lozenge. These dosage forms come in a variety of sizes, colors, and flavors, depending on the manufacturer or preparer, and on patient preference.

This type of dosage form is often used to increase patient compliance, especially in pediatric patients, as its sweetened contents are more palatable to children. While compounding is, in general, rather rare, it does occur, and you may be asked to compound hard lozenges—especially in a compounding pharmacy.

Procedure

In this lab, you will compound a lozenge. Your pharmacy has received a prescription for a 7.5% benzocaine lozenge compound to soothe a child's sore throat. Using the following steps, compound the product (and prepare a compounding log, if and as directed by your instructor, to record the steps and ingredients that you use). In this lab, a compounding formula is not needed; you will simply be given the recipe as the steps proceed.

1 Set your supplies on the workspace and arrange them in an easily accessible and organized manner. Visually inspect them to ensure that they are clean. If they are not, wash and dry them before use.

2 Wash your hands thoroughly, put on gloves and protective eyewear, and wear both throughout the procedure.

3 Using the balance or digital scale, carefully weigh out each of the four weighed ingredients in the recipe (2.5 oz [70 g] of sugar—or one of the suggested alternatives, 1.5 oz [45 g] of light corn syrup, 1 oz [30 mL] of distilled water, and 9 g of benzocaine powder). Clearly label each ingredient and have each weight verified by your instructor. Once the ingredients are weighed, labeled, and verified, set them aside for use later in the recipe.

4 Set out the lozenge mold and lightly spray it with cooking spray to prevent the hardened lozenges from sticking to the mold.

5 Switch on the hot plate and set the temperature to 155 °C (311 °F) or "high."

6 Pour tap water into the saucepan and place on the hot plate. You are creating a hot water bath (similar to working with a double boiler), which allows the contents of the beaker to melt without burning.

7 When the water begins to boil, place the beaker into the saucepan and add the powdered sugar or sugar substitute, corn syrup, and distilled water to the beaker.

8 Using the glass stirring rod, stir the contents of the beaker until the contents form a homogenous solution. Constantly check the solution's temperature as it approaches 149 °C (300 °F).

Tip: When sugar reaches 149 °C (300 °F), the

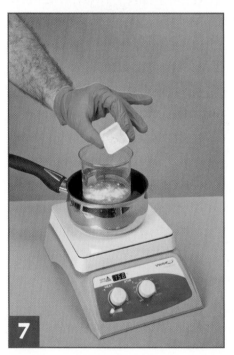

Pharmacy technician adding powdered sugar to liquid ingredients over a hot plate.

sugar molecules restructure and will cool into a hard-candy (or "hard crack") substance. Do not allow the solution to go above 155 °C (310 °F), or the sugar will caramelize.

9 At 149 °C (300 °F), add the desired flavoring, according to the manufacturer's specifications, and stir.

10 Stir in food coloring until desired color is reached.

11 Use the beaker tongs or heat-resistant gloves to hold the beaker and pour the contents of it into the unused beaker to a volume of 120 mL.

12 Add 9 g of benzocaine to the solution and stir until completely dissolved and homogenous.

13 Pour 5 mL of the solution into each cup of the lozenge mold and allow the lozenges to cool and firm up in the mold (approximately 5 to 8 minutes). Then place the lozenges in the freezer, where they will take approximately 120 minutes to harden completely.

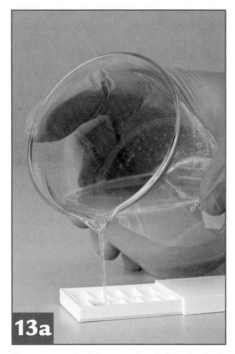
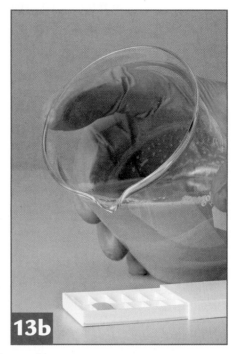

Pharmacy technician pouring finished solution into molds.

14 Once the lozenges have hardened, remove them from the mold and individually wrap them in aluminum wrappers to prevent them from sticking to each other.

15 While the lozenges cool, prepare the compounding log, if and as directed by your instructor. Wash, dry, and put away all supplies and clean up the work area.

16 **Conclusion:** Package and label the product and submit it with the compounding log, if created, to your instructor for final verification. On a separate sheet of paper, answer all questions in the following Lab Review section and turn in your answers to your instructor.

Lab Review

Check Your Understanding

1. A lozenge is also known as a _____.
   a. sucker
   b. lollipop
   c. troche
   d. medication stick

2. Creating a hot water bath ensures that the contents of the beaker are less likely to _____.
   a. burn
   b. melt
   c. boil
   d. curdle

3. Each lozenge will contain _____ of active ingredient.
   a. 7.5%
   b. 7.5 mg
   c. 7.5 gtts
   d. 7.5 fl. oz.

4. A sugar substitute, such as Splenda®, is best used for patients with what condition?
   a. hypertension
   b. diabetes
   c. influenza
   d. rhinovirus

5. Heating sugar to 149 °C (300 °F) causes the molecules to restructure and cool to a _____ form.
   a. caramelized
   b. pliable ball
   c. hard crack
   d. firm crack

Thinking Like a Pharmacy Tech

1. Explain why a lozenge is a viable alternative to tablets and capsules.

2. Perhaps more medications should come in this dosage form. Discuss any dangers you see in having sweetened dosage forms and any ideas you have to address or prevent those potential dangers.

3. While working as a pharmacy technician, you may encounter cultures that you have not previously interacted with. At times, these cultures have specific customs relating to medicine. Research a culture's beliefs on medicine, and write a short essay on how you would provide them with respectful care as a technician.

Unit 5

Aseptic Technique

A day in the life of a pharmacy technician...

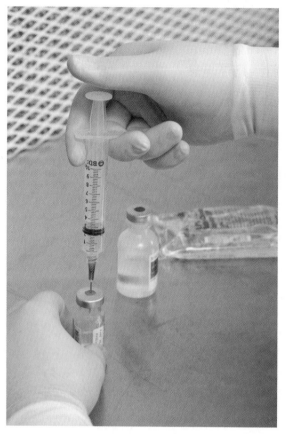

The stack of labels for the IV batch has grown to two inches high, there are four TPN solutions ready to be prepared, there is a new order for an investigational medication that is due in thirty minutes, and the pharmacist has just handed you three STAT IV medication labels through the pass-through window.

Are you prepared to work in the fast-paced, high-stress environment of sterile compounding?

Pharmacy technicians with special training in sterile compounding and aseptic technique prepare intravenous and parenteral medications for hospitalized patients. Patients requiring parenteral medications are often very sick and depend on these lifesaving medications for survival. Pharmacy technicians who prepare compounded sterile preparations must have excellent aseptic technique in compliance with guidelines set forth in Chapter <797> of the *United States Pharmacopeia* (USP Chapter <797>).

This unit will guide you in the essential tasks of the sterile compounding technician including aseptic garbing and hand-washing, hood cleaning, and large volume and small volume parenteral preparations. These tasks are the foundational aspects of sterile compounding and aseptic technique.

While speed and accuracy are essential when preparing compounded sterile preparations, you must also perform each step with careful adherence to USP Chapter <797> requirements in order to ensure that safe and effective medication is dispensed to the patient.

Take Note

The aseptic technique labs in the *Pharmacy Labs for Technicians, Second Edition* provide only a basic introduction to sterile compounding and aseptic technique. Students should refer to Paradigm's *Sterile Compounding and Aseptic Technique* by Lisa McCartney for in-depth instruction and training in sterile compounding and aseptic technique.

Garbing According to USP Chapter <797> Standards

Lab 28

Objectives

- Demonstrate proficiency in some of the processes and procedures related to garbing as defined in USP Chapter <797>.
- Discuss the procedures and rationale of the garbing procedures and related technique testing outlined in USP Chapter <797>.
- Understand how USP Chapter <797> affects the institutional pharmacy technician.

Supplies

- Sterile gown
- Sterile, powder-free gloves
- Hair cover or bouffant cap
- Shoe covers
- Face mask
- Sterile, Foamed alcohol
- Agar plates appropriate for glove-fingertip testing x 2
- Access to a tabletop or other surface that has been disinfected with 70% isopropyl alcohol or another suitable cleansing agent

"The United States Pharmacopoeia (USP) is the official public standards-setting authority for all prescription and over-the-counter medicines, dietary supplements, and other healthcare products manufactured and sold in the United States. USP sets standards for the quality of these products and works with healthcare providers to help them reach the standards," according to Chapter <797> of the USP as approved by *The United States Pharmacopoeial Convention*, 2007, page 1.

USP establishes policies regarding medication quality, patient safety, and healthcare personnel training, setting the standard of care to which all pharmacies in the United States conform. In 2007, USP revised Chapter <797> (referred to as USP Chapter <797>), the section of the book that outlines standards for "Pharmaceutical Compounding—Sterile Preparations."

USP Chapter <797> impacts your work as a pharmacy technician because it addresses many issues related to the preparation of compounded sterile preparations, including personnel training and evaluation in aseptic technique, hazardous drug preparation, environmental quality and control, verification of automated compounding devices such as total parenteral nutrition (TPN) compounders, medication storage, beyond-use dating, patient monitoring, and adverse events.

The sections of USP Chapter <797> that most directly affect the pharmacy technician address proper cleaning and preparation of the aseptic compounding environment and related products, including preparing your body, and donning aseptic garb, according to specific procedures governed by USP Chapter <797>, prior to entering the aseptic compounding area. Another area that will directly affect you concerns the training and testing of your skills and abilities as a qualified pharmacy technician.

Procedure

You will now garb according to strict USP Chapter <797> standards and undergo glove-fingertip sampling to verify that you have properly performed the procedure.

1 Read the instructions for agar plate fingertip testing prior to beginning this lab. Instructions are included in the agar plate package and will be provided to you by your instructor.

2 According to USP Chapter <797>, you should be free of cosmetics, jewelry, and visible body piercing, and your natural nails should be kept trimmed and clean—no false nails or nail polish. If you need to address these issues, do so now.
Tip: While body piercing cannot itself be removed, you should remove the jewelry from all body piercings that are visible outside your clothing.

3 Remove your personal outer garments (e.g., coats, hats, sweaters, jackets).

4 Apply foamed alcohol, or thoroughly wash your hands with soap and water before beginning this lab.

Take Note

It is considered "best practice" to apply foamed alcohol to your hands after donning each shoe cover, and after donning a hair cover. See step 10 for directions on the use of foamed alcohol.

5 Don each shoe cover by first identifying the toe-end (the longer end) of the cover and then slipping it over the toe of the shoe. Pull the shoe cover around the bottom of the shoe and up onto the heel. The shoe cover should completely envelop the entire shoe. Repeat the procedure with the other shoe.
Tip: You do not have to worry about "left" and "right" shoe covers; they are interchangeable.

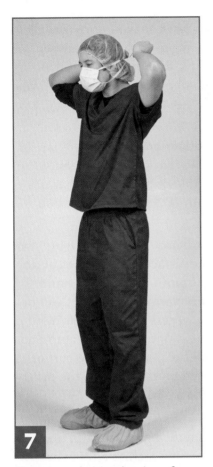

7

Pharmacy technician donning a face mask.

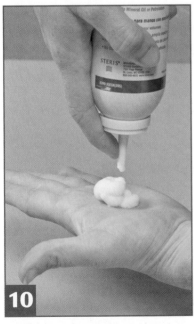

10

Proper procedure for dispensing foamed alcohol.

6 Put on the hair cover by gathering any loose hair and placing it into the hair cover so that the back of the hair cover contains the majority of the hair, and the elastic at the back of the hair cover is positioned against the back of the neck. Pull the front of the cap over your head until the elastic on the front of the hair cover is positioned against the forehead. Tuck any remaining hair under the hair cover. All hair must be covered by the hair cover.

Tip: People with long hair may find it helpful to put hair in a ponytail or otherwise tie it back prior to donning the hair cover.

7 Don a face mask by positioning it over the face with the top of the mask at the bridge of the nose. Pull the two uppermost ties around the sides of the face and then tie them behind the head with the ties resting just above the ears. Grasp the two lower ties and tie them behind the back of the neck. Adjust the mask so it is positioned securely over the nose, mouth, and chin.

*Tip: At this point in the procedure, USP Chapter <797> instructs the technician to complete a full aseptic hand-washing procedure, as taught in the next lab, Lab 29, before donning a sterile gown. Due to time constraints, your instructor **may** have you forgo that step during this training lab, instead having you use foamed alcohol to sterilize your hands. Be aware that in Step 10, below, you will be **required** to cleanse your hands using foamed alcohol, prior to gloving.*

8 Open the package containing a sterile gown, ensuring that the gown does not touch the floor or other surface at any time.

9 Insert one arm into the sleeve of the gown and pull it up onto the shoulder of that arm. Insert the other arm into the other sleeve and pull the gown up to the neck. Tie the neck ties of the gown behind the neck. Wrap the waist ties of the gown around the body and tie them behind the back.

10 Hold a can of foamed alcohol so that the tip is pointed down into the palm of the hand. Use the index finger of the hand that is holding the can to press against the tip of the dispenser, releasing a small amount (approximately golf-ball sized) of foamed alcohol onto the palm.

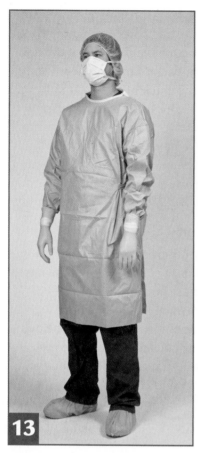

13

Pharmacy technician fully gowned and gloved.

11 Rub your hands together, making sure that the alcohol coats each finger—including between the fingers, the palms, and the backs of the hands. Allow the alcohol to evaporate until your hands are dry.

12 Open the outer wrapper on a package of sterile gloves. Place the inner package on a clean surface such as a table or countertop that has been disinfected with 70% isopropyl alcohol.

13 The gloves will be labeled "left" and "right." Do not touch the outer surface of the gloves at any time. Place the right glove on the right hand by grasping the inner part of the cuff (it will be folded over for easy access) with the left hand and carefully pulling it onto the right hand and up to the wrist. Pull the glove over the cuff of the gown. Repeat the procedure with the other glove using the opposite hand.

14 Remove the top from the agar plate and place it onto an aseptic surface such as a table or countertop that has been cleaned with 70% isopropyl alcohol.

15 Carefully press the gloved forefinger of the right hand onto the agar plate. Press the gloved right thumb onto a different section of the agar plate. Replace the cover on the agar plate.

16 Using a new agar plate, repeat the procedure in Step 15 with the left hand.

17 Label the plates as instructed and give both plates to your instructor for processing.

18 Unless otherwise instructed, remove, in this order: gloves, gown, face mask, hair cover, and shoe covers. All items should be disposed of in the pharmacy waste receptacle or designated area.

19 **Conclusion:** On a separate sheet of paper, answer all questions in the following Lab Review section and turn in your answers to your instructor.

Lab Review

Check Your Understanding

1. The abbreviation USP stands for _____.
   a. Under Sterile Preparation
   b. United States Pharmacies
   c. United States Pharmacopoeia
   d. Using Sterile Procedures

2. Which of the following statements best describes the contents of USP Chapter <797>?
   a. a set of standards and guidelines for procedures related to the compounding of nonsterile products
   b. a set of standards and guidelines for procedures related to the compounding of sterile preparations
   c. a set of standards and guidelines for procedures related to the compounding of narcotics
   d. All of the above

3. Which of the following best describes the proper order of garbing for working in the sterile compounding lab?
   a. shoe covers, hair cover, mask, gloves, gown
   b. hair cover, shoe covers, mask, gown, gloves
   c. shoe covers, hair cover, mask, gown, gloves
   d. shoe covers, hair cover, gown, mask, gloves

4. USP Chapter <797> addresses all of the following topics except _____.
   a. storage and beyond-use dating of commercially manufactured floor stock products
   b. procedures for the inspection and verification of TPN compounders
   c. training and testing of the pharmacy technician
   d. issues related to quality control

5. The purpose of gloved fingertip sampling is to verify that you _____.
   a. understand USP Chapter <797>
   b. are using proper sterile technique
   c. have garbed and gloved according to proper procedure
   d. have properly washed your hands

Thinking Like a Pharmacy Tech

1. Why is it important to garb in the order prescribed by USP Chapter <797> prior to working with sterile products?

2. USP Chapter <797> indicates that agar plate gloved fingertip sampling should be performed (with a negative or "no growth" result) to test the garbing and gloving of the newly trained pharmacy technician at least three times prior to allowing that person to compound sterile preparations. Why do you think that USP requires three negative samples as opposed to one?

3. One of the most important people to get along with in the workplace is, of course, your boss. What are some ways you can enjoy positive communication with your supervisor? What do you do if you and your boss don't see eye-to-eye?

Aseptic Hand Washing

Lab 29

Objectives

- Demonstrate excellence in aseptic hand-washing procedures.
- Discuss the procedures for and rationale behind aseptic hand washing.

Supplies

- Pre-packaged surgical scrub sponge/brush containing a suitable antimicrobial solution such as chlorhexidine 4% or Betadine
- Sink appropriate for aseptic hand washing
- Aseptic, lint-free paper towels dispensed from a container that does not compromise the cleanliness or integrity of the towels
- Garb (as required by your instructor)
- Sterile, powder-free gloves

Aseptic

Without infection; free of pathogens

Proper hand cleansing is the foundation of good aseptic technique. The word **aseptic** means "without infection," and aseptic hand washing is vital to keeping sterile products free from potentially infectious microorganisms. Pharmacy technicians must master aseptic hand washing, an essential skill when preparing sterile parenteral products such as intravenous (IV) solutions, total parenteral nutrition (TPN) solutions, and injectable solutions. Policy and procedures regarding hand washing vary slightly among hospitals in that you will sometimes do only a basic aseptic hand washing and at other times perform a complete aseptic hand washing, which requires the use of a surgical scrub sponge/brush.

A basic aseptic hand washing is achieved by vigorously washing both hands and forearms (spanning from the wrist to the elbow) for at least 30 seconds with an appropriate antimicrobial agent. Extra attention must be focused on areas that harbor multiple microorganisms, such as under the fingernails and in skin creases. A basic hand washing follows the same steps outlined in this lab for a complete aseptic hand washing; however, a

285

Minor contamination

A small amount or low level of contamination of the washed and scrubbed aseptic area

surgical scrub sponge/brush is not used. You may perform a basic hand washing—simply using antimicrobial soap or another hand-cleansing product such as foamed alcohol—any time there is the potential for **minor contamination**, such as after using a calculator or pen or inadvertently spilling a few drops of drug onto your hand.

Basic aseptic hand washing, just described, is an acceptable form of hand cleansing and meets all of the requirements set forth by USP Chapter <797>. However, many facilities that prepare parenteral products, such as compounded sterile preparations (CSPs), often require a more thorough type of aseptic hand washing that utilizes a surgical scrub sponge/brush. In these facilities, while basic aseptic hand washing is used upon minor hand contamination, there are circumstances in which a complete aseptic hand washing is desirable.

Major contamination

A large amount or significant level of contamination of the washed and scrubbed aseptic area

In particular, all personnel must perform a complete aseptic hand washing upon first entering the sterile compounding area and must repeat the entire procedure when re-entering the area; after eating, using the restroom, sneezing, or coughing; or on experiencing **major contamination** such as a large (greater than 5 mL) drug spill or a needle stick. A complete aseptic hand washing should take a *minimum* of 30 seconds. Spending 2 to 4 minutes is preferred, since the procedure contains many specific steps within these main categories: preparing the body; preparing the soap; scrubbing the nails; washing the fingers, palms, backs of the hands, and forearms; rinsing the hands and forearms; drying the hands and forearms; and gloving the hands.

Aseptic hand washing requires rigorous technique but simple tools—a sink and a few items kept nearby including aseptic, lint-free paper towels or a hot air hand dryer; sterile, powder-free gloves; and a surgical scrub sponge/brush pre-saturated with an appropriate antimicrobial solution. The sink itself should be located in the ante-room or just outside the door of the sterile compounding area and restricted to use for aseptic hand-washing procedures only. The sink should be deep, have a goose-neck faucet and hot and cold running water, and preferably be controlled by foot pedals. It should be clean and free of anything that might cause splashing.

A surgical scrub sponge/brush (which usually has both a sponge side and a brush side) is required for the complete aseptic hand-washing technique and is a very effective tool. Many facilities, especially those preparing medium risk compounded sterile preparations, and high-risk parenteral products compounded from nonsterile ingredients, prefer using a sterile, pre-packaged, surgical scrub sponge/brush that is pre-saturated with an approved antimicrobial soap.

Although the surgical scrub sponge/brush is a simple tool to use, you must take several precautions to ensure a contamination-free procedure. Do not use the brush side when scrubbing the skin. While the brush side scrubs effectively under the nails and around the cuticles, using it on the skin may cause skin particles to flake off into the clean environment. Do not reuse the scrub sponge/brush; it is intended for one-time use only and should then be thrown away immediately after use. Do not touch the sink or faucet with your fingers, hands, arms, or the scrub sponge/brush at any time. Do not apply lotion to your hands after completing the washing procedure. If you inadvertently do any of these things, you must repeat the entire hand-washing procedure with a *new* surgical scrub sponge/brush.

Procedure

In this lab, you will perform a complete aseptic hand-washing procedure using a sterile, pre-saturated surgical scrub sponge/brush.

1 Remove all jewelry. Because jewelry, makeup, nail polish, and false nails may not be worn in the compounding area, you should make adjustments as needed to comply with these rules.

2 Check with your instructor for guidance regarding garbing, and garb accordingly.
Tip: According to USP Chapter <797>, you should don hair cover, shoe covers, and mask prior to proceeding with this lab, and a sterile gown and gloves after completing the hand-washing procedure. However, because this is a training lab with time constraints, your instructor may have you eliminate one or more of these steps. In actual practice, all of the steps are mandatory.

3 Prior to opening the scrub packet, squeeze it several times to activate the soap suds. Carefully open the packet and throw away the outer wrapper.

4 Press the foot pedals to begin the flow of water and, when the water is warm, wet your hands and forearms.
Tip: If your sink is not equipped with foot pedals, you must let the water run throughout the entire hand-washing procedure and ignore any steps asking you to turn the water back on.

5 Without setting down the scrub sponge/brush, use the nail pick that is included in the scrub packet to clean under your fingernails. Throw away the pick when finished.

6 Apply a small amount of water to the scrub sponge/brush and then squeeze it several times so that it has ample, soapy lather. Manipulate the scrub sponge/brush so that you are using the *brush* side of the scrub, not the sponge side.
Tip: Throughout this lab's entire hand-washing procedure, you should squeeze the scrub sponge/brush or add a small amount of water as needed to maintain a good soapy lather.

7 Begin with the thumb and scrub under the thumbnail with the scrub brush. Go on to the next finger and scrub under the nail of that finger with the scrub brush, proceeding until you have scrubbed under all of the fingernails on the initial hand.

8 Continue to use the brush to clean under the thumbnail on the opposite hand, and continue scrubbing under the nail of each finger until you have cleaned under all the nails on that hand.

9 Manipulate the scrub brush to switch to its *sponge* side. Beginning with the thumb on the initial hand, clean each of the four surfaces of the thumb (the two sides and the top and bottom surfaces) with the sponge. *Tip: Remember not to use the brush side of the scrub sponge/brush on your skin because doing so may introduce skin cells into the environment, contaminating the aseptic procedure.*

10 Clean the webbing between the thumb and forefinger.

11 Proceed to clean all four surfaces of the forefinger and the webbing between it and the next finger. Continue this process of cleaning, in order, the next finger, the following webbing, the next finger, etc. until you have cleaned all fingers and webbings on that hand.

12 Move to the opposite hand and repeat the same process, Steps 7–11, beginning with the thumb and continuing through all the fingers and webbings on that hand.

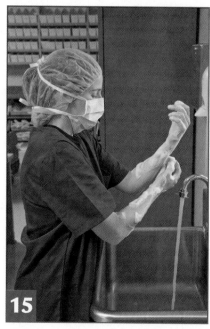

15

Pharmacy technician performing complete aseptic hand-washing procedure.

13 Move back to the initial hand and clean the palm with the sponge. Repeat the palm cleaning on the opposite hand.

14 Move back to the initial hand and clean the back of the hand with the sponge. Repeat the cleaning process on the back of the other hand.

15 Returning to the initial hand and, starting at the wrist, clean in a circular pattern, moving around the forearm as you work toward the elbow, where you stop. Repeat the procedure on the other forearm. This procedure is illustrated in Figure 29.1.

16 Throw the scrub sponge/brush away.

FIGURE 29.1
Proper aseptic hand-washing technique for forearms

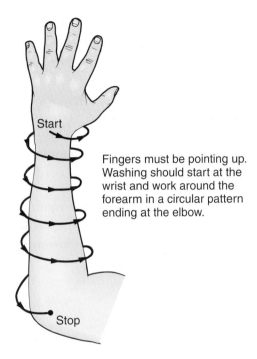

Start

Fingers must be pointing up. Washing should start at the wrist and work around the forearm in a circular pattern ending at the elbow.

Stop

17 Run the water until the flow is warm. On the side on which you began the hand-washing procedure, rinse the hand and forearm, rinsing the fingers first and keeping them pointing upward so that the water runs down toward the elbow.

Tip: Keep your fingers pointing upward throughout the entire rinsing and drying procedure. Do not allow the water to run down toward your fingers because this directional change will compromise the aseptic nature of the process.

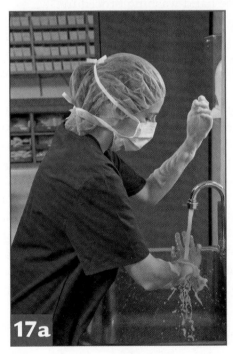

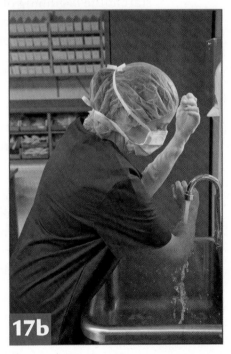

Pharmacy technician rinsing hands and forearms after aseptic hand-washing.

18 Repeat the hand and forearm rinsing process on the other side. Using aseptic, lint-free towels, dry your hands first and then throw the towels away. Using new towels, or a hot air hand dryer, dry the forearms and throw the towels away.

Tip: If you do not have foot pedals at your sink, use a paper towel to turn off the faucet before throwing the towel away.

19 Check with your instructor about gowning and gloving (as noted in the **Tip** for Step 2) and proceed accordingly.

20 **Conclusion:** Ask for instructor verification that you have properly completed the hand-washing procedure. On a separate sheet of paper, answer all questions in the following Lab Review section and turn in your answers to your instructor.

Lab Review

Check Your Understanding

1. What should you do if you accidentally drop the scrub sponge/brush in the sink while hand washing?
   a. Pick up the scrub sponge/brush and resume hand washing per protocol.
   b. Pick up the scrub sponge/brush and resume hand washing once you have thoroughly rinsed off the scrub sponge/brush.
   c. Discard the dropped scrub sponge/brush, open a new scrub packet, and restart at the beginning of the hand-washing procedure.
   d. Discard the dropped scrub sponge/brush, open a new one, and resume washing wherever you left off on the original hand-washing procedure.

2. Which statement most accurately describes the process of rinsing after an aseptic hand washing?
   a. A rinse should be performed so that the water runs down toward the fingertips.
   b. A rinse should be performed so that the water runs down toward the elbow.
   c. A rinse should be performed so that the water runs down toward the elbow, and then the hands should be shaken into the sink to remove excess water.
   d. It makes no difference how you rinse your hands since they are already clean.

3. Which of the following situations requires a complete aseptic hand washing?
   a. You enter the sterile compounding area after completing your lunch break.
   b. You suffer a small cut from a broken ampule.
   c. You contaminate your hands with 10 mL of IV penicillin.
   d. All of these situations require a complete aseptic hand washing.

4. How much time should you take to perform a complete aseptic hand washing?
   a. a minimum of 30 seconds, and more likely, 2 to 4 minutes
   b. exactly 30 seconds
   c. a minimum of 2 minutes
   d. It does not matter how long you scrub your hands as long as you are thorough.

5. What should you do if your hand accidentally touches the sink or faucet during the aseptic hand-washing procedure?
   a. Rinse your hand with water and continue the hand washing where you left off.
   b. Repeat the entire procedure with a new scrub sponge/brush.
   c. Provided that the sink and faucet have been cleaned recently, you do not have to do anything.
   d. Spray alcohol on your hands and start over with the same scrub sponge/brush.

Thinking Like a Pharmacy Tech

1. When working in a facility that has such requirements, why is it important to do a complete aseptic hand washing when first entering the sterile compounding area, or upon any major hand contamination, as opposed to simply washing your hands with antimicrobial soap?

2. Since you are wearing sterile gloves to prepare sterile products, why is there a need for proper aseptic hand washing?

3. When it comes to aseptic technique, there are different rules regarding dress and makeup. All sterile compounding labs will require you to wear no makeup, no jewelry, and to cover all hair, including beards. Why is it important to follow these rules?

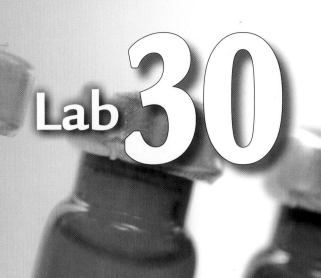

Hood Cleaning

Lab 30

Objectives

- Demonstrate proficiency in the cleaning of a standard horizontal laminar airflow hood.
- Explain the rationale and procedures for basic hood cleaning.

Supplies

- Sterile water for irrigation (in a pour bottle holding 250 mL or more)
- Sterile, 70% isopropyl alcohol (in a pour bottle holding 250 mL or more)
- Aseptic, lint-free, and non-shedding hood-cleaning pads or sterile gauze pads
- A hood appropriate for this procedure (any size horizontal, laminar airflow hood in which the HEPA filter is contained in the back wall of the cabinet)
- Hood-cleaning log sheet (attached to the hood)

Laminar airflow hoods are constructed to provide a constant flow of sterile air across a work surface that has been aseptically cleaned. The air is sterilized by being blown through a high-efficiency particulate air (HEPA) filter. As a pharmacy technician, you will probably work with several types of hoods, including the vertical laminar airflow hood (known as a biological safety cabinet or BSC), the self-contained laminar airflow barrier isolator hood, and the horizontal laminar airflow hood. All of these hoods are used to compound sterile preparations for parenteral administration using strict aseptic technique.

The vertical laminar airflow hood is primarily used to prepare chemotherapy drugs, chemotherapy medications, and other antineoplastic agents. (An antineoplastic agent inhibits or prevents the growth or development of malignant cells.) You will likely use this hood at some time in your work, but you must first receive specialized training. The self-contained laminar airflow barrier isolator hood, sometimes called a "glove box," is primarily used in environments where a relatively small number of sterile products are prepared at one time. Glove boxes are also sometimes used in small rural hospitals that do not have a dedicated pharmacy compounding room. However, pharmacies that prepare a large number of compounded sterile preparations usually use a standard horizontal laminar airflow hood because of its ease of use. Also referred to as a workbench or cabinet, the standard horizontal laminar airflow hood is the hood most frequently used in both hospital and compounding pharmacies and is the hood you will probably use most often as a pharmacy technician.

Because of the critical nature of the products prepared in a laminar airflow hood, the hood must be cleaned properly. Be aware that airflow in the hood should be left running at *all* times. If airflow in the hood somehow gets turned off, you must turn it back on and run it for a minimum of 30 minutes prior to using or cleaning the hood. Proper cleaning of the horizontal laminar airflow hood is generally performed with sterile, 70% isopropyl alcohol and aseptic, non-shedding wipes. Most facilities start the cleaning process by wiping down the interior surfaces of the cabinet using sterile water. Because some drugs are not soluble in alcohol, using water first allows those drugs to be dissolved and removed from the work surface prior to sterilizing it with alcohol. Proper hood cleaning requires several batches of cleaning pads because when you reach the **outer edge of the hood**—the border of the sterile zone—the pads become contaminated and must be discarded.

At times it may be appropriate to clean only the work surface of the hood, such as when a few drops of drug solution are spilled. However, most often a complete cleaning of the cabinet is required, such as when you begin each shift and every 30 minutes during continuous compounding periods. A complete hood cleaning should also be done when a large amount (greater than five milliliters) of drug is spilled, when drug has been aspirated into the hood, when the pre-filter is changed or the HEPA filter is recertified, or any time that major contamination (resulting from a needle stick or inadvertently sneezing or coughing into the hood) is suspected.

The hood-cleaning procedure requires strict recordkeeping for quality assurance. Thus, you should find a **hood-cleaning log sheet** for each hood, which is maintained inside a plastic sheet protector, in the anteroom. You must initial, date, and record the time on the log sheet each time you clean the hood. These records are kept for a minimum of two years and completed sheets may be reviewed by investigators from the Joint Commission, the State Board of Pharmacy, and other regulatory agencies. The hood-cleaning log sheet should reflect that the hood is being cleaned, at a minimum, at the beginning of every shift and every 30 minutes during continuous compounding periods, as well as upon any major contamination. You will likely need to clean each hood multiple times during your shift. Despite this frequency, it is imperative that you fill out the hood-cleaning log sheet every time you perform this task.

Outer edge of the hood

The outer six inches of the hood working surface, considered the "dirty edge" because sterile air mixes with room air

Hood-cleaning log sheet

A crucial document for recording who cleaned the hood, the date, and the time

Procedure

In this lab, you will clean a standard horizontal laminar airflow hood with sterile water and sterile, 70% isopropyl alcohol, according to standard USP Chapter <797> regulations.

1 Garb, hand wash, gown, and glove as directed by your instructor.

2 Remove everything (vials, syringe caps, and all other objects) from the hood, including anything hanging inside the hood, such as stock bottles.

3 Place an approximately 2-inch stack of aseptic, lint-free hood-cleaning pads on the work surface, at least 6 inches inside of the hood.

4 Pour an amount of sterile water onto the pads so that the entire stack is lightly saturated but *not* dripping with water.
Tip: *Do not let any liquid seep into the HEPA filter and do not touch the HEPA filter at any time.*

5 Take the top one-fourth of the stack of pads and clean the hang bar and, if present, the hooks. Then, beginning at the inside back corner of the cabinet, clean the ceiling of the cabinet. This cleaning should be done using overlapping *side-to-side* motions, moving from the interior of the cabinet to the outer edge of the cabinet. Once you have cleaned to the very outer edge of the hood, throw the used pads away.

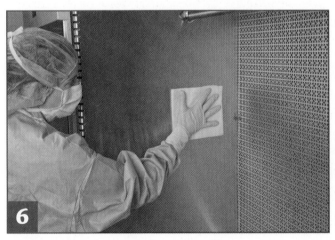

Pharmacy technician cleaning a side panel of a hood.

6 To begin cleaning the side panels, pick up the second one-fourth of the clean, water-saturated stack of pads. Beginning with the interior upper corner of one side panel, clean in a *down-and-up* motion, using overlapping strokes. Move from the interior upper corner of the cabinet toward the outer edge. This procedure is illustrated in Figure 30.1 on the next page. Once you have cleaned to the outer edge of the hood, throw the used pads away.

FIGURE 30.1
Horizontal laminar airflow hood: proper cleaning of side panels

Cleaning of side panels starts at the interior upper corner (X), close to the HEPA filter, and proceeds in sweeping, overlapping, down-and-up motions that move toward the outer edge of the hood.

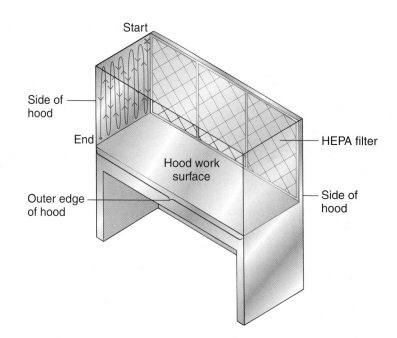

7 Pick up the third one-fourth of the clean, water-saturated stack of pads and repeat Step 6 on the other side panel. Once you have cleaned to the outer edge of the hood, throw the used pads away.

8 Take the remaining water-saturated pads and clean the work surface. Start in the back corner and clean with overlapping *side-to-side* strokes, working your way from the inside of the hood to the outer edge, as illustrated in Figure 30.2. Once you have cleaned to the outer edge of the hood, throw the used pads away.

FIGURE 30.2
Horizontal laminar airflow hood: proper cleaning of work surface

Cleaning of work surface starts at the interior, or back corner (X), close to the HEPA filter, and proceeds in sweeping, overlapping, side-to-side motions that move toward the outer edge of the hood.

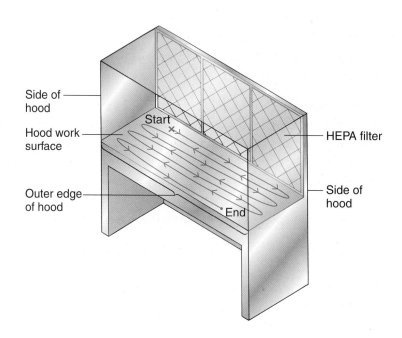

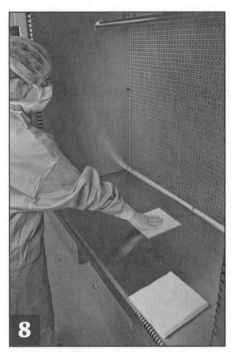

8

Pharmacy technician cleaning the work surface of a hood.

9 Repeat Steps 3–8 of the procedure, in the same order, using a new, approximately two-inch stack of hood-cleaning pads saturated this time with sterile, 70% isopropyl alcohol.

10 Initial, date, and record the time on the hood-cleaning log sheet that is attached to the hood. If you have questions about filling in this sheet, check with your instructor.

11 **Conclusion:** On a separate sheet of paper, answer all questions in the following Lab Review section and turn in your answers to your instructor.

Lab Review

Check Your Understanding

1. The components of a typical horizontal laminar airflow hood should be cleaned in what order?
   a. work surface, sides, ceiling
   b. HEPA filter, ceiling, sides, work surface
   c. ceiling, HEPA filter, work surface, sides
   d. ceiling, sides, work surface

2. At a minimum, a full hood cleaning should be performed ____.
   a. at the beginning of your shift, every 30 minutes during continuous compounding periods, and upon major contamination
   b. at the end of your shift, every 30 minutes during continuous compounding periods, and upon major contamination
   c. whenever it is dirty
   d. only when the filters are changed, cleaned, or recertified

3. When cleaning the hood you must wear the following: ____.
   a. mask and gloves
   b. hair cover and gown
   c. shoe covers
   d. All of the above

4. The type of pad or towel most appropriate for cleaning a horizontal laminar airflow hood is _____.
   a. nonsterile, lint-free, non-shedding hood-cleaning pads or nonsterile gauze
   b. regular paper towels
   c. aseptic, lint-free, non-shedding hood-cleaning pads or sterile gauze
   d. aseptic, lint-free, non-shedding hood-cleaning pads or nonsterile gauze

5. It is acceptable technique to use the *same* hood-cleaning pad to clean the entire hood.
   a. True. As long as it is clean, it is acceptable.
   b. False. You should only use the same pad to clean the ceiling and sides of the hood.
   c. True. As long as it has alcohol on it, it is acceptable.
   d. False. You should use a new pad with each section because the pad becomes contaminated when it reaches the outer edge of the hood.

Thinking Like a Pharmacy Tech

1. How does good hood-cleaning technique relate to patient care and safety?

2. *Scenario: While preparing a sterile IV solution, you realize that you accidentally cut yourself on a glass ampule. There is no visible blood on the work surface.* What, if any, procedures should you follow to clean the hood in this scenario?

3. IV technicians have a great deal of autonomy and often work alone–with the pharmacist only entering the IV room to perform the final check of the CSP. Considering the level of trust that is placed in an IV technician, what are some of the personal qualities that IV technicians must possess?

Preparing Large-Volume Parenteral Solutions

Lab 31

Objectives

- Demonstrate proficiency in aseptic technique as it relates to the preparation of large-volume parenteral products.
- Demonstrate accuracy in basic calculations related to the preparation of large-volume parenteral products.
- Discuss the procedures and rationale for the preparation of large-volume parenteral products.

Supplies

- Potassium chloride 2 mEq/1 mL, multi-dose, bulk vial 250 mL
- 0.9% Sodium chloride 1000 mL IV bag (with injection port)
- Sterile dispensing pin
- 20 mL syringe
- Regular needle $\times$ 1 (regular needle = no filter, no vent)
- Sharps container (dedicated for IV-room use only)
- Trash container (dedicated for IV-room use only)
- Alcohol swabs $\times$ 3
- Calculator

Introduction to Sterile Compounding for Labs 31–34

Previous labs in this aseptic technique section provide you with background and practice in garbing by USP Chapter <797> standards, aseptic hand washing, and hood cleaning. In the final four labs of this book, Labs 31–34, you will employ these techniques while preparing sterile products. Your instructor may provide you with more detailed guidelines for following aseptic technique, and you should ask for clarification on any points about which you are unsure.

You will find Labs 31–34 to be considerably longer than many others in the textbook. However, sterile compounding and aseptic technique skills are essential in pharmacy work and important to the healthcare field. In fact, this work is frequently performed by the pharmacy sterile compounding technician. Therefore, as you encounter a long series of steps in these labs, please take your time and follow each step to completion. Once you become familiar with the technique, the processes go very quickly.

The following lists basic terms that apply generally to sterile product preparation labs:

- **Aseptic technique:** A clean, "without infection," technique that is free of pathogens.
- **Clean room:** A space where sterile parenteral products are prepared and that is often referred to as the IV room or the sterile compounding room; the room where the laminar airflow hoods are located. Access to the clean room is restricted to trained and properly garbed personnel. Professional conduct is required in the clean room: eating, drinking, and gum chewing are prohibited. Only certain supplies are allowed and must first be wiped down with an antimicrobial solution.
- **Coring:** An undesired event that occurs when a needle is inserted incorrectly into a rubber stopper atop a solution vial, causing a small bit of the stopper to tear off and contaminate the solution inside the vial.
- **Critical areas:** Parts of equipment or supplies that must never be touched and to which airflow from the HEPA filter should never be interrupted. These parts include the vial top, needle, hub of the needle, hub of the syringe, tip of the syringe, ampule neck, dispensing pin spike, and IV bag injection port.
- **Dilution:** Injection of a liquid medication into an IV solution, or the mixing of a liquid medication with a fluid such as sterile water or normal saline, which results in a more dilute concentration of the drug.
- **Milking technique:** A process used to ease the negative pressure in a vial or other closed container by adding positive pressure to the system. This technique involves inserting a needle-and-syringe into the vial or container, adding a small amount of air to the vial, and then adding and removing small quantities of fluid and air as many times as necessary.
- **Negative pressure:** Applies to aseptic technique in being inherent to vials and some other closed systems, wherein negative pressure prohibits the withdrawal of fluid from the vial into a syringe. This situation is altered by equalizing the pressure inside of the vial by using a dispensing pin, vented needle, or the milking technique.
- **Parenteral:** Refers to medications administered by any route other than through the alimentary canal (the digestive tract), thus including every method of dispensation other than by mouth or rectum. The parenteral route of administration includes the intravenous, intramuscular, transdermal, intraocular, or intrathecal dispensation of drugs.
- **Pathogen:** An infectious agent that can cause disease or illness in a patient.
- **Positive pressure:** For the purposes of aseptic technique, this situation occurs when a small amount of air is introduced into a vial or other closed system, thereby easing the withdrawal of fluid from the vial into the syringe. (See the entry on milking technique for additional explanation.)
- **Shadowing:** A form of contamination that results when a worker's hands or supplies on the hood are incorrectly placed, disrupting sterile airflow from the HEPA filter to the critical area. Figure 31.1 shows airflow in a hood.
- **Six-inch rule:** Standard procedure whereby technicians must not work within the outer six inches of the hood's work surface. This area is considered the "dirty edge" because sterile air mixes with room air. However, for ease of access, pre-wrapped objects that are to be used shortly, such as needles, syringes, and alcohol swabs, are often placed in this outer-six-inch area.
- **Touch contamination:** A form of contamination that results when a critical area, or the hood surface itself, is contaminated through incorrect technique, needle stick, sneezing, or coughing.

FIGURE 31.1
Airflow in a horizontal laminar airflow hood

Downward view onto the hood work surface; items should be placed in the hood so as to receive uninterrupted airflow.

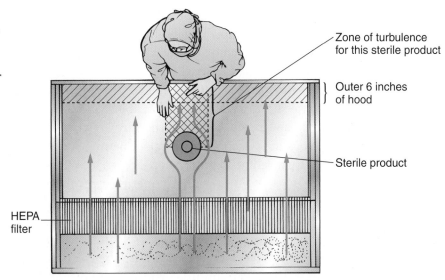

Zone of turbulence for this sterile product

Outer 6 inches of hood

Sterile product

HEPA filter

- **Zone of turbulence:** An area behind any item (e.g., vial, IV bag, syringe) on the hood where sterile airflow is interrupted; the zone or area is contaminated. Sterile parenteral products should never be prepared within a zone of turbulence.

Take Note

As a pharmacy technician, you are required to adhere to strict aseptic technique when preparing parenteral products. Why is that so crucial? Medications that are administered directly into the patient's bloodstream, internal organ, or internal tissue are considered to be the most dangerous to the patient—certainly more dangerous than are enteral (nonparenteral) products. Danger exists for a few reasons. First, because parenteral medications are administered directly into the bloodstream, organ, or tissue, the patient's only defense against potential pathogens is the patient's immune system, which is already compromised by fighting a primary infection or recovering from injury or surgery. In contrast, enteral products go through the digestive tract, where an abundance of flora defends against many pathogenic organisms. Second, once a medication is injected into the bloodstream, there is little to no chance of reversal; enteral medications can be reversed with ipecac or activated charcoal if a mistake is made (i.e., an incorrect drug or dose is administered). Third, parenteral agents introduce 100% of the drug into the bloodstream, whereas, with enteral administration, only a portion of the drug reaches the bloodstream.

Large-volume parenteral preparations are sterile solutions of 250 mL or larger volume that are administered parenterally. Many of the procedures performed while working in the sterile compounding room involve the aseptic preparation of large-volume parenteral products that are administered intravenously (often abbreviated IV). A large-volume IV solution is most often referred to as a "main" IV line, providing hydration for the patient and delivering electrolytes, such as potassium, directly into the patient's vein.

The most common large-volume parenteral preparations are intravenous solutions based on a standard solution such as 0.9% sodium chloride (which is called normal saline), dextrose 5% in water, dextrose 5% in normal saline, and lactated Ringer's solution. You will commonly see these base solutions referred to in abbreviated form (NS, D5W, D5NS, and LR, respectively) and find they are kept on hand at all times in the floor stock area of most hospitals. The most common volumes for large-volume intravenous solutions are 250 mL, 500 mL, and 1000 mL.

These base solutions are frequently a component of the sterile preparations prepared by pharmacy technicians. As a technician, you will compound large-volume parenteral solutions by aseptically injecting a medication into an intravenous base solution. Prior to preparing the solutions, however, you must execute the calculations most commonly used in sterile compounding—those based on ratio and proportion. Compounding large-volume parenteral solutions also requires familiarity with a dispensing pin, a syringe, and a needle. The **dispensing pin** is a specialized product that allows withdrawal of a large volume of fluid—in this case, potassium chloride—without concern for air pressure.

Dispensing pin

A specialized plastic device that includes a vent, a spike, and a syringe adaptor, and is inserted into the rubber stopper of a vial

Procedure

In this lab, you will perform a calculation related to the preparation of one large-volume parenteral product, demonstrate the correct use of a dispensing pin, and aseptically prepare a sterile solution for intravenous administration. The prepared intravenous solution will be composed of 1000 mL of 0.9% sodium chloride (NS) and 25 mEq of potassium chloride (KCl).

Take Note

"Eq" is the abbreviated form of "equivalent," a concentration unit used in chemistry. Since the amount is often very small, it is described as a milliequivalent (mEq) with the prefix "milli" indicating that it is divisible by one thousand. Interested students are referred to any basic chemistry text for further information.

1 In order to perform the necessary calculations for preparation of a 25 mEq dose of KCl solution, first verify the information provided on the KCl label. The KCl concentration should be stated as 2 mEq/1 mL.

Take Note

Potassium chloride is a commonly used electrolyte; however, it is also a "high alert" medication which, if administered incorrectly can cause immediate cardiac cessation leading to death.

2 Given this concentration, calculate how many milliliters you will need to withdraw from the vial in order to prepare the 25 mEq dose. Using the following formula, calculate the dose by cross-multiplying and then dividing to solve for x, the unknown volume. When your calculations are complete, write your answer for x here: _____ mL. This is the amount you must draw up and add to the IV bag to create your solution.

$$\frac{2 \text{ mEq}}{1 \text{ mL}} = \frac{25 \text{ mEq}}{x \text{ mL}}$$

3 Don aseptic garb, hand wash, don sterile gown and gloves, and clean the work area according to your instructor's direction.

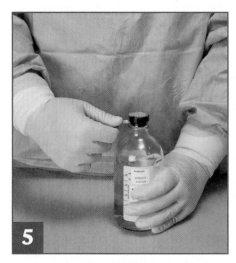

Pharmacy technician pulling the pull tab off of the aluminum cap on a bulk potassium chloride vial.

4 Remove and discard the outer wrapper from the IV bag and place the bag into the hood. Place the other necessary supplies in the hood, ensuring that supplies in an outer wrapper, such as syringes and needles, remain in the outer 6" zone closest to the edge of the hood until they are ready to be used.

Tip: *The waste container and the sharps container should be placed on the floor near the hood, but not within the hood itself.*

5 ***Tip:*** *Be very careful in this step when removing the aluminum cap from the KCl bulk vial. The cap is quite sharp.*

First, gently lift up the small pull tab on the top of the cap. Now grasp the pull tab and pull it

FIGURE 31.2 Cap removal from bulk vial

Correct technique for removing the aluminum cap from a bulk vial.

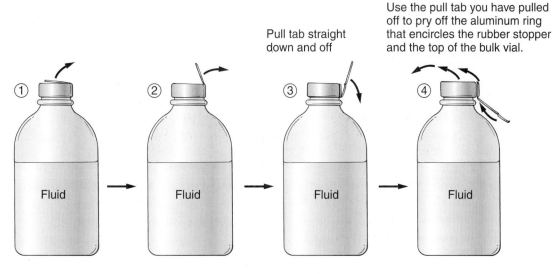

Pull tab straight down and off

Use the pull tab you have pulled off to pry off the aluminum ring that encircles the rubber stopper and the top of the bulk vial.

① Fluid → ② Fluid → ③ Fluid → ④ Fluid

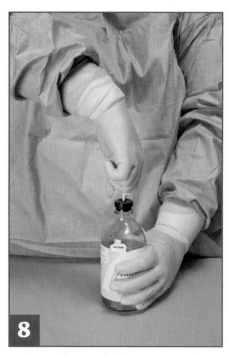

Correct technique for the insertion of a dispensing pin into a bulk potassium chloride vial.

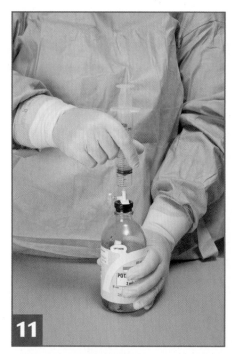

Pharmacy technician attaching a syringe to the open port of a dispensing pin.

down toward the bottom of the vial, pulling all the way down and removing it. Take care not to twist the tab, so that it does not break in two. Once the entire tab has been removed, use it as a tool for prying off the aluminum ring encircling the rubber stopper and vial top. Then lift off and discard the coin-like aluminum circle resting atop the rubber stopper. This technique is illustrated in Figure 31.2 and the accompanying photograph.

6   Swab the rubber stopper of the KCl vial with a sterile alcohol swab and place the swab on the hood in an area that is free of airflow obstruction.

7   Remove and discard the outer wrapper on the sterile dispensing pin. Hold the top of the dispensing pin in the dominant hand and, with the other hand, take the cap off the spike of the dispensing pin and discard the cap.

8   Hold the KCl vial steady against the hood surface with the non-dominant hand. Insert the spike of the dispensing pin straight into the rubber stopper of the KCl vial with the dominant hand.

9   Remove the cap from the top of the dispensing pin, taking care not to shadow or otherwise contaminate the dispensing pin, the top of the KCl vial, or the cap itself. Place the cap onto the sterile alcohol swab.

10   Remove and discard the outer wrapper of the syringe. If necessary, remove and discard the cap from the tip of the syringe.

Tip: Take care when removing the syringe from its outer wrapper. Some syringes have a cap on the tip; some do not. If there is a cap, it must be removed and discarded prior to attaching the syringe to the dispensing pin. If there is no cap, be careful not to shadow or otherwise contaminate the tip of the syringe. Never lay an uncapped syringe onto the work surface.

11   Without interrupting airflow to the KCl vial or the syringe, attach the tip of the syringe to the open port on the dispensing pin. Give the syringe a slight clockwise twist

FIGURE 31.3
Critical areas

Take care not to touch
or shadow any of the
critical areas.

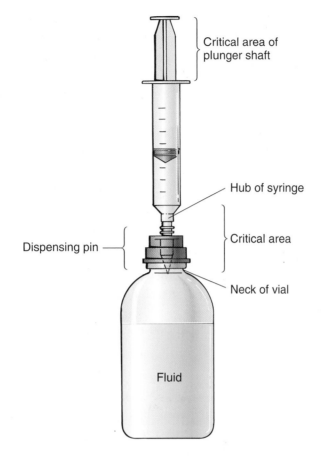

Critical area of
plunger shaft

Hub of syringe

Dispensing pin

Critical area

Neck of vial

Fluid

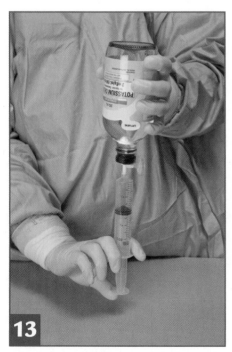

13

Correct technique for withdrawing fluid
using a 20 mL syringe, dispensing pin, and
inverted bulk vial.

to ensure that it is firmly attached to the
dispensing pin. Care must be taken to avoid
contaminating the critical areas, shown in
Figure 31.3

12 Invert the KCl vial such that the syringe is
located underneath it.

*Tip: Since the dispensing pin includes a vent,
there is no need to add air to the vial when withdrawing fluid.*

13 Holding the KCl vial with the non-dominant
hand, pull down on the plunger of the
syringe with the dominant hand until you
reach approximately the 15 mL graduation
mark on the syringe.

*Tip: Take care to hold the vial and syringe in such a
manner that airflow to the critical area—the area
from the hub of the syringe to the neck of the vial,
including the entire dispensing pin and the rubber vial
top—is unobstructed.*

14 Stabilize the syringe against the palm of your non-dominant hand and tap the syringe with the fingers or palm to force potential air bubbles toward the hub of the syringe. When all air bubbles have risen to the hub, gently push up on the plunger to expel any remaining air and continue slowly pushing up until the desired volume of 12.5 mL is reached. The configuration of the syringe and vial is shown in Figure 31.4.
Tip: Remember to take the syringe volume reading at the point where the shoulder of the rubber plunger meets the barrel of the syringe.

15 Invert the vial-and-syringe unit and return it to the work surface. Grasp the barrel of the syringe and twist counterclockwise to remove the syringe from the dispensing pin, taking care not to interrupt airflow to either the KCl vial or the syringe.

16 Without laying the syringe down or shadowing the hub, and without touching the needle hub, aseptically attach a regular needle, with cap, to the syringe.

17 Place the syringe, with capped needle, onto the work surface next to the KCl vial and the IV bag.

FIGURE 31.4
Filling a syringe from a bulk vial

Syringe measurement taken where the shoulder of the rubber plunger meets the barrel of the syringe.

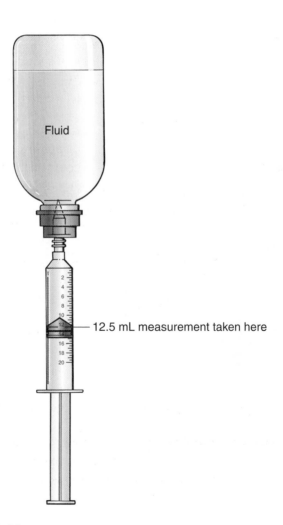

12.5 mL measurement taken here

FIGURE 31.5
Critical area during IV-bag preparation

Critical areas should not be touched or shadowed at any time.

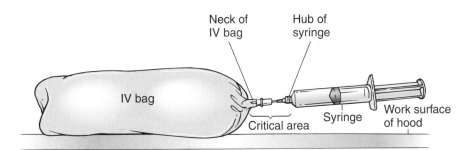

Neck of IV bag — Hub of syringe — IV bag — Critical area — Syringe — Work surface of hood

18 Recap the top of the dispensing pin with the cap that was earlier placed on the alcohol swab and ask for an instructor check.

19 Once your work has been approved, place the IV bag in a position to ensure that the injection port receives uninterrupted airflow. Swab the injection port of the IV bag with a new, sterile alcohol swab and place the swab on the hood surface such that it receives uninterrupted airflow. This process is shown in Figure 31.5.
Tip: Always keep the IV bag at least 6" from the outer edge of the hood.

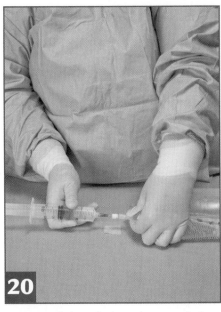

20

Correct technique for inserting a needle into the injection port of a large-volume parenteral solution.

20 Hold the barrel of the syringe in the dominant hand. Remove the cap of the needle and place it onto the alcohol swab. Hold the injection port steady with the non-dominant hand and insert the needle straight into the injection port.
Tip: The insertion should be smooth. If you encounter any resistance, the needle has likely entered the sidewall of the injection port stem, which is potentially dangerous. If this occurs, back out and repeat the insertion process with the same needle.

21 Inject the medication into the bag by pressing on the plunger of the syringe.

22 Holding only the barrel of the syringe, carefully remove the needle-and-syringe unit from the IV bag. Place the unit into the sharps container.

23 Without removing the IV bag from the hood, squeeze the bag to check for leaks and visually inspect the bag for precipitates.

24 **Conclusion:** Ask for a final check by the instructor. On a separate sheet of paper, answer all questions in the following Lab Review section and turn in your answers to your instructor.

Lab Review

Check Your Understanding

1. What is the best venting technique to use when preparing a parenteral solution by using a large-volume, or bulk, glass vial?
   a. Add a volume of air equal to what you will be withdrawing.
   b. Use a vented needle.
   c. Use the "milking" technique.
   d. Use a dispensing pin.

2. What is the correct venting technique to be used with a plastic or PVC bag such as normal saline 1000 mL?
   a. Allow air pressure to release into the syringe after the fluid is injected.
   b. There is no need to vent this product since it expands and contracts itself.
   c. Use negative pressure.
   d. Add a volume of air equal to the volume of solution that you wish to withdraw from the IV bag.

3. What concentration of sodium chloride is considered to be "normal saline"?
   a. 0.225% sodium chloride
   b. 0.33% sodium chloride
   c. 0.45% sodium chloride
   d. 0.9% sodium chloride

4. Which of the following describes the correct way to connect a syringe to a dispensing pin?
   a. The needle should be attached to the syringe, and the top of the dispensing pin should be swabbed with alcohol before attaching the syringe to the dispensing pin.
   b. The syringe, without a needle, should be attached directly to the dispensing pin after the top of the dispensing pin has been swabbed with alcohol.
   c. The syringe, without a needle, should be attached directly to the dispensing pin, and the top of the dispensing pin should not be swabbed.
   d. The needle should be attached to the syringe and then attached directly to the dispensing pin, without swabbing anything with alcohol.

5. Which of the following scenarios is an example of incorrect aseptic technique?
   a. laying an uncapped syringe onto the work surface
   b. placing an uncapped needle into the sharps container
   c. failing to insert the dispensing pin with the bevel pointed up
   d. failing to insert the needle into the IV bag with the bevel pointed up

Thinking Like a Pharmacy Tech

1. Why is it important that products administered parenterally be prepared using strict aseptic technique?

2. Intravenous KCl must be diluted in at least 100 mL of fluid. Why might this large fluid volume be necessary for the patient?

 3. As you progress in your career as a pharmacy technician, it is important to have goals in mind. Where do you see yourself in five years? Ten years? How will you go about accomplishing your goals?

Preparing Small-Volume Parenteral Solutions

Lab 32

Objectives

- Demonstrate proficiency in aseptic technique related to the preparation of small-volume parenteral products.
- Demonstrate accuracy in basic calculations related to the preparation of small-volume parenteral products.
- Discuss the procedures and rationale for the preparation of small-volume parenteral products.

Supplies

- Metoclopramide 10 mg/2 mL vials × 2
- D5W 50mL IVPB (with injection port) × 2
- Regular needles × 2 (regular needle = no filter, no vent)
- 3 mL syringes × 2
- Sharps container (dedicated for IV-room use only)
- Trash container (dedicated for IV-room use only)
- Alcohol swabs × 4
- Calculator

Introduction to Sterile Compounding for Labs 31–34

Note: If you have completed Lab 31, you may skip this introduction and begin after the first Take Note feature. Previous labs in this aseptic technique section provide you with background and practice in garbing by USP Chapter <797> standards, aseptic hand washing, and hood cleaning. In the final four labs of this book, Labs 31–34, you will employ these techniques while preparing compounded sterile preparations. Your instructor may provide you with more detailed guidelines for following aseptic technique, and you should ask for clarification on any points about which you are unsure.

You will find Labs 31–34 to be considerably longer than many others in the textbook. However, skills in sterile compounding and aseptic technique are essential in pharmacy work and important to the healthcare field. In fact, this work is frequently performed by the pharmacy sterile compounding technician. Therefore, as you encounter a long series of steps in these labs, please take your time and follow each step to completion. Once you become familiar with the technique, the processes go very quickly.

The following lists basic terms that apply generally to sterile product preparation labs:

- **Aseptic technique:** A clean, "without infection," technique that is free of pathogens.
- **Clean room:** A space where sterile parenteral products are prepared and that is often referred to as the IV room or the sterile compounding room; the room where laminar airflow hoods are located. Access to the clean room is restricted to trained and properly garbed personnel. Professional conduct is required in the clean room: eating, drinking, and gum chewing are prohibited. Only certain supplies are allowed and must first be wiped down with an antimicrobial solution.
- **Coring:** An undesired event that occurs when a needle is inserted incorrectly into a rubber stopper atop a solution vial, causing a small bit of the stopper to tear off and contaminate the solution inside the vial.
- **Critical areas:** On equipment or supplies, parts that must never be touched and to which airflow from the HEPA filter should never be interrupted. These parts include the vial top, needle, hub of the needle, hub of the syringe, tip of the syringe, ampule neck, dispensing pin spike, and IV bag injection port.
- **Dilution:** Injection of a liquid medication into an IV solution, or the mixing of a liquid medication with a fluid such as sterile water or normal saline, which results in a more dilute concentration of the drug.
- **Milking technique:** A process used to ease the negative pressure in a vial or other closed container by adding positive pressure to the system. This technique involves inserting a needle-and-syringe into the vial or container, adding a small amount of air to the vial, and then adding and removing small quantities of fluid and air as many times as necessary.
- **Negative pressure:** Applies to aseptic technique in being inherent to vials and some other closed systems, wherein negative pressure prohibits the withdrawal of fluid from the vial into a syringe. This situation is altered by equalizing the pressure inside of the vial by using a dispensing pin, vented needle, or the milking technique.
- **Parenteral:** Refers to medications administered by any route other than through the alimentary canal (the digestive tract), thus including every method of dispensation other than by mouth or rectum. The parenteral route of administration includes the intravenous, intramuscular, transdermal, intraocular, or intrathecal dispensation of drugs.
- **Pathogen:** An infectious agent that can cause disease or illness in a patient.
- **Positive pressure:** For the purposes of aseptic technique, this situation occurs when a small amount of air is introduced into a vial or other closed system, thereby easing the withdrawal of fluid from the vial into the syringe. (See the entry on milking technique for additional explanation.)
- **Shadowing:** A form of contamination that results when a worker's hands or supplies on the hood are incorrectly placed, disrupting sterile airflow from the HEPA filter to the critical area. Figure 32.1 shows airflow in a hood.
- **Six-inch rule:** Standard procedure whereby technicians must not work within the outer six inches of the hood's work surface. This area is considered the "dirty edge" because sterile air mixes with room air. However, for ease of access, pre-wrapped objects that are to be used shortly, such as needles, syringes, and alcohol swabs, are often placed in this outer-six-inch area.
- **Touch contamination:** A form of contamination that results when a critical area, or the hood surface itself, is contaminated through incorrect technique, needle stick, sneezing, or coughing.
- **Zone of turbulence:** An area behind any item (e.g., vial, IV bag, syringe) on the hood where sterile airflow is interrupted; the zone or area is thereby contaminated. Sterile parenteral products should never be prepared within a zone of turbulence.

Take Note

As a pharmacy technician, you are required to adhere to strict aseptic technique when preparing parenteral products. Why is that so crucial? Medications that are administered directly into the patient's bloodstream, internal organ, or internal tissue are considered to be the most dangerous to the patient—certainly more dangerous than are enteral (nonparenteral) products. Danger exists for a few reasons. First, because parenteral medications are administered directly into the bloodstream, organ, or tissue, the patient's only defense against potential pathogens is the patient's immune system, which is already compromised by fighting a primary infection or recovering from injury or surgery. In contrast, enteral products go through the digestive tract, where an abundance of flora defends against many pathogenic organisms. Second, once a medication is injected into the bloodstream, there is little to no chance of reversal; enteral medications can be reversed with ipecac or activated charcoal if a mistake is made (i.e., an incorrect drug or dose is administered). Third, parenteral agents introduce 100% of the drug into the bloodstream, whereas, with enteral administration, only a portion of the drug reaches the bloodstream.

Intravenous piggyback solution

An intermittent infusion containing a standard base solution plus an IV medication; delivered through a main IV line

Small-volume parenteral preparations are sterile solutions of 250 mL or smaller volume that are administered parenterally. The most common small-volume parenteral preparations compounded in the clean room are **intravenous** (IV) **piggyback** solutions, which are intermittent infusions that are delivered, or "piggybacked," through a main IV line. Intravenous piggybacks (often referred to in abbreviated form as IVPBs) consist of two components: a standard base solution and an IV medication that is added to that base.

Sterile compounding of small-volume parenteral solutions requires that you first execute calculations to determine the amount of medication to add to the base.

Some of the most common IVPB base solutions are: 0.9% sodium chloride (normal saline), dextrose 5% in water, and 0.45% sodium chloride. Again, abbreviations are popular, and those three base solutions are usually referred to, respectively, as NS, D5W, and 1/2 NS. IVPB base solutions are most commonly supplied in 50 mL and 100 mL volumes.

Procedure

In this lab you will first perform calculations related to small-volume parenteral preparation and then prepare two sterile solutions for intravenous piggyback administration using strict adherence to aseptic technique. The products you will prepare are:

> Metoclopramide 10 mg in 50 mL D5W
> Metoclopramide 7.5 mg in 50 mL D5W

1 First perform your necessary calculations based on the information provided on the metoclopramide label, which should indicate a concentration of 10 mg/2 mL. Given this concentration, separately calculate how many milliliters you need to withdraw from the vial in order to prepare the two doses, 10 mg and 7.5 mg. Using the following formulas, calculate the doses by cross multiplying and then dividing to solve for x, the unknown volume. When your calculations are complete, write your answer here: For the 10 mg dose, $x =$ _____ mL and for the 7.5 mg dose, $x =$ _____ mL . These are the amounts you must draw up and add to the IV bag to create your solutions.

$$\frac{10 \text{ mg}}{2 \text{ mL}} = \frac{10 \text{ mg}}{x \text{ mL}} \qquad \frac{10 \text{ mg}}{2 \text{ mL}} = \frac{7.5 \text{ mg}}{x \text{ mL}}$$

2 Don aseptic garb, hand wash, don sterile gown and gloves, and clean the hood according to your instructor's direction.

3 Remove the IVPBs from their outer wrapper. Place the wrappers in the trash, and place the IVPBs onto the hood surface, at least six inches inside the hood. Place the other supplies into the outer six inch edge of the hood.

4 Remove the cap from the top of the metoclopramide vial and swab the rubber stopper with a sterile alcohol swab. Place the swab on the hood in an area that is free of airflow obstruction.

FIGURE 32.1
Critical areas of needle and syringe

Always be cautious and avoid touching or shadowing the critical areas.

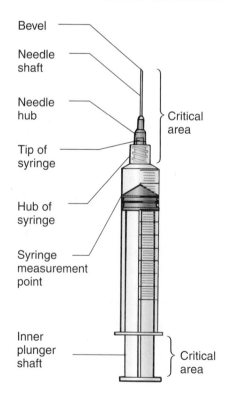

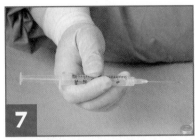

Correct technique for holding a syringe in preparation for insertion into a vial or bag.

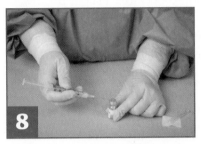

Correct placement of a needle onto the surface of the vial top. The beveled end of the needle should face upward.

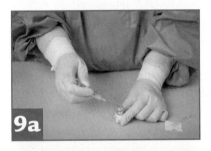

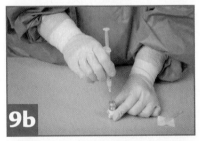

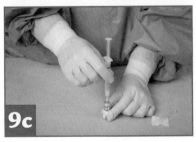

Correct technique for inserting a needle into a vial. Note the slight bending of the needle and the technician's arm motion (upward) as the needle is inserted into the vial.

5 Aseptically attach a regular needle to a 3 mL syringe. Details of a syringe are shown in Figure 32.1.

Tip: Take care when removing the syringe from its outer wrapper. Some syringes have a cap on the tip; some do not. If there is a cap, it must be removed prior to attaching the syringe to the dispensing pin. If there is no cap, be careful not to shadow or otherwise contaminate the tip of the syringe. Never lay an uncapped syringe onto the work surface.

6 Prepare the syringe by adding an amount of air that is equal to the amount of diluent to be withdrawn. (When preparing your first dose, 2 mL will be withdrawn and thus you should pull the plunger down to the 2 mL volume mark on the syringe.)

7 Hold the syringe with the thumb and the index and middle finger of the dominant hand in a manner similar to how you might hold a pencil or dart. Remove the cap from the needle and place the cap onto the alcohol swab with the open end facing toward the hood filter.

8 Using the non-dominant hand, brace the diluent vial against the work surface. Lay the tip of the needle onto the rubber vial top of the diluent such that your palm is facing upward and the tip of the needle is facing bevel up and is located at the center of the top of the vial.

9 Insert the needle into the vial using a slight upward rotation of the wrist (rotating in a counterclockwise direction if the right hand holds the syringe or a clockwise direction if the left hand holds the syringe.) Keep the tip of the needle in contact with the rubber vial top at all times to ensure smooth insertion into the vial.

Tip: There should be a very slight—almost imperceptible—bend in the needle from the gentle downward pressure as it enters the vial. Correct needle insertion will help to prevent coring of the vial's rubber top.

10 Hold the metoclopramide vial in the non-dominant hand and the barrel of the syringe in

the dominant hand and, while keeping the needle completely inserted into the diluent vial, invert the vial so that the needle-and-syringe unit is now below the vial.

Tip: Take care to hold the vial and syringe in such a manner that airflow to the critical area—the area from the tip of the syringe to the neck of the vial, including the entire needle and the rubber vial top—is unobstructed.

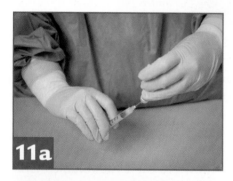

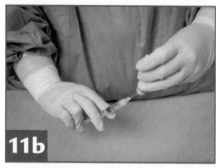

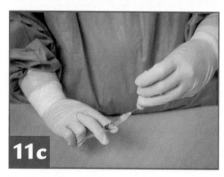

Creation of positive pressure within a vial using the milking technique. Notice positioning of the technician's fingers and that the syringe volume changes from empty (top) to actively filling (middle) to mostly full (bottom).

11 Gradually push up on the plunger to add a small amount—approximately 1 mL—of air to the vial. This addition creates a slight positive-pressure environment within the vial and will assist you in withdrawing fluid from the vial. Release the plunger to allow some fluid to flow into the syringe. Repeat this process of adding a small amount of air and removing a small amount of fluid (often called the "milking" technique) until all of the pre-measured air is added to the vial and an equal amount of diluent has been drawn into the syringe.

Tip: As you withdraw liquid from the vial, be sure to keep the tip of the needle within the fluid to avoid drawing air into the syringe.

12 Verify that the syringe now contains the desired amount of medication (in the case of the first dose, 2 mL). If necessary, tap the syringe to force air bubbles to the tip of the syringe and then expel any excess air by gently pressing upward on the plunger. Verify again that the desired amount of medication is present, and if it is not, pull down on the plunger to draw more fluid into the syringe.

Tip: Be sure that you have drawn up the correct amount of fluid and that there are no large bubbles in the syringe before proceeding to Step 13.

13 While keeping the needle firmly inserted into the vial, return the vial and syringe to the original starting position, with the upright vial braced against the work surface and the dominant hand correctly holding the barrel of the inverted syringe. Slowly remove the needle-and-syringe unit from the medication vial. Remember to avoid touching the plunger of the syringe at any time while removing it from the vial.

Take Note

The **scoop method** of recapping involves laying the needle cap on the hood surface with the non-dominant hand while carefully holding the syringe at the barrel with the dominant hand. Slowly move the tip of the needle inside the empty cap until enough of the needle is inside of the cap such that you can use the dominant hand, holding the syringe, to lift the syringe and cap off the hood into a vertical, or upright, position. Once the syringe and needle are in an upright position, use the non-dominant hand to snap the cap firmly back onto the needle. Take care not to touch the needle to the work surface, your fingers, or other contaminant while recapping the needle. If, by using the scoop method, the needle is inadvertently contaminated by touch or shadowing, you must dispose of the needle-and-syringe and repeat the entire procedure starting at step 4, using new supplies.

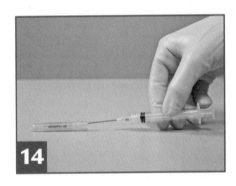

14 Carefully recap the needle using the "scoop," or other appropriate, method.

15 Repeat Steps 4 through 14 with the other 3 mL syringe, withdrawing the amount you calculated as necessary for the 7.5 mg dose.

16 Place both filled syringes, with capped needles, on the work surface next to the metoclopramide vial and IVPBs and ask for an instructor check.

17 Once your work has been approved, place the first IVPB, to which you will add the 10 mg dose, in a position to ensure that the injection port receives uninterrupted airflow. Swab the injection port of the IV bag with a new, sterile alcohol swab.

18 Place the swab on the hood surface such that it receives uninterrupted airflow.

19 Hold the barrel of the syringe in the dominant hand. Remove the cap of the needle and place it onto the alcohol swab.

20 Hold the injection port steady with the non-dominant hand, taking care to avoid shadowing the injection port.

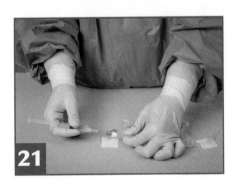

21 Insert the needle straight into the injection port. *Tip: The insertion should be smooth. If you encounter any resistance, the needle has likely entered the sidewall of the injection port stem, which is potentially dangerous. If this occurs, back out and repeat the insertion process with the same needle.*

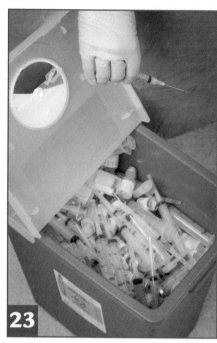

23

Technician placing a needle and syringe into the sharps container.

22 Inject the medication into the bag by pressing on the plunger of the syringe.
Tip: When inserting a needle into the injection port of an IVPB, it is not necessary to consider the direction of the bevel. The needle should be inserted straight into the bag, without angle and without bending the needle.

23 Holding only the barrel of the syringe, carefully remove the needle-and-syringe unit from the IV bag. Place the unit into the sharps container.

24 Repeat Steps 17 through 23 for the 7.5 mg dose, using the second IVPB.

25 Squeeze each IVPB to check for leaks and visually inspect each bag for precipitates.

26 **Conclusion:** Ask for a final check from your instructor. On a separate sheet of paper, answer all questions in the following Lab Review section and turn in your answers to your instructor.

Lab Review

Check Your Understanding

1. Which of the following correctly describes the characteristics of an intravenous piggyback?
   a. an intermittent infusion of medication administered through a main IV line
   b. a continuous infusion of medication administered through a main IV line
   c. an intermittent injection of medication given intramuscularly
   d. a continuous infusion of medication administered through a peripheral IV line

2. Incorrect placement of the vial on the hood can lead to a type of contamination commonly referred to as what?
   a. touch contamination
   b. shadowing
   c. incorrect volume
   d. coring

3. Which of the following volumes is considered to be a small-volume parenteral?
   a. 25 mL
   b. 50 mL
   c. 500 mL
   d. a and b only

4. Forcing into a vial an amount of air that is equal to or slightly less than the volume you wish to withdraw from the vial creates _____.
   a. negative pressure
   b. positive pressure
   c. low pressure
   d. high pressure

5. Which of the following best describes the correct way to hold a syringe when inserting the needle into a vial?
   a. It does not matter how the syringe is held provided that the airflow is uninterrupted.
   b. like a knife with the bevel pointing up
   c. like a dart with the bevel pointing down
   d. like a dart with the bevel pointing up

Thinking Like a Pharmacy Tech

1. Why is it important to perform any necessary calculations at the beginning of the compounding process as opposed to right before the solution needs to be drawn up?

2. First describe some of the "critical areas" of the IVPB and the syringe-and-needle unit. Then describe at least three specific, different examples of poor technique that might potentially contaminate any compounded sterile preparation should a technician fail to follow the rules of strict aseptic technique.

3. USP Chapter <797> guidelines require initial and annual competency assessments, which include a written exam, process validation, and media-fill aseptic technique testing. Why is it important for the technician to undergo such rigorous testing? Why is it important to be retested annually?

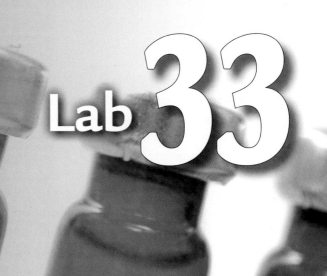

Preparing Sterile Powder Drug Vials

Lab 33

Objectives

- Demonstrate proficiency in aseptic technique as it relates to the preparation of sterile powder drug vials.
- Demonstrate accuracy in basic calculations related to the preparation of sterile powder drug vials.
- Discuss the procedures and rationale for the preparation of sterile powder drug vials.

Supplies

- Ampicillin 1 gram vial (powder, for parenteral administration)
- Sterile water vial for injection 10 mL
- 10 mL syringe
- 5 mL syringe $\times$ 2
- Regular needle $\times$ 3 (regular needle = no filter, no vent)
- Vented needle
- Sharps container (dedicated for IV-room use only)
- Trash container (dedicated for IV-room use only)
- Alcohol swabs $\times$ 3
- Calculator

Introduction to Sterile Compounding for Labs 31–34

Note: If you have completed Lab 31, you may skip this introduction and begin after the first Take Note feature. Previous labs in this aseptic technique section provide you with background and practice in garbing by USP Chapter <797> standards, aseptic hand washing, and hood cleaning. In the final four labs of this book, Labs 31–34, you will employ these techniques while preparing sterile products. Your instructor may provide you with more detailed guidelines for following aseptic technique, and you should ask for clarification on any points about which you are unsure.

You will find Labs 31–34 to be considerably longer than many others in the textbook. However, skills in compounding and aseptic technique are essential in pharmacy work and important to the healthcare field. In fact, this work is frequently performed by the pharmacy sterile compounding technician. Therefore, as you encounter a long series of steps in these labs, please take your time and follow each step to completion. Once you become familiar with the technique, the processes go very quickly.

The following lists basic terms that apply generally to sterile product preparation labs:

- **Aseptic technique:** A clean, "without infection," technique that is free of pathogens.
- **Clean room:** A space where sterile parenteral products are prepared and that is often referred to as the IV room or the sterile compounding room; the room where the laminar airflow hoods are located. Access to the clean room is restricted to trained and properly garbed personnel. Professional conduct is required in the clean room: eating, drinking, and gum chewing are prohibited. Only certain supplies are allowed and must first be wiped down with an antimicrobial solution.
- **Coring:** An undesired event that occurs when a needle is inserted incorrectly into a rubber stopper atop a solution vial, causing a small bit of the stopper to tear off and contaminate the solution inside the vial.
- **Critical areas:** On equipment or supplies, areas that must never be touched and to which airflow from the HEPA filter should never be interrupted. These areas include the vial top, needle, hub of the needle, hub of the syringe, tip of the syringe, ampule neck, dispensing pin spike, and IV bag injection port.
- **Dilution:** Injection of a liquid medication into an IV solution, or the mixing of a liquid medication with a fluid such as sterile water or normal saline, which results in a more dilute concentration of the drug.
- **Milking technique:** A process used to ease the negative pressure in a vial or other closed container by adding positive pressure to the system. This technique involves inserting a needle-and-syringe into the vial or container, adding a small amount of air to the vial, and then adding and removing small quantities of fluid and air as many times as necessary.
- **Negative pressure:** Applies to aseptic technique in being inherent to vials and some other closed systems, wherein negative pressure prohibits the withdrawal of fluid from the vial into a syringe. This situation is altered by equalizing the pressure inside of the vial by using a dispensing pin, vented needle, or the milking technique.
- **Parenteral:** Refers to medications administered by any route other than through the alimentary canal (the digestive tract), thus including every method of dispensation other than by mouth or rectum. The parenteral route of administration includes the intravenous, intramuscular, transdermal, intraocular, or intrathecal dispensation of drugs.
- **Pathogen:** An infectious agent that can cause disease or illness in a patient.
- **Positive pressure:** For the purposes of aseptic technique, this situation occurs when a small amount of air is introduced into a vial or other closed system, thereby easing the withdrawal of fluid from the vial into the syringe. (See the entry on milking technique for additional explanation.)
- **Shadowing:** A form of contamination that results when a worker's hands or supplies on the hood are incorrectly placed, disrupting sterile airflow from the HEPA filter to the critical area. Figure 33.1 shows airflow in a hood.
- **Reconstitution:** Dissolving a powder drug into its liquid, injectible form by mixing it with a diluent such as sterile water or normal saline.
- **Six-inch rule:** Standard procedure whereby technicians must not work within the outer six inches of the hood's work surface. This area is considered the "dirty edge" because sterile air mixes with room air. However, for ease of access, pre-wrapped objects that are to be used shortly, such as needles, syringes, and alcohol swabs, are often placed in this outer-six-inch area.
- **Touch contamination:** A form of contamination that results when a critical area, or the hood surface itself, is contaminated through incorrect technique, needle stick, sneezing, or coughing.

- **Zone of turbulence:** An area behind any item (e.g., vial, IV bag, syringe) on the hood where sterile airflow is interrupted; the zone or area is thereby contaminated. Sterile parenteral products should never be prepared within a zone of turbulence.

Take Note

As a pharmacy technician, you are required to adhere to strict aseptic technique when preparing parenteral products. Why is that so crucial? Medications that are administered directly into the patient's bloodstream, internal organ, or internal tissue are considered to be the most dangerous to the patient—certainly more dangerous than are enteral (nonparenteral) products. Danger exists for a few reasons. First, because parenteral medications are administered directly into the bloodstream, organ, or tissue, the patient's only defense against potential pathogens is the patient's immune system, which is already compromised by fighting a primary infection or recovering from injury or surgery. In contrast, enteral products go through the digestive tract, where an abundance of flora defends against many pathogenic organisms. Second, once a medication is injected into the bloodstream, there is little to no chance of reversal; enteral medications can be reversed with ipecac or activated charcoal if a mistake is made (i.e., an incorrect drug or dose is administered). Third, parenteral agents introduce 100% of the drug into the bloodstream, whereas, with enteral administration, only a portion of the drug reaches the bloodstream.

Working in the clean room often requires the pharmacy technician to prepare medications involving reconstitution of a sterile powder drug. While many medications for parenteral use are supplied by the manufacturer in the form of an injectable liquid, others are supplied in a powder form that requires reconstitution prior to use. Some medications are supplied in powder form primarily because the drug has a longer shelf life or stability as a powder than it would in liquid form. Reconstitution of sterile powder drugs demands strict adherence to aseptic technique and the execution of calculations commonly used in sterile compounding.

Hospital pharmacy technicians reconstitute many powder medications to be administered as intravenous, intravenous piggyback, and intramuscular injections. Many of these types of products are antibiotics that are given to the patient to treat infection from pathogenic microorganisms such as bacteria, protozoa, or fungi. Hospital inpatients are commonly too ill to take medications orally, either because of nausea or because of poor digestive system function. In addition, some infections require treatment by antibiotics that are available only in injectable form.

The two most common diluents used to reconstitute sterile powder drugs are sterile water and 0.9% sodium chloride (known as normal saline). Both of these diluents are available with or without preservatives. Diluents with preservatives are commonly referred to as **bacteriostatic**—indicating that they contain an agent or preservative that inhibits the growth of bacteria within the diluent vial. Two commonly used preservatives are methylparaben and benzyl alcohol, and diluents containing them are used to dilute most powders in the sterile compounding lab. Diluents without preservatives are referred to as preservative free (PF) and are generally used

Bacteriostatic

Containing an agent or preservative to inhibit bacterial growth only in special situations, such as for neonatal patients or for intrathecal administration, or upon a physician's request.

Procedure

In this lab you will perform calculations related to drug reconstitution, use correct venting technique to reconstitute a sterile powder drug, and aseptically prepare two syringes with injectable antibiotic doses of the following:

Ampicillin 450 mg   Ampicillin 375 mg

Preparatory Steps

1 Perform your calculations based on the following information: Once reconstituted, the vial will contain 1 gram of ampicillin in 10 mL of solution. You need to draw up one dose of 450 mg and one dose of 375 mg. Use the following formula (cross multiply and then divide to solve for x, the unknown volume) to separately calculate how many milliliters you must withdraw from the vial in order to prepare the two doses. For the 450 mg dose, $x =$ _____ mL and for the 375 mg dose, $x =$ _____ mL .

$$\frac{1000 \text{ mg}}{10 \text{ mL}} = \frac{450 \text{ mg}}{x \text{ mL}} \qquad \frac{1000 \text{ mg}}{10 \text{ mL}} = \frac{375 \text{ mg}}{x \text{ mL}}$$

2 Don aseptic garb, hand wash, don sterile gown and gloves, and clean the hood according to your instructor's direction.

Drawing Up the Diluent

3 Remove the cap from the top of the diluent vial and swab the rubber stopper with a sterile alcohol swab. Place the swab on the hood in an area that is free of airflow obstruction.

4 Aseptically attach a regular needle to a 10 mL syringe.

5 Prepare the syringe by adding an amount of air that is equal to the amount of diluent to be withdrawn, in this case 10 mL. Do this by pulling the plunger down to the 10 mL volume mark on the syringe.

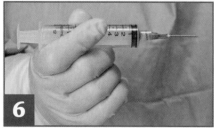

6

6 Hold the syringe with the thumb and the index and middle finger of the dominant hand in a manner similar to how you might hold a pencil or dart. Remove the cap from the needle and place it onto the alcohol swab with the open end of the cap facing toward the hood filter.

Correct technique for holding a syringe in preparation for insertion into a vial or bag.

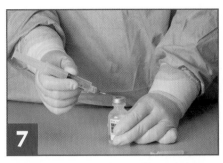

Correct placement of a needle onto the surface of the vial top. The beveled end of the needle should face upward.

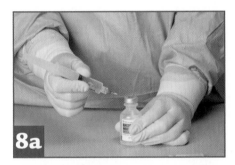

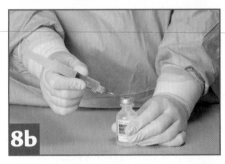

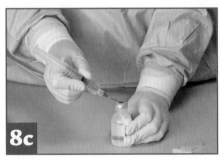

Correct technique for inserting a needle into a vial. Note the slight bending of the needle and the technician's arm motion (upward) as the needle is inserted into the vial.

7 Using the non-dominant hand, brace the diluent vial against the work surface. Lay the tip of the needle onto the rubber vial top of the diluent such that the tip of the needle is facing bevel up and located at the center of the top of the vial.

8 Insert the needle into the vial using a slight upward rotation of the wrist (rotating in a counterclockwise direction if the right hand holds the syringe or a clockwise direction if the left hand holds the syringe.) Keep the tip of the needle in contact with the rubber vial top at all times to ensure smooth insertion into the vial.

Tip: There should be a very slight—almost imperceptible—bend in the needle from the gentle downward pressure as it enters the vial. Correct needle insertion will help to prevent coring of the vial's rubber top.

9 Hold the diluent vial in the non-dominant hand and the barrel of the syringe in the dominant hand, and while keeping the needle completely inserted into the diluent vial, invert the vial so that the needle-and-syringe unit are now below the vial as shown in Figure 33.1 on the next page.

Tip: Take care to hold the vial and syringe in such a manner that airflow to the critical area (the area from the tip of the syringe to the neck of the vial, including the entire needle and the rubber vial top) is unobstructed.

10 Gradually push up on the plunger to add a small amount (approximately 2 mL) of air to the vial. This will create a slight positive pressure in the vial which will assist you in withdrawing the fluid. Release the plunger to allow some fluid to flow into the syringe. Repeat this process of adding a small amount of air and removing a small amount of diluent (often called the "milking" technique) until all the air that was in the syringe is added to the vial and the required amount of diluent has been drawn into the syringe. This technique is shown in the photos on the next page.

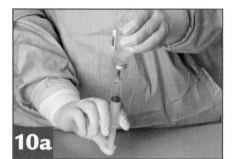
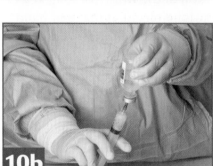

10a

10b

10c

Creation of positive pressure within a vial using the milking technique. Notice positioning of the technician's fingers and that the syringe volume changes from empty (top) to actively filling (middle) to mostly full (bottom).

FIGURE 33.1 **Critical areas for vial, needle, and syringe.**

Take special care not to touch critical areas.

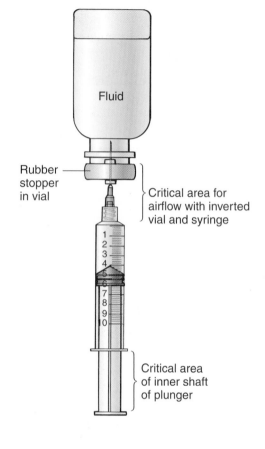

Fluid

Rubber stopper in vial

Critical area for airflow with inverted vial and syringe

Critical area of inner shaft of plunger

11 Verify that the syringe now contains the desired amount of diluent, in this case 10 mL. If necessary, tap the syringe to force air bubbles to the tip of the syringe and then expel any excess air by gently pressing upward on the plunger. Verify again that the desired amount of diluent is present, and if it is not, pull down on the plunger to draw more fluid into the syringe.

12 While keeping the needle firmly inserted into the vial, return the vial and syringe to the original starting position, with the vial braced against the work surface and the dominant hand correctly holding the barrel of the syringe.

13 Slowly remove the needle-and-syringe unit from the diluent vial. Carefully recap the needle using the "scoop" or other appropriate method.

Tip: *Be sure to avoid touching the plunger of the syringe at any time while removing it from the vial. Also take care not to touch the needle to the work surface or other contaminant while recapping it. If needed, review the "scoop" method as described above Step 14 of the previous lab, Lab 32.*

14 Hold the syringe so that the capped needle is pointing up and gently pull the plunger down approximately one-half milliliter. This pulling action will draw fluid from the needle into the syringe.

15 Remove the regular needle and place it into the sharps container.

Attaching the Vented Needle and Diluting the Ampicillin

16 Aseptically attach a capped, vented needle to the syringe. While holding the syringe with the needle pointing up, slowly push up on the plunger to expel any air that may be in the syringe. Tap the barrel of the syringe to dislodge air bubbles and move them up, toward the needle (see Figure 33.2a). Pull down on the plunger to clear fluid from the needle (see Figure 33.2b). Gently push up on the plunger until the fluid enters the colored part of the needle hub, thus expelling the air pocket (see Figure 33.2c).

Tip: *Avoid getting fluid into the needle cap by always pulling down on the plunger to remove fluid from the needle **after** tapping the syringe to dislodge air bubbles. Pulling down must be the **last** thing you do before expelling the air from the syringe; do not tap the syringe again.*

FIGURE 33.2 Bubble expulsion from a syringe

Procedure for expelling bubbles and air pocket from a filled syringe.

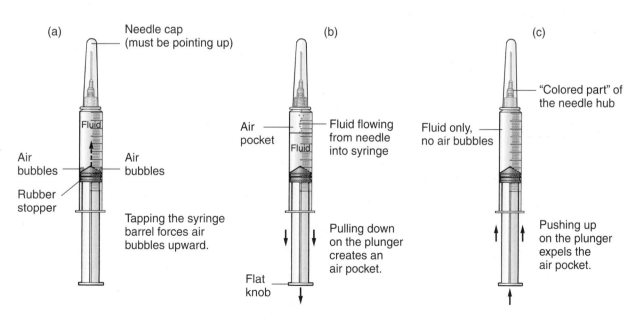

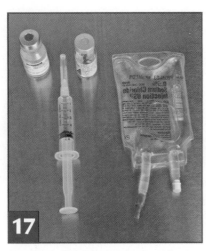

17 Place the filled syringe (with the vented needle capped) onto the work surface next to the diluent vial.

18 Ask for an instructor check on the filled syringe, diluent vial, and calculations.

19 Once your work has been approved, remove the cap of the ampicillin vial and swab it with a new sterile alcohol swab.

20 Correctly grasp the barrel of the syringe and remove the cap of the vented needle.
Tip: Vented needles can be used **only to inject** a diluent into a vial containing a powder drug.

Filled syringe, capped vented needle, and vials set on the work surface, awaiting an instructor check.

FIGURE 33.3

Correct use of a vented needle

Procedure for inserting vented needle and diluting powder drug vial.

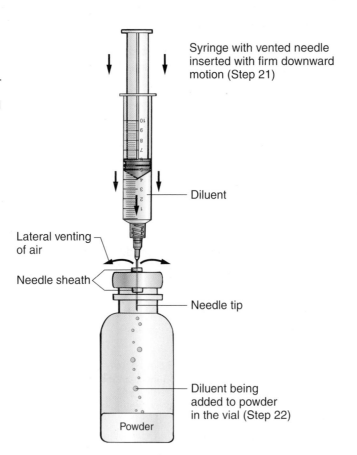

Syringe with vented needle inserted with firm downward motion (Step 21)

Diluent

Lateral venting of air

Needle sheath

Needle tip

Diluent being added to powder in the vial (Step 22)

Powder

21 Use the non-dominant hand to hold the ampicillin vial against the work surface. With the dominant hand, insert the vented needle directly into the top of the vial with a firm downward motion (see Figure 33.3).

Tip: Apply enough downward pressure so that the aluminum sheath surrounding the needle is firmly seated into the rubber vial top. If correctly inserted, the needle itself should be able to move up and down freely while the sheath remains stuck in the rubber vial top.

22 While maintaining the needle in the vial at such a depth that the hub of the needle stays approximately one-eighth inch above the rubber vial top, inject the diluent into the ampicillin vial (see Figure 33.3).

Tip: Two common errors might occur at this point in the procedure. First, if there was a noticeable amount of fluid pooling on top of the rubber vial top while using the vented needle, it is likely that the syringe was held too far above the vial top. Second, if the vented needle failed to vent the vial adequately, it is likely that the syringe was held too close to the vial top, which prohibited adequate venting. If either of these errors occurs, notify your instructor.

23 Correctly grasp the barrel of the syringe, taking care not to touch the plunger, and remove the needle from the vial. Place the needle-and-syringe unit into the sharps container.

24 Shake the reconstituted ampicillin vial to dissolve the drug in the diluent. Continue shaking until the powder is completely dissolved. Then wait long enough for any foam or bubbles to dissipate.

Withdrawing the Correct Dose Volume

25 Aseptically attach a regular needle to a 5 mL syringe.

26 Swab the top of the ampicillin vial with a new alcohol swab and place the swab on the hood surface such that it receives uninterrupted airflow.

27 Uncap the needle and place it on top of the swab such that the cap faces the hood filter.

28 Hold the barrel of the syringe according to standard procedures. Insert the needle, bevel up, using appropriate technique to prevent coring.

Tip: Take care to avoid inserting this needle into the hole left in the rubber vial top by the vented needle. Also, because the vial was previously vented by the vented needle, there is no need to add air to the vial or use the milking technique at this point in the procedure.

29 Invert the vial, taking care to avoid blocking airflow, and withdraw 450 mg of diluted drug by pulling down on the plunger to the volume calculated earlier in the lab for the 450 mg dose.

Tip: Be sure to keep the tip of the needle inside the fluid within the vial so that you do not withdraw from the air pocket within the vial.

30 Remove any bubbles or excess air using the technique mentioned earlier, in Step 11. Verify again that the desired amount of medication is present, and if it is not, pull down on the plunger to draw more fluid into the syringe.

31 Return the vial and syringe to the original starting position with the vial braced against the hood surface and the dominant hand holding only the barrel of the syringe.

32 Remove the needle-and-syringe unit from the ampicillin vial and carefully recap the needle. Place the capped syringe on the work surface.

33 Repeat the withdrawal procedure, Steps 25 through 32, with the other 5 mL syringe, withdrawing the amount calculated for the 375 mg dose.

34 Place both filled syringes, with capped needles, on the work surface next to the ampicillin vial and ask for a final check by your instructor.

35 **Conclusion:** On a separate sheet of paper, answer all questions in the following Lab Review section and turn in your answers to your instructor.

Lab Review

Check Your Understanding

1. Why is it important to have a check of the diluent prior to reconstituting the sterile powder drug?
   a. to verify that the drug's dosage volume is correct
   b. to verify that the correct diluent is used to prepare the desired drug concentration
   c. to verify that the correct drug is reconstituted
   d. It is not important to have the diluent checked, only the final drug dose.

2. If it is difficult to pull the plunger back to the desired volume of diluent, what is the likely cause?
   a. Too much air was injected into the diluent vial.
   b. Too much water was injected into the powder drug vial.
   c. Too little air was injected into the diluent vial.
   d. Too little air was injected into the powder drug vial.

3. If too much diluent is forced into the syringe when using the milking technique, what will be the likely result?
   a. leakage of fluid from the vial due to the excessive pressure
   b. difficulty withdrawing fluid due to negative pressure in the vial
   c. It will be necessary to change to a vented needle.
   d. None of the above

4. What is the correct technique for inserting a vented needle into a vial top?
   a. The needle should be bevel up and there should be a slight bend upon insertion.
   b. The needle should be bevel down and there should be no bend upon insertion.
   c. The needle should be directly inserted into the vial without bending it and without regard to the position of the bevel.
   d. The needle should be directly inserted into the vial without bending it, and the bevel should be pointed up.

5. Which of the following situations has the potential to contaminate the compounded sterile preparation?
   a. touching the needle to the work surface
   b. blocking the airflow to the critical area
   c. failing to swab the rubber vial top
   d. All of the above are potentially contaminating situations.

Thinking Like a Pharmacy Tech

1. Verifying the concentration of the medication is vital to the process of determining the necessary volume to draw up for the desired dose. If the 1 gram ampicillin had been reconstituted with 5 mL of sterile water instead of 10 mL, how would this have affected the amount that was calculated for each of the two doses?

2. Why might it be important to use a preservative-free diluent for neonatal patients or for intrathecal administration?

3. One key to being a successful pharmacy technician is continuing to learn about the field and practice. A mentor can be an excellent way to do this—a more experienced technician or a pharmacist can answer your questions, challenge your ideas, and help you succeed in your career. Who in your life has been a mentor to you? What qualities are necessary in a mentor?

Using Ampules

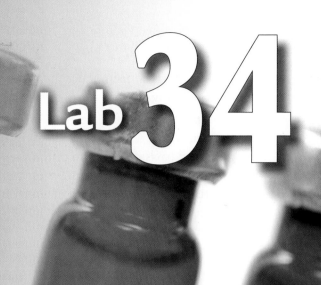

Lab 34

Objectives

- Demonstrate proficiency in the aseptic preparation of an intravenous medication withdrawn from a glass ampule.
- Demonstrate accuracy in basic calculations related to the preparation of an intravenous medication withdrawn from a glass ampule.
- Discuss the procedures and rationale for the use of medications supplied in ampule form.

Supplies

- Promethazine ampule
- 3 mL syringe × 1
- 1 mL syringe × 1
- Filter needle × 2
- Regular needle × 2 (regular needle = no filter, no vent)
- Alcohol swabs × 4
- Dextrose 5% in water 50 mL IVPB × 2
- Calculator
- Trash container (dedicated for IV-room use only)
- Sharps container (dedicated for IV-room use only)

Introduction to Sterile Compounding for Labs 31–34

Note: If you have completed Lab 31, you may skip this introduction and begin after the first Take Note feature. Previous labs in this aseptic technique section provide you with background and practice in garbing by USP Chapter <797> standards, aseptic hand washing, and hood cleaning. In the final four labs of this book, Labs 31–34, you will employ these techniques while preparing sterile products. Your instructor may provide you with more detailed guidelines for following aseptic technique, and you should ask for clarification on any points about which you are unsure.

You will find Labs 31–34 to be considerably longer than many others in the textbook. However, sterile compounding and aseptic technique skills are essential in pharmacy work and important to the healthcare field. In fact, this work is frequently performed by the pharmacy sterile compounding technician. Therefore, as you encounter a long series of steps in these labs, please take your time and follow each step to completion. Once you become familiar with the technique, the processes go very quickly.

The following lists basic terms that apply generally to sterile product preparation labs:

- **Aseptic technique:** A clean, "without infection" technique that is free of pathogens.
- **Clean room:** A space where sterile parenteral products are prepared and that is often referred to as the IV room or the sterile compounding room; the room where the laminar airflow hoods are located. Access to the clean room is restricted to trained and properly garbed personnel. Professional conduct is required in the clean room: eating, drinking, and gum chewing are prohibited. Only certain supplies are allowed and must first be wiped down with an antimicrobial solution.
- **Coring:** An undesired event that occurs when a needle is inserted incorrectly into a rubber stopper atop a solution vial, causing a small bit of the stopper to tear off and contaminate the solution inside the vial.
- **Critical areas:** On equipment or supplies, areas that must never be touched and to which airflow from the HEPA filter should never be interrupted. These areas include the vial top, needle, hub of the needle, hub of the syringe, tip of the syringe, ampule neck, dispensing pin spike, and IV bag injection port.
- **Dilution:** Injection of a liquid medication into an IV solution, or the mixing of a liquid medication with a fluid such as sterile water, or normal saline, which results in a more dilute concentration of the drug.
- **Milking technique:** A process used to ease the negative pressure in a vial or other closed container by adding positive pressure to the system. This technique involves inserting a needle-and-syringe into the vial or container, adding a small amount of air to the vial, and then adding and removing small quantities of fluid and air as many times as necessary.
- **Negative pressure:** Applies to aseptic technique in being inherent to vials and some other closed systems, wherein negative pressure prohibits the withdrawal of fluid from the vial into a syringe. This situation is altered by equalizing the pressure inside of the vial by using a dispensing pin, vented needle, or the milking technique.
- **Parenteral:** Refers to medications administered by any route other than through the alimentary canal (the digestive tract), thus including every method of dispensation other than by mouth or rectum. The parenteral route of administration includes the intravenous, intramuscular, transdermal, intraocular, or intrathecal dispensation of drugs.
- **Pathogen:** An infectious agent that can cause disease or illness in a patient.
- **Positive pressure:** For the purposes of aseptic technique, this situation occurs when a small amount of air is introduced into a vial or other closed system, thereby easing the withdrawal of fluid from the vial into the syringe. (See the entry on milking technique for additional explanation.)
- **Reconstitution:** Dissolving a powder drug into its liquid, injectible form by mixing it with a diluent such as sterile water or normal saline.
- **Shadowing:** A form of contamination that results when a worker's hands or supplies on the hood are incorrectly placed, disrupting sterile airflow from the HEPA filter to the critical area. Figure 29.1 shows airflow in a hood.
- **Six-inch rule:** Standard procedure whereby technicians must not work within the outer six inches of the hood's work surface. This area is considered the "dirty edge" because sterile air mixes with room air. However, for ease of access, pre-wrapped objects that are to be used shortly, such as needles, syringes, and alcohol swabs, are often placed in this outer-six-inch area.
- **Touch contamination:** A form of contamination that results when a critical area, or the hood

surface itself, is contaminated through incorrect technique, needle stick, sneezing, or coughing.

- **Zone of turbulence:** An area behind any item (e.g., vial, IV bag, syringe) on the hood where sterile airflow is interrupted; the zone or area is thereby contaminated. Sterile parenteral products should never be prepared within a zone of turbulence.

Take Note

As a pharmacy technician, you are required to adhere to strict aseptic technique when preparing parenteral products. Why is that so crucial? Medications that are administered directly into the patient's bloodstream, internal organ, or internal tissue are considered to be the most dangerous to the patient—certainly more dangerous than are enteral (nonparenteral) products. Danger exists for a few reasons. First, because parenteral medications are administered directly into the bloodstream, organ, or tissue, the patient's only defense against potential pathogens is the patient's immune system, which is already compromised by fighting a primary infection or recovering from injury or surgery. In contrast, enteral products go through the digestive tract, where an abundance of flora defends against many pathogenic organisms. Second, once a medication is injected into the bloodstream, there is little to no chance of reversal; enteral medications can be reversed with ipecac or activated charcoal if a mistake is made (i.e., an incorrect drug or dose is administered). Third, parenteral agents introduce 100% of the drug into the bloodstream, whereas, with enteral administration, only a portion of the drug reaches the bloodstream.

Ampule

A small, sealed glass vial used to contain a fluid

Historical records verify the use of glass **ampules** to hold important fluids beginning around the fourth century CE, though it's possible that ampules originated thousands of years earlier. For example, records indicate that some early Christians had a small ampule of their own blood entombed with them—a special ceremonial tradition originally reserved for martyrs. The association of ampules with ceremonies of death and honor carries on today in some areas of Europe, where religious pilgrims place ampules of oil next to the tombs of well-known saints and martyrs to honor them in annual ceremonies.

Your use of ampules links you, as a modern pharmacy technician, with ancient practices of careful storage, transport, and use of valuable liquids. Patients today receive life-sustaining liquid medications that you prepare by aseptically processing the contents of glass ampules into compounded sterile preparations. Although many of these medications are available in glass or plastic vials, some are provided only in ampule form because they must be protected from air during storage. Ampules are airtight because they are flame sealed after filling—providing an optimum environment for certain drugs.

Incompatibility

An undesired chemical reaction between two drugs, or between a drug and its container, negatively affecting drug composition, efficacy, or stability

The most common motivation for drug manufacturers to supply a medication in ampule form is the drug's **incompatibility** with plastic, rubber, or polyvinyl chloride (PVC). In fact, most parenteral drug vials contain one of these components and incompatibility arises from an undesired reaction between the medication and part of the drug vial. These undesired chemical reactions can affect the drug's composition or efficacy, or drastically reduce the medication's shelf stability. By using ampules made entirely of glass, you eliminate incompatibility problems.

Ampule preparation requires excellent aseptic technique, with special attention focused on correctly breaking the ampule and on several specific processes for withdrawing and injecting its contents. Unlike other medications, drugs withdrawn from ampules must be filtered. A filter needle is used to prevent the transfer of tiny glass shards from the ampule to the patient. The same needle must not be used both to withdraw medication from an ampule and to inject it. Rather, you *must change the needle* prior to injecting the medication into the patient or the IVPB. Once ampules are broken and thus open to the air, you will not need to create a positive pressure environment, as is necessary when working with vials. You will use a syringe to withdraw liquid from ampules, and since air bubbles will float to the top of the liquid— regardless of the direction in which the syringe is initially pointed—you must remove air bubbles from the syringe once you take it out of the ampule. Used ampules should be disposed of in the sharps container because of potential injury from the broken glass.

Procedure

In this lab you will perform basic calculations and aseptically prepare these two doses of intravenous medication from a glass ampule:

Promethazine 25 mg

Promethazine 10 mg

1 Perform calculations based on the concentration that is provided on the ampule label. For example, the label on the promethazine ampule states that it is 50 mg/2 mL. Based on this concentration, how many milliliters will you need to withdraw from the ampule to separately prepare the following two doses?

25 mg × **1** dose   and   **10 mg** × **1** dose

$$\left.\frac{50 \text{ mg}}{2 \text{ mL}} = \frac{25 \text{ mg}}{x \text{ mL}}\right\}$$ Cross-multiply and then divide to solve for x, the unknown volume:

$$25 \times 2 = 50$$

$$\frac{50}{50} = \textbf{1 mL} \text{ required for the 25 mg dose.}$$

$$\left.\frac{50 \text{ mg}}{2 \text{ mL}} = \frac{10 \text{ mg}}{x \text{ mL}}\right\}$$ Cross-multiply and then divide to solve for x, the unknown volume:

$$10 \times 2 = 20$$

$$\frac{20}{50} = \textbf{0.4 mL} \text{ required for the 10 mg dose.}$$

FIGURE 34.1
Glass ampule

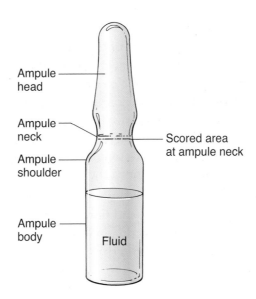

Ampule head

Ampule neck

Ampule shoulder

Ampule body

Scored area at ampule neck

Fluid

2 Don aseptic garb, hand wash, don sterile gown and gloves, and clean the hood according to your instructor's direction.

3 Gently tap or swirl the ampule so that the head and neck are free of fluid and all of the medication is in the body of the ampule. Swab the neck of the ampule with a sterile alcohol swab. A glass ampule is illustrated in Figure 34.1.

4 Prepare the syringe by aseptically attaching a regular needle.

5 Gently but firmly hold the body of the ampule with the thumb and index finger of the non-dominant hand, curling the remaining three fingers around the body of the ampule to help stabilize it. Verify that the fingers of this hand are situated below the neck of the ampule.
Tip: Hold the ampule firmly but avoid crushing it; the glass walls are quite thin.

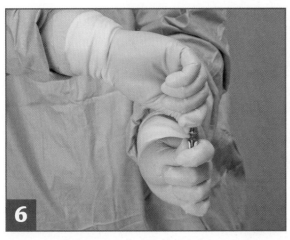

Correct hand placement for breaking a glass ampule.

6 Place the dominant hand such that the thumb and forefinger have a firm grasp of the head of the ampule.

Tip: Because you will shortly be snapping the neck of the ampule, take care both to verify that the fingers of both hands are positioned away from the neck of the ampule, avoiding potential injury, and to aim toward the side of the hood, not toward the back, avoiding damage to the hood filter from glass shards.

7 Use the dominant hand to apply pressure to the neck of the ampule with a quick snapping motion of the wrist. The ampule should break at the neck.
*Tip: Be sure to keep hold of the head of the ampule with the thumb and index finger of the dominant hand so that it does not dislodge when broken off. Keep your arms and fingers steady and use a snapping motion **at the wrist** to break the ampule. Always snap away from your body, never toward yourself.*

8 Put the head of the ampule into the sharps container and place the body of the ampule onto the hood surface in an area that ensures uninterrupted airflow.

9 Open a new sterile alcohol swab and place it on the work surface such that it receives uninterrupted airflow.

10 Hold the barrel of the syringe with the dominant hand, remove the cap of the needle, and place the cap onto the swab with the opening pointing toward the hood filter.

11 Rotate the barrel of the syringe such that the bevel of the needle is pointing down. Stabilize the ampule with the non-dominant hand and carefully insert the needle into the ampule.
Tip: Be sure that the tip of the needle has entered the fluid inside the ampule.

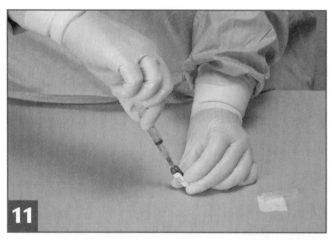

Correct technique for inserting a needle into a glass ampule.

12 Pull the plunger back until the syringe contains approximately 0.5 mL more than what is desired (in the case of the 25 mg dose, approximatey 1.5 mL).
Tip: As you draw up fluid into the needle and the ampule becomes emptier, it may be necessary to tip the ampule slightly to bring the fluid into the shoulder of the ampule where the tip of the needle can more easily remain in the fluid.

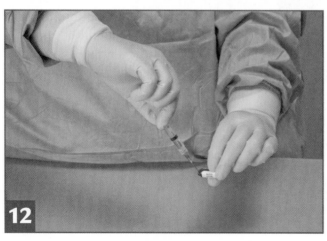

Withdrawal of fluid from the shoulder of a glass ampule.

13 Keep hold of the ampule in your non-dominant hand. With the fingers of the dominant hand, keep hold of the barrel of the syringe, release the plunger, and then carefully remove the syringe from the ampule. Place the ampule on the work surface such that it receives uninterrupted airflow. Turn the syringe so the needle points upward and recap the needle.

14 Tap the syringe to force air bubbles up toward the hub. Pull down slightly on the plunger to draw fluid from the needle down into the syringe. (The procedure for expelling bubbles and excess air from a filled syringe is shown in the previous lab in Figure 33.2.)
*Tip: Avoid fluid flow into the needle cap by always pulling down on the plunger to remove fluid from the needle **after** tapping the syringe to dislodge air bubbles. Pulling down must be the **last** thing you do before expelling the air from the syringe; do not tap the syringe again.*

15 Slowly push up on the plunger to expel all of the air from the syringe. Release the plunger and hold the barrel of the syringe in the dominant hand.

16 Remove the needle cap and place it on the alcohol swab.

17 Carefully insert the needle back into the ampule and use the plunger to push any excess fluid into the ampule. Keeping your eye on the graduations on the syringe barrel, push the plunger down slowly and stop when you reach the correct volume (in the case of the 25 mg dose, 1 mL).

18 While grasping only the barrel of the syringe, remove it from the ampule. Recap the needle.

19 Pull down on the plunger to clear the needle of fluid. Remove the needle and place it in the sharps container.

20 Aseptically attach a filter needle to the syringe.

21 Slowly push up on the plunger to expel all of the air from the syringe and place the capped syringe on the work surface.

22 Repeat the entire procedure, Steps 4 through 21, for the 10 mg dose. However, note that you should *ignore Steps 5–8* because you have already broken open the ampule.

23 Ask for an instructor check of the syringes, the IVPBs, and the promethazine ampule.

24 Swab the injection port of a D5W 50 mL IVPB and inject the 25 mg dose of promethazine according to accepted protocol (as described in Lab 30, Steps 19–23, pages 297–298).

25 Place the empty needle-and-syringe unit into the sharps container.

26 Squeeze the IVPB to check for leaks and set it aside.

27 Repeat the IVPB injection procedure, Steps 24 through 26, using the second IVPB for the 10 mg dose.

28 Place the empty needle, syringe, and broken ampule into the sharps container and clean your work area according to your instructor's direction. *Tip: Use caution when cleaning the work surface to avoid injury or product contamination from small shards of glass that may be present.*

29 **Conclusion:** On a separate sheet of paper, answer all questions in the following Lab Review section and turn in your answers to your instructor.

Lab Review

Check Your Understanding

1. Considering correct technique and safety when breaking an ampule, you should apply force so that breaking occurs at the _____ of the ampule.
   a. body
   b. neck
   c. shoulder
   d. head

2. At what point should the air bubbles be removed from the syringe when working with ampules?
   a. prior to removing the syringe from the ampule
   b. prior to removing the syringe from the vial
   c. after removing the syringe from the ampule
   d. There is no need to remove air bubbles from the syringe when working with ampules.

3. When working with ampules, why is it important to remove the regular needle and to change to a filter needle prior to injecting the medication into the IVPB or the patient?
   a. Because the filter needle traps potential glass fragments, changing needles ensures that those glass fragments are not injected into the IVPB or patient.
   b. The regular needle traps potential glass fragments, so it is not necessary to change needles before injecting.
   c. Since all IVPBs are administered through an in-line filter, the use of a filter needle is unnecessary.
   d. None of the above

4. Why is it important to verify correct hand placement prior to breaking an ampule?
   a. to ensure correct aseptic technique
   b. to ensure the safety of the pharmacy technician
   c. to correctly break the ampule at the neck
   d. All of the above

5. Which items should be placed into the sharps container upon the completion of this lab?
   a. everything used during the course of this lab
   b. only the needles, syringes, and broken ampule
   c. only the needles and broken ampule
   d. only broken glass

Thinking Like a Pharmacy Tech

1. Why is it *not* necessary to inject air into an ampule prior to drawing up its contents, as you would need to do when drawing up the contents of a vial?

2. Some facilities prefer that the technician draw up the solution through a filter needle and then change to a regular needle prior to injecting the prepared solution into the IVPB. Discuss whether this option ensures that glass is sufficiently filtered from the solution.

3. How can you further your education as a pharmacy technician? How do you plan to continue your education even after you have landed a job?

Appendix A

Most Commonly Prescribed Drugs

Generic Name	Pronunciation	Classification	Brand Name
acetaminophen/ codeine	a-seat-a-MIN-oh-fen KOE-deen	opioid analgesic	Tylenol/ codeine
acyclovir	ay-SYE-kloe-veer	antiviral	Zovirax
albuterol	al-BYOO-ter-ole	beta-2 agonist	Ventolin HFA
albuterol (nebulizer solution)	al-BYOO-ter-ole	beta-2 agonist	AccuNeb
albuterol HFA	al-BYOO-ter-ole	beta-2 agonist	Pro-Air
alendronate	a-LEN-droe-nate	bisphosphonate	Fosamax
allopurinol	al-o-PURE-i-nole	antigout agent xanthine oxidase inhibitor	Zyloprim
alprazolam	al-PRAY-aoe-lam	benzodiazepine	Xanax
amitriptyline	a-mee-TRIP-ti-leen	antidepressant tricyclic	Elavil
amlodipine	am-LOE-di-peen	antianginal calcium channel blocker	Norvasc
amlodipine	am-LOE-di-peen	antianginal calcium channel blocker	Norvasc
amoxicillin	a-moks-i-SIL-in	antibiotic penicillin	Amoxil
amoxicillin ER	a-moks-i-SIL-in	antibiotic penicillin	Moxatag
aripiprazole	ay-ri-PIPra-zole	antipsychotic	Abilify
aspirin (EC)	AS-pir-in	antiplatelet	Bayer Aspirin EC
atenolol	a-TEN-oh-lole	beta blocker	Tenormin
atorvastatin	a-TORE-va-sta-tin	antilipemic	Lipitor
azithromycin	az-ith-ro-MYE-sin	antibiotic macrolide	Zithromax, Z-Pak
baclofen	BAK-loe-fen	skeletal muscle relaxant	Lioresal

Generic Name	Pronunciation	Classification	Brand Name
benazepril	ben-AY-ze-pril	ACE inhibitor	Lotensin
benzonatate	ben-ZO-em-tate	antitussive	Tessalon
bisoprolol-hydrochlorothiazide	bis-OH-proe-lol hye-droe-klor-oh-THYE-a-side	beta blocker/diuretic	Ziac
budesonide/formoterol	byoo-DES-oh-nide/fo-MOH-te-rol	beta-2 agonist/corticosteroid	Symbicort
buprenorphine/naloxone	byoo-pre-NOR-feen/nor-OKS-on	opioid analgesic	Suboxone
bupropion	byoo-PROE-pee-on	antidepressant	Budeprion, Wellbutrin, Zyban
bupropion SR	byoo-PROE-pee-on	antidepressant	Budeprion SR, Wellbutrin SR
bupropion XL	byoo-PROE-pee-on al-byoo-ter-ole	antidepressant	Budeprion XL, Wellbutrin XL
butalbital acetaminophen-caffeine	byoo-TAL-bi-tal a-seat-a-MIN-oh-fen KAF-een	barbiturate	Fioricet, Esgic Plus
carisoprodol	kar-eye-soc-PROE-dle	skeletal muscle relaxant	Soma
carvedilol	KAR-ve-dil-ole	beta blocker	Coreg
cefdinir	SEF-di-ner	antibiotic cephalosporin	Omnicef
celecoxib	sele-KOKS-ib	NSAID	Celebrex
cephalexin	sef-a-LEKS-in	antibiotic cephalosporin	Keflex
chlorhexidine gluconate	klor-heks-i-deen GLOO-ko-nate	antiseptic	Peridex
ciprofloxacin	sip-roe-FLOK-a-sin	antibiotic quinolone	Cipro
citalopram	sye-TAL-oh-pram	antidepressant SSRI	Celexa
clarithromycin	kla-RITH-ree-my-e-sin	antibiotic macrolide	Biaxin
clobetasol	kloe-BAY-ta-sol	corticosteroid	Temovate, Olux
clonazepam	kloe-NA-ze-pam	benzodiazepine	Klonopin
clonidine	KLON-i-dine	alpha-2 adrenergic agonist	Catapres
clopidogrel	klok-PID-oh-grel	antiplatelet agent	Plavix
clotrimazole-betamethasone	klo-TRIM-a-zole bay-ta-METH-a-sone	antifungal/corticosteroid	Lotrisone
colchicine	KOL-chi-seen	antigout	Colcrys

Generic Name	Pronunciation	Classification	Brand Name
cyclobenzaprine	sye-kloe-BEN-za-preen	skeletal muscle relaxant	Flexeril
dextroamphetamine-amphetamine XR	deks-troe-am-FET-a- min am-FET-a-min	stimulant	Adderall XR
dextroamphetamine-amphetamine	deks-troo-am-FET-a-mine	stimulant	Adderall
diazepam	dye-AZ-e-pam	benzodiazepine	Valium
diclofenac	dye-KLOE-fen-ak	NSAID	Cataflam
dicyclomine	dye-SYE-kloe-meen	anticholinergic	Bentyl
digoxin	di-JOKS-in	antiarrhythmic	Lanoxin
diltiazem CD	dil-TYE-a-zem	antianginal calcium channel blocker	Cardizem
divalproex	dye-VAL-pro-ex	anticonvulsant	Depakote
donepezil	doh-NEP-e-zil	acetylcholinesterase inhibitor	Aricept
doxazosin	doks-AY-zoe-sin	alpha-1 blocker	Cardura
doxycycline	doks-i-SYEkleen	antibiotic tetracycline	Vibramycin
duloxetine	doo-LOKS-e-teen	antidepressant SSRI	Cymbalta
dutasteride	do-TAS-teer-ide	5-alpha-reductase inhibitor	Avodart
enalapril	e-NAL-a-pril	ACE inhibitor	Vasotec
escitalopram	es-sye-TAL-oh-pram	antidepressant SSRI	Lexapro
esomeprazole	es-oh-MEpray-zol	proton pump inhibitor	Nexium
estradiol	es-tra-DYE-ole	estrogen	Estrace, Climara, Femrin-
estrogens (conjugated)	ES-troe-jenz	estrogen	Premarin
eszopiclone	es-zoe-PIK-lone	hypnotic	Lunesta
ethinyl estradiol-drospirenone	ETH-in-yl-es-tra-DYE-ole droh-SPYE-re-none	contraceptive	Ocella
ethinyl estradiol-drospirenone	ETH-in-yl-es-tra-DYE-ole droh-SPYE-re-none	contraceptive	Yaz
ethinyl estradiol-etonogestrel	ETH-in-yl-es-tra-DYE-ole et-noe-JES-trel	contraceptive	NuvaRing
ethinyl estradiol-levonorgestrel	ETH-in-il-es-tra-DYE-ol LE-voe-nor-jes-trel	contraceptive	Aviane

Generic Name	Pronunciation	Classification	Brand Name
ethinyl estradiol–norethindrone	ETH-in-il-es-tra-DYE-ole nor-eth-IN-drone	contraceptive	Loestrin 24 FE
ethinyl estradio–norgestimate	ETH-in-il-es-tra-DYE-ole nor-JES-ti-mate	contraceptive	Tri-Sprintec
ethinyl estradiol–norgestimate	ETH-in-il-es-tra-DYE-ole nor-JES-ti-mate	contraceptive	Ortho Tri-cyclen Lo
ethinyl estradiol–norgestimate	ETH-in-il-es-tra-DYE-ole nor-JES-ti-mate	contraceptive	Sprintec
ethinyl estradiol–norgestimate	ETH-in-il-es-tra-DYE-ol nor-JES-ti-mate	contraceptive	TriNessa
ezetimibe	ez-ET-i-mibe	antilipemic	Zetia
ezetimibe-simvastatin	ez-ET-i-mbe SIM-va-stat-in	antilipemic	Vytorin
famotidine	fa-MOE-ti-dine	h-2 antagonist	Pepcid
fenofibrate	fen-oh-FYE-brate	antilipemic	TriCor
fenofibric acid	fen-oh-FYE-brik-ASid	antilipemic	Trilipix
fentanyl (transdermal)	FEN-ta-nil	opioid analgesic	Duragesic
ferrous sulfate	FER-us-SUL-fate	iron supplement	Feosol, Slow FE
fexofenadine	feks-oh-FEN-a-deen	Antihistamine h-1 agonist	Allegra
finasteride	fi-NAS-teer-ide	5-alpha-reductase inhibitor	Proscar
fluconazole	flu-KOE-na-zole	antifungal	Diflucan
fluoxetine	floo-OKS-e-teen	antidepressant SSRI	Prozac
fluticasone (HFA)	floo-TIK-a-sone	corticosteroid	Flovent
fluticasone (nasal spray)	floo-TIK-a-son	corticosteroid	Flonase
fluticasone/salmeterol	floo-TIK-a-sone	beta-2 agonist/ corticosteroid	Advair
folic acid	FOE-lik-AS-id	vitamin	Folate
furosemide	fyoor-OH-se-mide	diuretic	Lasix
gabapentin	GA-ba-pen-tin	anticonvulsant	Neurontin
glimepiride	GLYE-me-pye-ride	antidiabetic sulfonylurea	Amaryl
glipizide	GLIP-i-zide	antidiabetic, sulfonylurea	Glucotrol
glipizide ER	GLIP-i-zide	antidiabetic	Glucotrol XL

Generic Name	Pronunciation	Classification	Brand Name
glipizide XL	GLIP-i-zide	antidiabetic sulfonylurea	Glucotrol XL
glyburide	GLYE-byoor-ide	antidiabetic sulfonylurea	DiaBeta, Glynase
glyburide/metformin	GLYE-byoor-ride met-FOR-man	antidiabetic biguanide/sulfonylurea	Glucovance
guaifenesin/codeine	guye-FEN-e-sin/KOE-deen	antitussive	Cheratussin AC
hydralazine	hye-DRAL-a-zen	vasodilator	Apresoline
hydrochlorothiazide	hye-droe-klor-oh-THYE-e-zide	diuretic	Microzide
hydrocodone/ acetaminophen	hye-droe-KOE-done a-seat-a-MIN-oh-fen	opioid analgesic	Lortab, Vicodin, Norco
hydroxyzine	hy-DROKS-i-zeen	h-1 agonist	Vistaril, Atarax
ibandronate	eye-BAN-droh-nate	bisphosphonate derivative	Boniva
ibuprofen	eye-byoo-PROE-fen	NSAID	Advil, Motrin
insulin aspart	IN-soo-lin-AS-part	antidiabetic	NovoLog
insulin lispro	IN-soe-lin-LYE-sproe	antidiabetic	Humalog
insulin, glargine	in-soo-lin-GLAR-jeen	antidiabetic	Lantus
ipratropium-albuterol	i-pra-TROE-pee-um/ al-byoo-ter-ole	anticholinergic beta-2 agonist	Combivent
irbesartan	ir-be-SAR-tan	angiotensin II receptor blocker	Avapro
isosorbide	eye-soe-SOR-bide	antianginal vasodilator	Imdur
lamotrigine	la-MOE-tri-jeen	anticonvulsant	Lamictal
latanoprost	la-TA-noe-prost	antiglaucoma prostaglandin	Xalatan
levetiracetam	lee-va-tyre-RA-se-tam	anticonvulsant	Keppra
levothyroxine	lee-voe-thye-ROKS-een	thyroid produce	Synthroid
levothyroxine	lee-voe-thye-ROKSeen	thyroid product	Levoxyl
lisdexamfetamine	les-dex-am-FET-a-meen	stimulant	Vyvanse
lisinopril	lyse-IN-oh-pril	ACE inhibitor	Prinivil, Zestril
lisinopril-hydrochlorothiazide	lyse-IN-o-pril hye-droe-klo-roh-THYE-a-side	ACE inhibitor/diuretic	Prinzide, Zestoretic
lorazepam	lor-AZE-pam	benzodiazepine	Ativan
losartan	loe-SAR-tan	angiotensin II receptor blocker	Cozaar

Generic Name	Pronunciation	Classification	Brand Name
losartan-hydrochlorothiazide	loe-SAR-tan hye-droe-klor-oh-THYE-e-zide	angiotensin II receptor blocker	Hyzaar
lovastatin	LOE-va-sta-tin	antilipemic agent	Mevacor
meclizine	MEK-li-aeen	antiemetic h-1 antagonist	Antivert, Boniva
meloxicam	mel-OKS-a-kam	NSAID	Mobic
memantine	me-MAN-tine	n-methyl-d-aspartate receptor agonist	Namenda
metformin	met-FOR-min	antidiabetic biguanide	Glucophage
methocarbamol	meth-oh-KAR-ba-mole	skeletal muscle relaxant	Robaxin
methotrexate	meth-oh-TREKS-ate	antineoplastic	Rheumatrex
methylphenidate	meth-il-FEN-i-date	stimulant	Concerta
methylprednisolone	meth-il-pred-NIS-o-lone	corticosteroid	Medrol
metoclopramide	met-oh-KLOE-pro-mide	antiemetic	Reglan
metoprolol (succinate)	me-toe-PROE-lole	beta blocker	Toprol XL
metoprolol (tartrate)	me-toe-PROE-lole	antianginal	Lopressor
metronidazole	met-roe-NYE-da-zole	antibiotic and amebicide	Flagyl
mirtazapine	mir-TAZ-a-peen	antidepressant	Remeron
mometasone	moe-MET-a-sone	corticosteroid	Nasonex
montelukast	mon-te-LOO-kast	leukotriene receptor agonist	Singulair
moxifloxacin	moks-i-FLOKS-a-sin	antibiotic quinolone	Vigamox
nabumetone	na-BYOO-me-tone	NSAID	Relafen
naproxen	na-PROKS-en	NSAID	Aleve, Anaprox
nebivolol	ne-BIV-oh-lole	beta blocker	Bystolic
niacin	nye-a-sin	antilipemic	Niaspan
nifedipine ER	nye-FED-ipeen	antianginal calcium channel blocker	Adalat, Procardia
nitroglycerin	nye-tro-GLIS-er-in	antianginal vasodilator	Minitran, Nitro-Dur
nortriptyline	nor-TRIP-ti-len	antidepressant tricyclic	Pamelor
nystatin (topical)	nye -STAT-in	antifungal	Nystop
olanzapine	OH-lan-a-peen	antipsychotic	Zyprexa
olmesartan	ole-me-SAR-tan	angiotensin II receptor blocker	Benicar

Generic Name	Pronunciation	Classification	Brand Name
omega 3 acid	oh-MEG-a-three ASID	antilipemic	Lovaza
omeprazole	oh-MEP-ra-zole	proton pump inhibitor	Prilosec
oxycodone ER	oks-i-KOE-done	opioid analgesic	OxyContin
oxycodone-acetaminophen	oks-i-KOE-done a-seat-a-MIN-oh-fen	opioid analgesic	Percocet, Tylox
pantoprazole	pan-TOE-pra-zole	proton pump inhibitor	Protonix
paroxetine	pa-ROKS-e-teen	antidepressant SSRI	Paxil
phenazopyridine	fen-az-oh-PEER-i-deen	urinary analgesic	Pyridium, Azo-Standard
phentermine	FEN-ter-meen	anorexiant	Adipex-P
pioglitazone	pye-oh-GLI-ta-zone	antidiabetic thiazolidine	Actos
polyethylene glycol	pol-i-ETH-i-leen GLY-col	laxative	MiraLAX
potassium chloride	poe-TASS-e-um KLOR-ide	electrolyte supplement	Klor-Con
potassium chloride	poe-TASS-e-um-KLOR-ide	electrolyte supplement	Klor-Con
pravastatin	prav-s-STAT-in	antilipemic agent	Pravachol
prednisolone	pred-NISS-oh-lone	corticosteroid	Orapred, Pediapred
pregabalin	pre-GAB-a-lin	analgesic anticonvulsant	Lyrica
promethazine	pro-METH-a-zeen	antiemetic	Phenergan
promethazine-codeine	pro-METH-a-zeen KOE-deen	opioid analgesic	Phenergan/codeine
propranolol	proe-PRAN-oh-lol	beta blocker	Inderal
quetiapine	kwe-TYE-a-peen	antipsychotic	Seroquel
quinapril	KWIN-a-pril	ACE inhibitor	Accupril
rabeprazole	ra-BEP-ra-zole	proton pump inhibitor	AcipHex
raloxifene	ral-OKS-i-feen	estrogen receptor modulator	Evista
ramipril	RA-mipril	ACE inhibitor	Altace
ranitidine	ra-NI-ti-deen	h-2 antagonist	Zantac
risperidone	ris-PER-i-done	antipsychotic	Risperdal
rosuvastatin	roe-soo-va-STAT-in	antilipemic	Crestor
sertraline	SER-tra-leen	antidepressant SSRI	Zoloft

Generic Name	Pronunciation	Classification	Brand Name
sildenafil	sil-DEN-a-fil	phosphodiesterase-5-enzyme inhibitor	Viagra
simvastatin	sim-va-STAT-in	antilipemic	Zocor
sitagliptin	sit-a-GLIP-tin	antidiabetic DPP-4 inhibitor	Januvia
spironolactone	speer-on-oh-LAK-tone	diuretic	Aldactone
sumatriptan	soo-ma-TRIP-deen	serotonin-5-h agonist	Imitrex
tadalafil	tah-DA-la-fil	phosphodiesterase 5 enzyme inhibitor	Cialis
tamsulosin	tam-SOO-loe-sin	alpha-1 blocker	Flomax
temazepam	te-MAZ-e-pam	benzodiazepine	Restoril
terazosin	ter-AY-zoe-sin	alpha-1 blocker	Hytrin
tiotropium	ty-oh-TRO-pee-um	anticholinergic	Spiriva
tizanidine	tye-ZAN-i-deen	alpha-2 adrenergic agonist	Zanaflex
tolterodine LA	tole-ER-oh-deen	anticholinergic	Detrol LA
topiramate	toe-PYRE-a-mate	anticonvulsant	Topamax
tramadol	TRA-ma-dole	opioid analgesic	Ultram
trazodone	TRAZ-oh-done	antidepressant SSRI	Desyrel
triamcinolone	try-am-SIN-oh-lone	corticosteroid	Kenalog
triamterene-hydrochlorothiazide	trye-AM-ter-en hye-droe-klor-oh-THYE-e-zide	diuretic	Dyazide, Maxzide
trimethoprim-sulfamethoxazole	trye-METH-oh-prim sul-fa-meth-OKSa-zole	antibiotic sulfa	Bactrim
valacyclovir	val-ay-SYE-kloe-veer	antiviral	Valtrex
valsartan	val-SAR-tan	angiotensin II receptor blocker	Diovan
valsartan-hydrochlorothiazide	val-SAR-tan hye-droe-klor-oh-THYE-e-zide	angiotensin II blocker/ diuretic	Diovan/HCT
venlafaxine XR	ven-la-FAX-een	antidepressant SSRI	Effexor XR
warfarin	WAR-fa-in	anticoagulant	Coumadin
zolpidem	zole-PI-dem	hypnotic	Ambien
zolpidem CR	zole-PI-dem	hypnotic	Ambien CR

Appendix B

Appendix B: Suggested Alternative Ingredients for Unit 4, Labs 22 to 27, and Unit 5, Lab 31

	Original Ingredient	Alternative Ingredient
Lab 22 — Reconstituting Powders	Augmentin 125mg/5mL, 100mL bottle	Placebo bottles, 125mg/5mL 100mL bottle, 250mg/5mL or 400mg/5mL KoolAid or Crystal Light drink powder in an amber vial
Lab 23 — Filling Capsules	Metronidazole 500mg tablets	Placebo 500mg tablets Vitamin C 500mg tablets Smarties
	Syrpalta	Simple Syrup (See included recipe) Ora-Sweet Syrup/Ora Plus
Lab 24 — Creating Suspensions from Tablets	Amoxicillin 250mg capsules	Placebo 250mg capsules Milk Thistle 250mg capsules
Lab 25 — Creating Suspensions from Capsules	Syrpalta or OraPlus	Simple Syrup (See included recipe) Ora-Sweet Syrup/Ora Plus
Lab 26 — Preparing Creams, Ointments, Gels, and Pastes	Surgical lubricant	KY Jelly Aloe Vera gel Hair gel
Lab 27 — Making Lozenges	Lozenge mold	Mini cupcake liners Miniature silicone ice cube tray
	Benzocaine powder	Corn starch Baking soda
Lab 31 — Preparing Large-Volume Parenteral Solutions	Potassium cholride bulk vial, 250 mL	Potassium chloride, 40 mL vial Dextrose 50%

Suggested Product Sources

Amazon.com   Paddock Laboratories, Inc.   Healthcare Logistics
MockMeds   Pocket Nurse   Your local drug or grocery store
Moore Medical   Wallcur

351

Acne Skin Astringent

Tea tree oil	1 mL
Witch hazel solution	qs 8 oz
Amber vial, 8 oz in volume	1
1 mL dropper or pipette	1

1. Add 1mL tea tree oil to amber vial
2. Using witch hazel solution, fill amber vial to 8 ounces
3. Shake well
4. Label

Beyond use date: 50% of shortest shelf life of ingredients

Alprazolam 1 mg/mL Syrup

Alternative Ingredients

Rx Alprazolam 2 mg tablets	#60	Miniature Altoid mints
Syrup vehicle	qs 120 mL	Simple syrup
Amber vial, 120 mL in volume	1	
4 oz or 6 oz mortar and pestle	1	

1. Triturate alprazolam tablets using a mortar and pestle
2. Carefully pour triturated tablet powder into the amber vial
3. Using the syrup vehicle as a rinse for the mortar and pestle, gently swish approximately 20 to 30 mL of syrup around the mortar, and pour the contents into the amber vial
4. Rinse the mortar two more times using the syrup vehicle
5. Fill the amber vial to 120 mL with syrup vehicle

Beyond use date: 6 weeks

Benzocaine 5% Ointment

Alternative Ingredients

Benzocaine	5 grams	Kosher salt
White petrolatum	qs 100 grams	Petroleum jelly
100 gram ointment container	1	
Digital scale	1	
Mortar and pestle	1	
Stainless steel spatula	1	
Ointment slab	1	

1. Accurately weigh each ingredient
2. Reduce the particle size of the benzocaine to a fine powder
3. Spatulate a small quantity of the petrolatum into the benzocaine and work until very smooth
4. Incorporate the remainder of the petrolatum geometrically and mix well
5. Package and label

Beyond use date: 50% of shortest shelf life of ingredients

Lip Balm

Beeswax	8 oz
Coconut oil	1 pint
Vitamin E 400IU capsules	#45
Preferred flavoring oil	7 to 10 mL
Lip balm containers	#45
Self-stirring hot plate	1
Double boiler or	
500 mL beaker	1
Water for hot bath	1 pint

Prepares: approximately 45 units

1. In a double boiler, or a beaker in heated water bath, melt beeswax. Do NOT boil
2. Once beeswax is melted, gradually stir coconut oil into melted wax
3. Empty contents of vitamin E capsules into solution
4. Stir until mixture is homogenous
5. Add flavoring oil and stir
6. Carefully pour solution into lip balm containers and allow to cool

Beyond use date: 50% of shortest shelf life of ingredients

Progesterone 5% Cream

		Alternative Ingredients
Progesterone, micronized	5 grams	Corn starch
Glycerin	qs	Mineral oil
Dermabase	95 grams	White petrolaum (i.e. Aquaphor®)
100 gram ointment container	1	
Ointment slab	1	
1 mL dropper	1	
Stainless steel spatula	1	

1. Levigate the micronized progesterone with a small quantity of glycerin to form a smooth paste
2. Geometrically, incorporate the Dermabase and mix until uniform and smooth
3. Package and label

Beyond use date: 50% of shortest shelf life of ingredients

Simple Syrup

Sucrose	85 grams
Distilled water	100 mL
Amber vial, 120 mL in volume	1
4 oz or 6 oz mortar and pestle	1

1. Geometrically dilute sucrose and water in a mortar and pestle, triturating until dissolved
2. Pour contents into 120 mL amber vial
3. Label

Beyond use date: 30 days from date of preparation

Zinc Oxide Paste

Zinc oxide powder	25 grams
Cornstarch	25 grams
White petrolatum	50 grams
Mineral oil	2 mL
4 oz mortar and pestle	1
Ointment slab	1
Digital scale	1
1 mL oral syringe	1
Stainless steel spatula	1
Ointment jar, 1 oz	4

Prepares: up to 4, 1 oz jars

1. Weigh ingredients
2. Geometrically dilute zinc oxide using a mortar and pestle
3. Levigate zinc oxide powder and cornstarch powder using mineral oil
4. Spatulate the zinc oxide/cornstarch powder and white petrolatum into a paste
5. Ensure a homogenous mixture by thorough spatulation
6. Weigh and tare the empty ointment container
7. Package the product to 30 grams
8. Label and prepare product

Beyond Use Date: 30 days from date of preparation

Glossary

Page numbers are included at the end of each entry.

A

active ingredient the medication that is added to the base ingredient during compounding

ADSDS discrepancy a disagreement between the actual count of a medication in the ADSDS and the amount displayed on the verification screen

ampule a small, sealed glass vial used to contain a fluid

aseptic without infection; free of pathogens

B

bacteriostatic containing an agent or preservative to inhibit bacterial growth

base ingredient an inert substance, such as a cream, ointment, gel, or paste, to which an active ingredient is added during compounding

best practice a highly effective process, technique, or activity designed to deliver the best results with little or no margin of error

C

capturing successfully submitting and obtaining payment on an insurance claim

cash price the price patients must pay when they do not have insurance coverage or their insurance plan is not accepted

chronic condition a health concern that recurs frequently or lasts for an extended time

code a life-threatening situation when a patient is in cardiac or respiratory arrest

compounding preparing individualized medications per prescription order

compounding log an official record of the processes and materials used to compound a prescription

confidentiality the ethical practice of keeping patients' personal and private information safe and secure

control number unique number assigned to any monitored prescription for management and tracking purposes

copay the set price often paid by patients having third-party insurance coverage

cross-reference directs a reader to another part of the text for related information

crushing a method of removing air bubbles from a syringe

current edition published within the most current year

D

diluent the liquid added to a powder during reconstitution

dispensing pin a specialized plastic device that includes a vent, a spike, and a syringe adaptor, and is inserted into the rubber stopper of a vial

drug diversion stealing or otherwise taking or using drugs from the facility illegally

E

8-point check a systematic approach to verifying prescription data during the filling process, often done first by a pharmacy technician and again by a pharmacist

enteral a route of administration (oral, buccal, or rectal) delivering medication through a patient's gastrointestinal tract

F

filling technician pharmacy technician responsible for prescription counting or pouring, packaging, and labeling during the filling process

floor stock a small supply of medications kept on each floor or unit

355

H

hood-cleaning log sheet a crucial document for recording who cleaned the hood, the date, and the time

I

incompatibility an undesired chemical reaction between two drugs, or between a drug and its container, negatively affecting drug composition, efficacy, or stability

intravenous piggyback solution an intermittent infusion containing a standard base solution plus an IV medication; delivered through a main IV line

L

lozenge a dosage form that resembles hard candy and is administered orally; also known as a troche or pastille

M

major contamination a large amount or significant level of contamination of the washed and scrubbed aseptic area

medication therapy management collaborative oversight of a patient's medications and their delivery to promote a safe, effective plan and encourage targeted outcomes

minor contamination a small amount or low level of contamination of the washed and scrubbed aseptic area

monograph a detailed document containing specific information about a drug product

N

narcotic cabinet a double-locked location in the pharmacy where narcotic medications are securely stored; page181

narcotic discrepancy a disagreement between the actual count of a narcotic and the amount listed in the perpetual log or narcotic record

O

outer edge of the hood the outer six inches of the hood working surface, considered the "dirty edge" because sterile air mixes with room air

P

parenteral any route of administration other than enteral or topical, such as intravenous or intramuscular

particulate a powder or fine-textured material

perpetual log an official, legal record of all activity relating to medications in the narcotic cabinet

pharmacopoeia an official compendium of drug products

profit margin the difference between the pharmacy's prescription cost and the amount charged to the patient or insurance provider

punch method a technique for filling capsules from a leveled cake of drug powder

R

recipe a listing of the exact quantity of each ingredient and the processes required to compound a particular prescription

reconstitute to change into liquid form by adding water or other fluid to a powder

S

signa a series of abbreviations to communicate prescription and patient directions

spatulation a method of mixing ingredients together into a homogeneous mixture by combining and smoothing them on a slab with a spatula

suspension a dispersion of fine solid particles in a liquid

T

third-party adjudication an insurance company determination to pay the pharmacy an amount on behalf of the patient's account

transcribing transferring information between documents, in electronic or other form

triturate to break up or grind into smaller pieces

U

unit dose a medication packaged in a single dose, one-time-use container

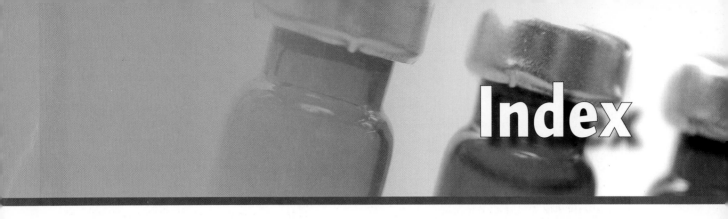

Index

Page numbers followed by i. indicate an illustration.

A

active ingredient, defined, 266

ADSDS discrepancy, defined, 216

ampules, 335–336

antineoplastic agents, 293

aseptic, defined, 285

aseptic hand washing, 285–287

aseptic technique, defined, 300, 312, 322, 334

audit log, described, 164

automated drug storage and dispensing system (ADSDS), 215–216, 216i.

Average Wholesale Price (AWP), defined, 19

B

bacteriostatic, defined, 323

base ingredient, defined, 266

basic aseptic hand washing, 285–286

best practice, defined, 38

biological safety cabinets (BSCs), 293

C

Canadian drug names, 5

capsules
    compounding oral solutions from, 260
    filling, 246

capturing, defined, 138

Cart Fill Forms, information on, 176

cart fills, 175–176

cash price, 153–154

Centers for Medicare and Medicaid (CMS), reimbursement amounts, 19

checked by (floor stock term), described, 182

children, patient information for, 38

chronic conditions, defined, 113

claims, submitting insurance, 137–138

clean room, described, 300, 312, 322, 334

code carts, 205–206

code/code blue/code zero, defined, 205

color coding prescription profiles, 114

communication lapse prevention process, 223–226

compounding. *See also* compounding sterile
    preparations
    defined, 237, 245, 251, 259, 265, 272
    filling capsules, 246
    lozenges, 272
    nonsterile preparations, 237–238, 245–246
    oral solutions, 252, 260
    safety requirements, 238, 260
    topical preparations, 266

compounding log
    defined, 238, 246, 252, 260, 266, 272
    example of page, 239i.

compounding sterile preparations
    drugs in ampules and, 335–336
    hand washing procedure, 285–287
    providing sterile air, 293–294
    terms used, 300
    USP Chapter <797> standards, 279–280

confidentiality, defined, 38

contamination, defined, 286

controlled substances
    cabinet holding, 189, 191
    DEA numbers and, 29–30, 49–50
    filling prescriptions for, 50, 64
    floor stock and, 182
    form for ordering, 190i.
    monitoring prescriptions for, 96
    pharmaceutical duties, 189–190
    refilling prescriptions for, 64, 113–114, 126
    required record keeping, 190–191, 191i.

control number, defined, 96

copay, defined, 137–138

coring, described, 300, 312, 322, 334

crash, defined, 205

crash carts/trays, 205–206

critical areas, described, 300, 312, 322, 334

cross-references, 5–6

current edition, defined, 6

D

DEA numbers
    decoding, 29–30

357